HOW TO EAT

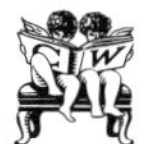

HOW TO EAT

THE PLEASURES AND PRINCIPLES OF GOOD FOOD

NIGELLA LAWSON

Chatto & Windus
LONDON

2 4 6 8 10 9 7 5 3 1

This edition first published in Great Britain in 1999 by Chatto & Windus
Random House, 20 Vauxhall Bridge Road, London SW1V 2SA

First published in hardback
in 1998 by Chatto & Windus

Random House Australia (Pty) Limited
20 Alfred Street, Milsons Point, Sydney,
New South Wales 2061, Australia

Random House New Zealand Limited
18 Poland Road, Glenfield,
Auckland 10, New Zealand

Random House South Africa (Pty) Limited
Endulini, 5A Jubilee Road, Parktown 2193, South Africa

Random House UK Limited Reg. No. 954009

A CIP record for this book is available from the British Library.

ISBN 0 7011 6576 6 (hardback)
ISBN 0 7011 6911 7 (paperback)

Papers used by Random House UK Limited are natural, recyclable products made from wood grown in sustainable forests. The manufacturing processes conform to the environmental regulations of the country of origin.

Printed and bound in Great Britain by
Butler & Tanner Ltd, Frome and London

IN MEMORY OF MY MOTHER, VANESSA (1936–1985)

AND MY SISTER THOMASINA (1961–1993)

AND FOR JOHN, COSIMA AND BRUNO

WITH LOVE

contents

Cooking is not about just joining the dots, following one recipe slavishly and then moving on to the next. It's about developing an understanding of food, a sense of assurance in the kitchen, about the simple desire to make yourself something to eat. And in cooking, as in writing, you must please yourself to please others. Strangely it can take enormous confidence to trust your own palate, follow your own instincts. Without habit, which itself is just trial and error, this can be harder than following the most elaborate of recipes. But it's what works, what's important.

There is a reason why this book is called *How to Eat* rather than *How to Cook*. It's a simple one: although it's possible to love eating without being able to cook, I don't believe you can ever really cook unless you love eating. Such love, of course, is not something which can be taught, but it can be conveyed – and maybe that's the point. In writing this book, I wanted to make food and my slavering passion for it the starting point; indeed for me it *was* the starting point. I have nothing to declare but my greed.

The French, who've lost something of their culinary confidence in recent years, remain solid on this front. Some years ago in France, in response to the gastronomic apathy and consequent lowering of standards nationally – what is known as *la crise* – Jack Lang, then Minister of Culture, initiated *la semaine du goût*. He set up a body expressly to go into schools and other institutions not to teach anyone how to cook, but how to eat. This group might take with it a perfect baguette, an exquisite cheese, some local speciality cooked *comme il faut*, some fruit and vegetables grown properly and picked when ripe, in the belief that if the pupils, if people generally, tasted what was good, what was right, they would respect these traditions; by eating good food, they would want to cook it. And so the cycle continues.

I suppose you could say that we, over here, have had our own unofficial version of this. Our gastronomic awakening – or however, and with whatever degree of irony, you want to describe it – has been to a huge extent restaurant-led. It is, you might argue, by tasting food that we have become interested in

preface

cooking it. I do not necessarily disparage the influence of the restaurant: I spent twelve years as a restaurant critic, after all. But restaurant food and home food are not the same thing. Or, more accurately, eating in restaurants is not the same thing as eating at home. Which is not to say, of course, that you can't borrow from restaurant menus and adapt their chefs' recipes – and I do. This leads me to the other reason this book is called *How to Eat*.

I am not a chef. I am not even a trained or professional cook. My qualification is as an eater. I cook what I want to eat – within limits. I have a job – another job, that is, as an ordinary working journalist – and two children, one of whom was born during the writing of this book. And during the book's gestation, I would sometimes plan to cook some wonderful something or other, then work out a recipe, apply myself in anticipatory fantasy to it, write out the shopping list, plan the dinner – and then find that when it came down to it I just didn't have the energy. Anything that was too hard, too fiddly, filled me with dread and panic or, even if attempted, didn't work or was unreasonably demanding, has not found its way in here. And the recipes I do include have all been cooked in what television people call Real Time: menus have been made with all their component parts, together; that way, I know whether the oven settings correspond, whether you'll have enough hob space, how to make the timings work and how not to have a nervous breakdown about it. I wanted food that can be made and eaten in a real life, not in perfect, isolated laboratory conditions.

Much of this is touched upon throughout the book, but I want to make it clear, here and now, that you need to acquire your own individual sense of what food is about, rather than just a vast collection of recipes.

What I am not talking about, however, is strenuous originality. The innovative in cooking all too often turns out to be inedible. The great Modernist dictum, Make It New, is not a helpful precept in the kitchen. 'Too often,' wrote the great society hostess and arch foodwriter Ruth Lowinsky, as early as 1935, 'the inexperienced think that if food is odd it must be a success. An indifferently roasted leg of mutton is not transformed by a sauce of hot raspberry jam, nor a plate of watery consommé improved by the addition of three glacé cherries.' With food, authenticity is not the same thing as originality; indeed they are often at odds. So while much is my own here – insofar as anything can be – many of the recipes included are derived from other writers. From the outset I wanted this book to be, in part, an anthology of the food I love eating and a way of paying my respects to the foodwriters I've loved reading. Throughout I've wanted, on principle as well as to show my gratitude, to credit honestly wherever appropriate, but I certainly wish to signal my thanks here as well. And if at any time a recipe has found its way onto these pages without having its source properly documented, I assure you and the putative unnamed originator that this is due to ignorance rather than villainy.

But if I question the tyranny of the recipe, that isn't to say I take a cavalier attitude. A recipe has to work. Even the great abstract painters have first to learn figure drawing. If many of my recipes seem to stretch out for a daunting number of pages, it is because brevity is no guarantee of simplicity. The easiest way to learn how to cook is by watching; and bearing that in mind I have tried more to talk you through a recipe than bark out instructions. As much as possible, I have wanted to make you feel that I'm there with you, in the kitchen, as you cook. The book that follows is the conversation we might be having.

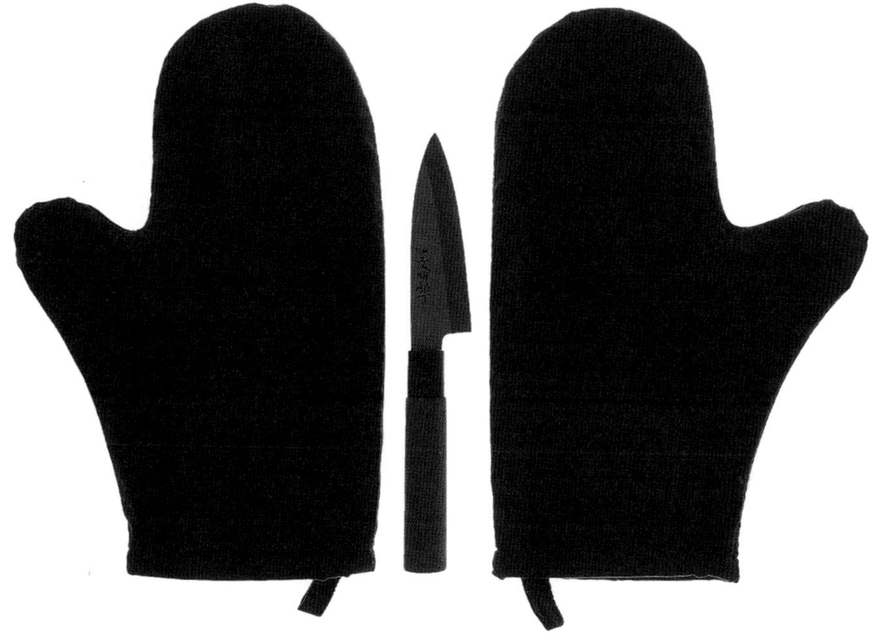

OVEN TEMPERATURES

gas mark	°C	description
1	140	very cool
2	150	cool
3	160	warm
4	180	moderate
5	190	fairly hot
6	200	fairly hot
7	210	hot
8	220	very hot
9	240	very hot

ROASTING CHART

	Starting temperature		After 15 minutes		Minutes per 500g	
	°C	gas	°C	gas		
Beef	250	9	180	4	Rare:	15
					Medium:	18
					Well done:	25
Chicken	200	6	200	6		20+30 overall
Farmed Duck	210	7	180	4		20
Goose	200	6	200	6		15+30 overall
Lamb and venison	250	9	200	6	Rare:	12
					Medium:	16
					Well done:	20
Pork	200	6	180	4		30
Veal	210	7	180	4		20
Turkey	See page 63					

charts & conversions

There is more than one way to skin a rabbit: you may well find that throughout this book instructions are given for cooking various meats in the oven at temperatures or for times which differ from those given above. There are many variables in roasting, as in cooking generally, but the chart opposite, drawn up with my butcher, David Lidgate, should provide a clear and reliable guide to roasting times. If it's possible to switch off the fan on your oven, do so in order to reduce evaporation: 75 per cent of lean meat is water, so it's no wonder that fan ovens can make even good joints dry and tough. The other important factor in following these timings is the temperature of the meat before it goes into the oven. If it's fridge-cold the guidelines are irrelevant, inadequate, all bets are off. Let the meat stand, out of the fridge, to get to room temperature before you cook it as instructed. After the meat has had its advised cooking time, test it: either press it (if it feels soft it's rare, bouncy it's medium, hard it's well-done) or pierce with a knife to see. With chicken, stick a knife in between the thigh and the body; if the juices run clear, it's cooked. And always let meat rest out of the oven for at least 10 minutes before carving.

FISH

Go to a fishmonger while they still exist to get good advice and wise information, and to ensure, please, their continuing existence. Going to a fishmonger, like going to a butcher, makes life easier where it matters – in the kitchen. I go for good fish, good meat, no funny stuff. But once there I make the most of it: butchers and fishmongers have skills that we don't. Don't feel apologetic about asking a fishmonger to fillet or a butcher to bone. When I order fish or meat I practically hold a conference to discuss every possibility, every eventuality; I pick brains, ask for advice on cooking and relentlessly exploit the expertise on offer. So should you.

For those times you can't get to a fishmonger I suggest you check the advice offered by the Canadian Department of Fisheries concerning cooking times: for every 1 inch of thickness, cook the fish, by whatever means – frying, grilling, poaching, baking – for 10 minutes; for a whole fish, measure at its thickest point and multiply accordingly. I heed this advice, but I alter it; I reckon that 8–9 minutes per inch will do, so I recommend translating the 1 inch as 3 centimetres, thus giving myself extra ½ centimetre for the Canadians' ten minutes. When baking fish, whether wrapped in buttered foil or not, I use a gas mark 5/190°C oven. Obviously there are exceptions. (See page 321 for notes on cooking a whole salmon.) And there are times when I ignore these rules altogether.

CONVERSION TABLES

All recipes in this book are given in metric measurements and to tell the truth, it is much easier to try and get used to this without always translating back to or from pounds and ounces. It's only if you use metric scales and make yourself think metrically that you can begin to get a sense of what 100g of something looks or feels like – which is important, imperative even, if you're to feel comfortable while cooking. And really, I'm not sure the two systems easily and accurately translate; any recipe tends to work better in the system in which it was first cooked. Of course it's also true that with most recipes the exact quantities, the odd few grams here or there, don't really matter: the thing is to be consistent, but relaxed; only in baking do you need to worry about precise weights.

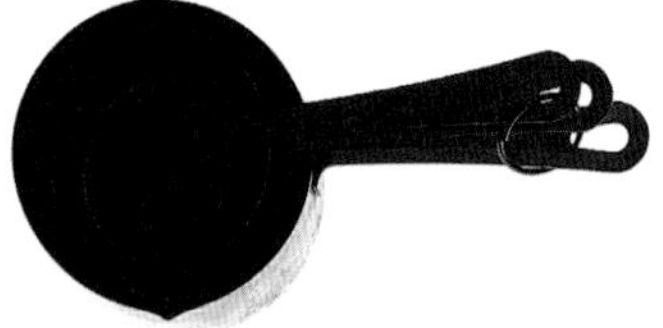

WEIGHTS

Construed accurately, 1 ounce equals 28 grams: in practice, the convention is to express an ounce as 25 or 30 grams; either makes the sums easier and you can choose which you like. Because I have now trained myself to think metrically, and therefore have actually formulated recipes in grams and litres and so on, I cannot honestly say which is the convention you should apply here. It makes sense, then, to give all three – the two rough, the one precise – equivalents.

ounces	grams		
1	25	28	30
2	50	56	60
3	75	84	90
4	100	112	120
5	125	140	150
6	150	168	180
7	175	196	210
8	200	224	240
9	225	252	270
10	250	280	300
11	275	308	330
12	300	336	360
13	325	364	390
14	350	392	420
15	375	420	450
16/1lb	400	448	480

VOLUME & LIQUID MEASUREMENTS

Because a standard tablespoon has a capacity of 15ml it makes more sense, although it's not entirely accurate, to settle for the conversion of 1 fluid ounce as 30ml (in other words 2 tablespoons). Again, though, it will help if you start thinking in terms of metric units, and once manufacturers stop packaging their products in imperial units which have been translated into metric (e.g. a 284ml tub of cream) this will be easier. For the time being, if I do, for example, specify 300ml cream, you should use said 284ml container; I don't mean for you to go out and buy another tub just for the extra 16 millilitres.

For smaller amounts, then, I suggest using tablespoons for measuring. For larger amounts, jugs are calibrated in both metric and imperial, but it's worth knowing that

2 fl oz is approximately	60ml
3	90
5 (¼pt)	150
10 (½pt)	300
15 (¾pt)	450
1 pint	600
1¼	750
1¾	1 litre
2	1.2
2½	1.5

If it helps you when seeing stipulations of 1¼ litres, 1½ litres and so on, you should know that

1¼ litres is just over 2 pints
1½ litres is approximately 2½ pints

Throughout the book, there are references to tablespoons and teaspoons. A tablespoon indicates a specific 15ml measuring spoon (and see above); a teaspoon one of 5ml. These spoons are sold in sets comprising ¼ teaspoon, ½ teaspoon, teaspoon and tablespoon and are incredibly useful. I also find I use more and more my set of American measuring cups which come in sets of cup (250ml), ½ cup (125ml), ⅓ cup (80ml) and ¼ cup (60ml).

Americans tend to use their cups for dry ingredients and, bafflingly, for specifying quantities of chopped vegetables and the like (which must make shopping difficult sometimes) whereas I find them most useful (and consistent) for liquids – oil, wine, whatever. I never seem to come up with the same weight of flour per cup measurement twice, and since it is with baking that one reasonably desires consistency and precision, I prefer to weigh. Still, for making white sauce, for example, the slight differences in weight you might get here or there, depending on the airiness of the flour or how packed it is on the spoon, are easily accommodated. It is useful, therefore, to have some idea of how much a tablespoon of some common ingredients weighs.

	1 level tablespoon
rice	15g
sugar	15g
butter	15g
flour, unsifted	8g
grated parmesan	5g
breadcrumbs	3–4g

I give the weight of a level tablespoon of freshly-grated parmesan, but for large quantities I find it simplest to weigh the chunk of parmesan before grating, then plonk it back on the scales at regular intervals during grating.

It is also helpful to know that a cupful of sugar or rice comes in at 200g. Flour, as I said, can alter hugely: a cupful of plain flour, sifted is about 115g, unsifted but lightly spooned into the cup, is 120g and if you lower the cup into the bag of flour and dredge out said amount, it is likely to hit the 140g mark. As far as I can see from tables in my American books, 1 cup of their all-purpose flour is generally taken to mean 4oz, which I translate here as 120g. And while we're on US terms, it should help you to know that a stick of butter weighs 4oz or 120g.

SOME OTHER USEFUL WEIGHTS AND MEASURES

garlic	1 finely chopped clove = 1 teaspoon
onion	1 average onion = 130g
citrus fruits	Using a zester and an electric juicer you should find, give or take, that you get the following amounts: 1 lime — 1 teaspoon zest 2 tablespoons juice (30ml) 1 lemon — 2 teaspoons zest 8 tablespoons juice (120ml) 1 orange — 1 tablespoon zest 10 tablespoons juice (150ml)
nuts	Reckon on nuts weighing twice as much in their shells as shelled, and adapt recipes and shopping lists accordingly.
peas and beans	Peas-in-the-pod weigh about three times as much as they do podded; the weight of shelled broad beans is about a third of the weight in the pod. Again, adapt shopping lists and recipes accordingly.
shellfish	10 palourdes clams = 154g (i.e. 6–7 palourdes per 100g) 30 mussels = 500g
rhubarb	There are a lot of rhubarb recipes in this book, so it may be useful to know that when cooked in the oven with sugar as on page 122, but with no liquid added, 800g untrimmed = 475g trimmed = 275g puréed (i.e. cooked and drained of excess juice), producing, on average, 225ml juice.

Unless otherwise specified, throughout this book:

- all eggs are large, free-range (and see below)
- all milk is full-fat
- all olive oil is extra virgin: if 'best olive oil' is itemised, that too indicates extra virgin
- flour is usually Italian 00, and an explanation for this is generally given with the recipe; ordinary plain flour can easily be used in its place.

I always use Martin Pitt eggs (and see Gazetteer) since they are extremely good and the hens that lay them are checked regularly for salmonella. I thus have no anxieties about raw eggs, but you should know that because of possible infection from salmonella, the old, the ill, the vulnerable, the pregnant, babies and children are advised not to eat anything with uncooked egg in it.

See page 276 for a fuller discussion of beef regulations and safety, but as with the eggs, so with any foodstuff, especially meat: buy from shops where the produce is traceable; that's to say, you can find out where it comes from and what's happened to it along the way.

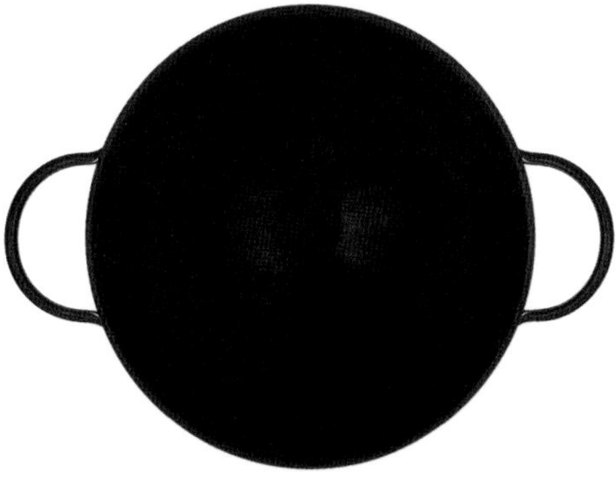

basics etc.

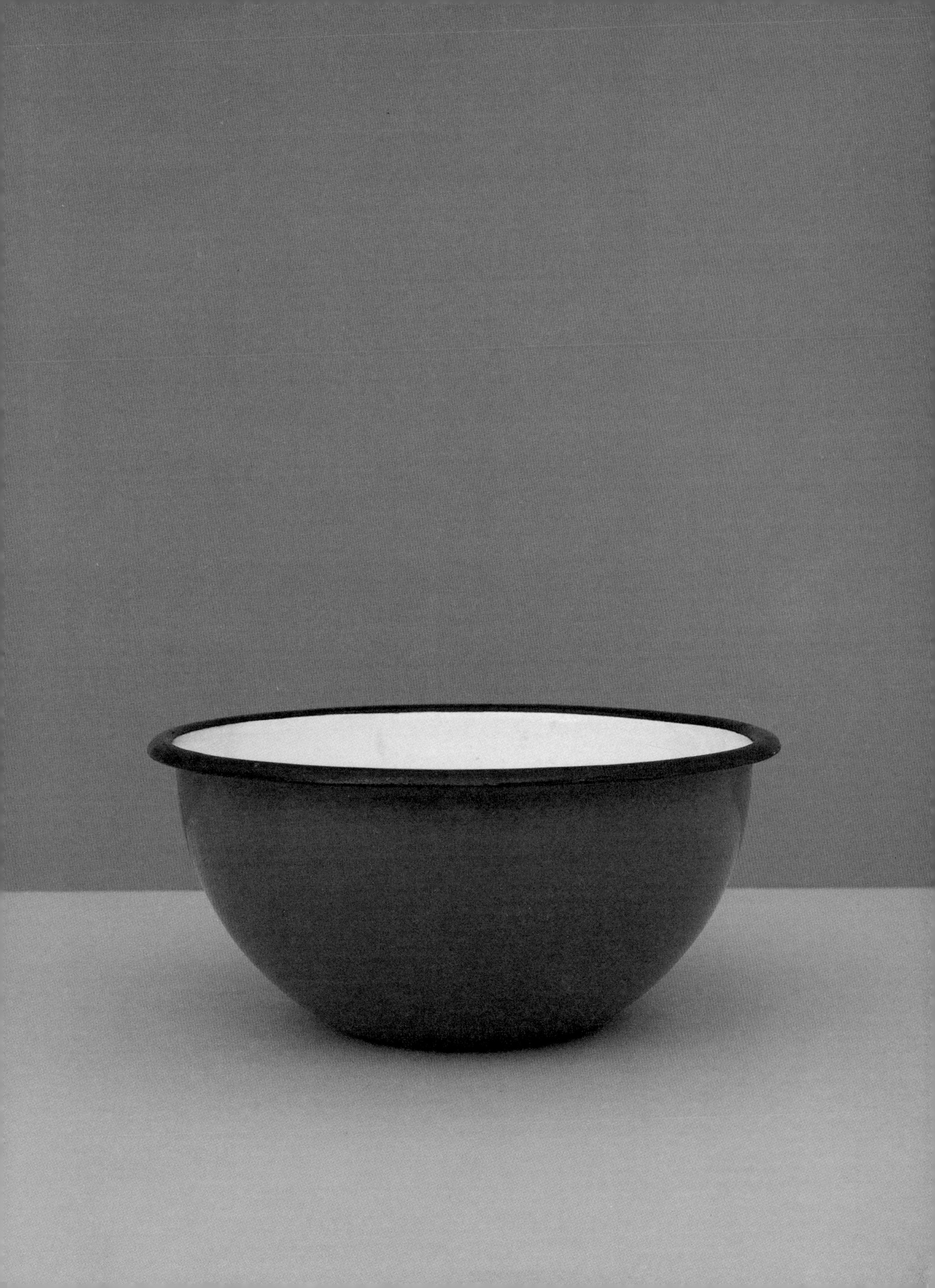

The Great Culinary Renaissance we hear so much about has done many things – given us extra virgin olive oil, better restaurants and gastroporn – but it hasn't taught us how to cook.

Of course standards have improved. Better ingredients are available to us now, and more people know about them. Food and cookery have become more than respectable: they are fashionable. But the renaissance of British cookery, as it was relentlessly tagged in the late 1980s, started in the restaurant and filtered its way into the home. This is the wrong way round. Cooking is best learned at your own stove: you learn by watching and by doing. Chefs themselves know this. The great chefs of France and Italy learn about food at home: what they do later, in the restaurants that make them famous, is use what they have learnt. They build on it, they start elaborating. They take home cooking to the restaurant, not the restaurant school of cookery to the home. Inverting the process is like learning a vocabulary without any grammar. The analogy is pertinent. In years as a restaurant critic, I couldn't help noticing that however fine the menu, some chefs, for all that they seem to have mastered the idiom, have no authentic language of their own. We are at risk, here, of becoming a land of culinary mimics. There are some things you just cannot learn from a professional chef. I am not talking of home economics – the rules that govern what food does when you apply heat or introduce air or whatever – but of home cooking, and of how experience builds organically. For there is more to cooking than being able to put on a good show. Of course there are advantages in an increased awareness of and enthusiasm for food, but the danger is that it excites an appetite for new recipes, new ingredients: follow a recipe once and then – on to the next. Cooking isn't like that. The point about real-life cooking is that your proficiency grows exponentially. You cook something once, then again, and again. Each time you add something different (leftovers from the fridge, whatever might be in the kitchen or in season) and what you end up with differs also.

basics etc.

You can learn how to cook fancy food from the colour supplements, but you need the basics. And anyway, it is better to be able to roast a chicken than to be a dab hand with focaccia. I would be exhausted if the cooking I did every day was recipe-index food. I don't want to cook like that all the time, and I certainly don't want to eat like that.

Nor do I want to go back to some notional golden age of nursery food. I wasn't brought up on shepherd's pie and bread-and-butter pudding and I'm not going to start living on them now. It is interesting though, that these homely foods have not been revived in our homes – they have been rediscovered by restaurants. And, even if I don't wish to eat this sort of thing all the time, isn't it more appropriate to learn how to cook it at home than to have to go to a restaurant to eat it?

By invoking the basics I certainly don't mean to evoke a grim, puritanical self-sufficiency, with austere recipes for home-made bread and stern admonishments against buying any form of food ready cooked. I have no wish to go on a crusade. I doubt I will ever become someone who habitually bakes her own bread – after all, shopping for good food is just as much of a pleasure as cooking it can be. But there is something between grinding your own flour and cooking only for special occasions. Cooking has become too much of a device by which to impress people rather than simply to feed them pleasurably.

In literature, teachers talk about key texts: they exist, too, in cooking. That's what I mean by basics.

Everyone's list of basics is, of course, different. Your idea of home cooking, your whole experience of eating, colours your sense of what foods should be included in the culinary canon. Cooking, indeed, is not so very different from literature: what you have read previously shapes how you read now. And so we eat; and so we cook.

If I don't include your nostalgic favourite in this chapter, you may find a recipe for it elsewhere in the book (see Index). And it is impossible to write a list without being painfully aware of what has been missed out: cooking is not an exclusive art, whatever its grander exponents might lead you to think. Being familiar with making certain dishes – so familiar that you don't need to look in a book to make them (and much of this chapter should eventually make itself redundant) – doesn't preclude you from cooking other things.

So what are basic dishes? Everyone has to know how to roast chicken, pork, beef, game, lamb: what to do with slabs of meat (and turn to the roasting chart on page xii). This is not abstruse knowledge, but general information so basic that many books don't bother to mention it. I am often telephoned by friends at whose houses I have eaten something more elaborate than I would ever cook, to be asked how long their leg of lamb needs to be in the oven and at what temperature.

The key texts constitute the framework of your repertoire: stews, roasts, white sauce, mayonnaise, stocks, soups. You might also think of tackling pastry.

Because the English don't any longer have a firmly based culinary tradition – and even at its solid best English cookery never had anything like the range and variation of, say, regional French cooking – we tend to lack an enduring respect for particular dishes. It's not so much that we hunger to eat whatever is fashionable as that we drop anything that is no longer of the moment. The tendency is not exclusively English – if you were to go to a grand dinner party in France or Italy, you might be served whatever was considered the culinary *dernier cri* – but what makes our behaviour more emphatic, more ultimately sterile, is that we don't seem to cook any food other than style-conscious dinner-party food.

I think it is true, too, that we are quick to despise what once we looked at so breathlessly in colour supplement and delicatessen. Just because a food is no longer flavour of the month, it shouldn't follow that it is evermore to be spoken of as a shameful aberration. It is important always to judge honestly and independently. This can be harder than it sounds. Fashion has a curious but compelling urgency. Even those of us who feel we are free of fashion's diktats are, despite ourselves, influenced by them. As what is seemingly desirable changes, so our eye changes. It doesn't have to be wholesale conversion for this effect to take place: we just begin to look at things differently.

Of course, fashion may lead us to excesses. It is easy to ascribe the one-time popularity of nouvelle cuisine – which fashion decrees we must now treat as hootingly risible – to just such an excess. And to some extent that would be correct. But what some people forget is that the most ludicrous excesses of nouvelle cuisine were not follies committed by its most talented exponents but by the second and third rank. It is important to distinguish between what is fashionable and good and what is fashionable and bad.

With food it should be easier to maintain your integrity: you must, after all, always know whether you enjoy the taste of something or not. And in cooking as in eating, you just have to let your real likes and desires guide you.

My list of basics – and the recipes that constitute it – are dotted throughout this book. The list is eclectic. And in this chapter I have tried, in the main, to stay with the sort of food most of us anyway presume we can cook; it's only when we get started that we realise we need to look something up, check times, remind ourselves of the quantities. I want to satisfy those very basic demands without in any way wishing to make you feel as if there were some actual list of recipes which you needed to master before acquiring some notional and wholly goal-oriented culinary expertise. My aim is not to promote notions of uniformity or consistency – or even to imply that either might be desirable – but to suggest a way of cooking which isn't simply notching up recipes. In short, cooking in context.

First, you have to know how to do certain things, things that years ago it was taken for granted would be learned at home. These are ordinary kitchen skills, such as how to make pastry or a white sauce.

I learned some of these things with my mother in the kitchen when I was a child, but not all of them. So I understand the fearfulness that grips you just as you anticipate rolling out some shortcrust, say. We ate no puddings at home, my mother didn't bake and nor did my grandmothers. I didn't acquire early in life that lazy confidence, that instinct. When I cook a stew I have a sense, automatically, of whether I want to use red or white wine, of what will happen if I add anchovies or bacon. But when I bake I feel I lack that instinct, though I hope I am beginning to acquire it.

And of course I have faltered, made mistakes, cooked disasters. I know what it's like to panic in the kitchen, to feel flustered by a recipe which lists too many ingredients or takes for granted too much expertise or dexterity.

I don't think the answer, though, is to avoid anything that seems, on first view, complicated or involves elaborate procedures. That just makes you feel more fearful. But what is extraordinarily liberating is trying something – say, pastry – and finding out that, left quietly to your own devices, you can actually do it. What once seemed an arcane skill become second nature. It does happen.

And how it happens is by repetition. If you haven't made pastry before, follow the recipe for shortcrust on page 41. Make a flan. Don't leave it too long to make another one. Or a pie or a savoury tart. The point is to get used gradually to cooking something in the ordinary run of things. I concede that it might mean having to make more of a conscious effort in the beginning, but the time and concentration needed will recede naturally, and the effort will soon cease altogether to be conscious. It will just become part of what you do.

You could probably get through life without knowing how to roast a chicken, but the question is, would you want to?

BASIC ROAST CHICKEN

When I was a child we had roast chicken at Saturday lunch, and probably one evening a week, too. Even when there were only a few of us, my mother never roasted just one chicken; she cooked two, one to keep in the fridge, cold and whole, for picking at during the week. It's partly for that reason that a roast chicken, to me, smells of home, of family, of food that carries some important, extra-culinary weight.

My basic roast chicken is the same as my mother's: I stick half a lemon up its bottom, smear some oil or butter on its breast, sprinkle it with a little salt, and put it in a gas mark 6/200°C oven for about 20 minutes per 500g plus 30 minutes.

My mother could make the stringiest, toughest flesh – a bird that had been intensively farmed and frozen since the last Ice Age – taste as if it were a lovingly reared poulet de Bresse. She, you see, was a product of her age, which believed that cooking lay in what you did to inferior products (and I expect she did no more in this case than use much more butter than anyone would now); I, however, am a product of mine, which believes that you always use the best, the freshest produce of the highest quality you can afford – and then do as little as possible to it. So I buy organic free-range chickens and anoint them with the tiniest amount of extra virgin olive oil or butter – as if I were putting on very expensive handcream – before putting them in the oven. I retain the lemon out of habit – and to make my kitchen smell like my mother's, with its aromatic, oily-sharp fug.

I can't honestly say that my roast chicken tastes better than hers, but I don't like eating intensively farmed, battery-reared meat. However, if you know you've got an inferior bird in front of you, cook it for the first hour breast side down. This means you don't, at the end, have quite that glorious effect of the swelling, burnished breast – the chicken will have more of a flapper's bosom, flat but fleshy – but the white meat will be more tender because all the fats and juices will have oozed their way into it.

If you want to make a good gravy – and I use the term to indicate a meat-thick golden juice or, risking pretentiousness here, *jus* – then put 1 tablespoon of olive oil in the roasting dish when you anoint the bird before putting it in the oven, and about half an hour before the end add another tablespoon of oil and a spritz from the lemon half that isn't stuffed up the chicken. By all means use butter if you prefer, but make sure there's some oil in the pan, too, to stop the butter from burning.

When you remove the chicken, let it stand for 5 or 10 minutes before carving it, and make gravy by putting the roasting dish on the hob (remove, if you want, any excess fat with a spoon, though I tend to leave it as it is). Add a little white wine and boiling water or chicken stock, letting it all bubble away till it's syrupy and chickeny. If you don't have to hand any home-made stock a stock cube, or portion thereof, would be fine. In fact, Italians sometimes put a stock cube inside the chicken along with or instead of the lemon half before roasting it.

ROASTED GARLIC AND SHALLOTS

My basic chicken recipe also includes garlic and shallots; this is the easy way to have dinner on the table without doing much. About 50 minutes before the end of the cooking time, pour 2 tablespoons olive oil either into the same pan or another one and add, per 2kg chicken (which is for 4 people), the unpeeled cloves of 2 heads of garlic and about 20 unpeeled shallots. They don't roast, really, but steam inside their skins, which on the garlic are like boiled-sweet wrappers, on the shallots like twists of brown paper. Eat them by pressing on them with a fork, and letting the soft, mild – that's to say intensely flavoured and yet wholly without pungency – creamy interior squeeze out on to your plate. Put some plates on the table for the discarded skins, and if not finger bowls then napkins or a roll of paper towel. My children adore garlic and shallots cooked like this, and sometimes, when I don't want to cook a whole chicken for them, I roast a poussin instead and put the shallots and garlic and poussin in all at the same time. And if you want to make this basic recipe feel a little less basic, then you can sprinkle some toasted pine nuts and flat-leaf parsley, chopped at the last minute, over the food before serving.

If you've managed to fit the garlic and shallots in the tray with the chicken, you can roast a tray of potatoes in the same oven at the same time. Dice the potatoes, also unpeeled, into approximately 1cm cubes, or just cut new potatoes in half lengthways, and anoint them with oil (or melted lard, which fries them fabulously crisp). Sprinkle them with a little dried thyme (or freshly chopped rosemary) before cooking them for 1 hour to 1 hour 10 minutes.

All of which leads us to the next basic recipe:

STOCK

Do not throw away the chicken carcass after eating the chicken. Go so far, I'd say, as to scavenge from everyone's plate, picking up the bones they've left. I'm afraid I even do this in other people's houses. You don't need to make stock now – and indeed you couldn't make anything very useful from the amount of bones from one bird – but freeze them. Indeed freeze whatever bones you can, whenever you can, in order to make stock at some later date (see page 78 for further, passionate, adumbration of this thesis).

An actual recipe for stock would be hard to give with a straight face; boiling remains up to make stock is as far from being a precise art as you can get. Look at the recipes for broth and consommé (see pages 94–5) if you want something highfalutin', but if you're looking for what I call chicken stock (but which classically trained French chefs, who would use fresh meat and raw bones, boiled up specifically to make stock, would most definitely not), then follow my general instructions. At home, I would use the carcasses of 3 medium, cooked chickens.

Break the bones up roughly and put them in a big pan. Add a stick of celery broken in two or a few lovage leaves, 1 or 2 carrots, depending on size, peeled and halved, 1 onion stuck with a clove, 5 peppercorns, a bouquet garni, some parsley stalks and the white of a leek. Often I have more or less everything to hand without trying, except for that leek; in which case I just leave it out. (At the time of writing, it is still permitted to buy veal shin, and I sometimes add a couple of discs if I want a deeper-toned broth of almost unctuous mellowness.) Cover with cold water, add 1 teaspoon of salt and bring to the boil, skimming off the froth and scum that rises to the surface. Lower the heat and let the stock bubble very, very gently, uncovered, for about 3 hours. Allow to cool a little, then strain into a wide, large bowl or another pan. When cold, put in the fridge without decanting yet. I like to let it chill in the fridge so that I can remove any fat that rises to the surface, and the wider that surface is, the easier.

When I've removed the fat, I taste the stock and consider whether I'd prefer it stronger flavoured. If so, I put it back in a pan on the hob and boil it down till I've got a smaller amount of rich, intensely flavoured stock.

I then store it in differing quantities in the freezer. On the whole, the amount of stock I find most useful is in packages of 150ml and 300ml. For the smaller amount, I just ladle ten tablespoons into a freezer bag or small tub with a lid; for the larger, I line a measuring jug with a freezer bag and pour it in till I've got, give or take, 300ml (it's difficult, because of the baggy lining, to judge with super-calibrated accuracy). I then twist on the tie-up and put the whole thing, jug and all, into the freezer. This is why I own so many plastic measuring jugs. I am constantly forgetting about them once they're buried in the freezer. But, in principle, what you should do is leave the stock till solid, then whisk away the jug, leaving the jug-shaped cylinder of frozen liquid, which you slot back into the deep-freeze. You may need to run hot water over the jug for a minute in order to let the stock in its bag just slip out. This is a useful way to freeze any liquid. Although it's a bore, it pays to measure accurately and to label clearly at the time of freezing. Later you can take out exactly the quantity you need.

Poussins make wonderful, strong, easily jellied stock; it must be the amount of zip and gelatin in their poor young bones. So if ever you need to make a stock from scratch, with fresh meat, not cooked bones (in other words the way you're supposed to), and you can't find a boiling fowl, then buy some poussins, about 4, cut each in half, use vegetables as above, cover with cold water and proceed as normal.

I do not disapprove of stock cubes, if they're good. (See page 506.)

CELERY AND LOVAGE

One of the most useful things an Italian friend once showed me was how important even half a stick of celery is in providing base-note flavour, not just to stocks, but to tomato and meat sauces, to pies, in fact to almost anything savoury. The taste is not boorishly celery-like; it just provides an essential floor of flavour.

In Italy, when you buy vegetables from the greengrocer you can ask for a bunch of *odori*, which is a bunch of those herbs which breathe their essential scent into sauces and is given, gratis. Included in it will be one stick of celery.

And I wish we could buy, let alone get for free, celery by the single stick in Britain. You need so little of it when cooking, and most of what's on sale anyway – white, limp and waterlogged – scarcely repays the eating. If I can get huge, leafy, green Spanish or Italian celery, I mind less about having to buy a whole bunch; apart from anything else it looks beautiful in a vase in the kitchen. But those leaf-stripped, bendy-stalked clumps of waxy-white celery that are normally on sale, especially in the supermarkets, are the saddest of dismal forced-hand purchases.

In summer or even from spring onwards, if you've got a garden or bit of yard, you can grow some lovage, the leaves and stalks of which fabulously impart the scent of a grassy, slightly more aromatic celery. You just pick a bit as you need it. I often use lovage as a replacement for celery; if I'm chopping some onion, carrot and garlic to make a base for a shepherd's pie or a thick soup, I chop in some lovage leaves at the same time.

LETTUCE AND LOVAGE SOUP

Naturally, you can use more if you want the lovage to be the subject, the actual focus. To make a lettuce and lovage soup, soften a handful of finely chopped lovage leaves along with 4 finely chopped spring onions in about 30g of butter, then add 2 shredded cos lettuces and let them wilt in the buttery heat. Stir in ½ teaspoon sugar and some salt if the stock you're using is not very salty itself. Add about 1 litre of stock – a light chicken stock, possibly from your freezer, or vegetable stock made with Marigold granules – or ½–¾ stock and the rest milk. Gently simmer, uncovered, for about 10 to 15 minutes, then either blend in a machine, or push through a sieve or a mouli. Taste again for seasoning. Add a good grating of fresh nutmeg. If you want a velvety cream rather than a light, pale broth, stir an egg yolk beaten with 100ml cream, double or single, into the soup over the heat, but make sure it doesn't boil. Remove and serve, sprinkling over some more choppped lovage leaves.

You can grow lovage from seed, but I bought a little pot from a garden centre some years back and planted it out; now each spring it grows back huge, its bushy, long-stalked arms outstretched, magnificently architectural.

You should grow your own herbs if you can and want to, but don't spread yourself, or your plants, too thinly. It is counter-productive if you have so little of each herb that you never pick much of it for fear of totally denuding your stock. In my own garden, I stick to rosemary, flat-leaf parsley, rocket and sorrel. I like to grow lots of parsley – at least two rows, the length of the whole bed – and even more rocket. Some years I've planted garlic so that I can use the gloriously infused leaves, as they grow, cut up freshly in a salad. In pots I keep bay, marjoram and mint. This year I'm going to try some angelica – to flavour custards – and Thai basil, so that I don't have to go to the Thai shop to buy huge bunches of the stuff, wonderfully aromatic though it is, only to see it go off before I've had a chance to use it all. I have never had any success with coriander (from seed). I can manage basil easily, but then I suddenly feel overrun. And I have to say, I find watering pots excruciatingly effortful.

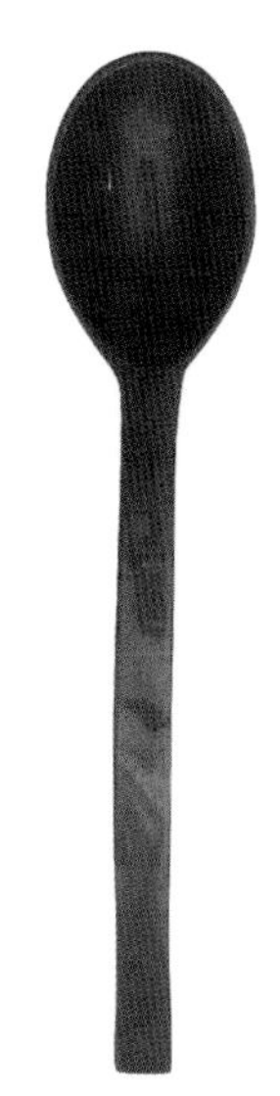

As with so much to do with food, a lot of a little rather than a little of a lot is the best, most comforting and most useful rule. You can always buy herbs growing in pots, in season, at good supermarkets and garden centres, and herbs cut in big bunches in specialist shops and good greengrocers.

MAYONNAISE

Stock is what you may make out of the bones of your roasted chicken, but mayonnaise, real mayonnaise, is what you might make to eat with the cold, leftover meat. There is one drawback: when you actually make mayonnaise you realise, beyond the point of insistent denial, how much oil goes into it. But since even the best bottled mayonnaise – and I don't mean the one you think I mean, but one manufactured by a company called Cottage Delight (see Gazetteer, page 506) – bears little or no relation to real mayonnaise, you may as well know how to make it.

When I was in my teens, I loved Henry James. I read him with uncorrupted pleasure. Then, when I was eighteen or so, and had just started *The Golden Bowl*, someone – older, cleverer, whose opinions were offered gravely – asked me whether I didn't find James very difficult, as she always did. Until then, I had no idea that I might, and I didn't. From that moment, I couldn't read him but self-consciously; from then on, I did find him difficult. I do not wish to insult by the comparison, but I had a similar, Jamesian mayonnaise experience. My mother used to make mayonnaise weekly, twice weekly; we children would help. I had no idea it was meant to be difficult, or that it was thought to be such a nerve-racking ordeal. Then someone asked how I managed to be so breezy about it, how I stopped it from curdling. From then on, I scarcely made a mayonnaise which didn't split. It's not surprising: when confidence is undermined or ruptured, it can be difficult to do the simplest things, or to take any enjoyment even in trying.

I don't deny that mayonnaises can split, but please don't jinx yourself. Anyway, it's not a catastrophe if it does. A small drop of boiling water can fix things, and if it doesn't, you can start again with an egg yolk in a bowl. Beat it and slowly beat in the curdled mess of mayo you were previously working on. Later add more oil and a little lemon juice. You should, this way, end up with the smoothly amalgamated yellow ointment you were after in the first place. I hate to say it, but you may have to do this twice. You may end up with rather more mayonnaise than you need, but getting it right in the end restores your confidence, and this is the important thing.

I make mayonnaise the way my mother did: I warm the eggs in the bowl (as explained more fully later) then beat and add oil just from the bottle, not measuring, until the texture feels right, feels like mayonnaise. I squeeze in lemon juice, also freehand, until the look and taste feel right. If you make a habit of making mayonnaise, you will inevitably come to judge it instinctively too. I don't like too much olive oil in it: if it's too strong it rasps the back of the throat, becomes too invasive. I use a little over two-thirds groundnut oil and a little under one-third olive oil, preferably that lovely mild stuff from Liguria. If you prefer, do use half and half and a mild French olive oil, which is probably more correct, anyway, than the Italian variety.

By habit, and maternal instruction, I always used to use an ordinary whisk. This takes a long time (and I can see why my mother used us, her children, as *commis* chefs). Now I use my KitchenAid (similar to a Kenwood Chef, but American) with the wire whip in place. You can equally well use one of those electric hand-held whisks, which are cheap and useful. Please, whatever you do, don't use a food processor: if you do, your finished product tastes just like the gluey bought stuff. And then, hell, you might as well just go out and buy it.

2 egg yolks (but wait to separate the eggs, and see below)
225ml groundnut or sunflower oil
75ml extra virgin olive oil
juice of 1/2 lemon

Put the eggs, in their shells, in a large bowl. Fill it with warm water from the tap and leave for 10 minutes. (This brings eggs and bowl comfortably to room temperature, which will help stop the eggs from curdling, but is optional, as long as you remember to take the eggs out of the fridge well before you need them.) Then remove the eggs, get rid of the water and dry the bowl thoroughly. Wet and then wring out a tea towel and set the bowl on it; this stops it slipping and jumping about on the worksurface.

Separate the eggs. Put aside the whites and freeze them for another use (and see page 19), and let the yolks plop into the dried bowl. Start whisking the yolks with a pinch of salt. After a few minutes very, very gradually and drop by mean drop, add the groundnut oil. You must not rush this. It's easier to let the oil seep in gradually if you pour from a height, holding the measuring jug (or bottle with a spout attached, if you're not actually using measured quantities) well above the bowl. Keep going until you see a thick mayonnaise form, about 2–3 tablespoons' worth, then you can relax and let the oil drip in small glugs. When both oils have been incorporated (first the groundnut, then the olive oil) and you have a thick, smooth, firm mayonnaise, add a few squeezes of lemon juice, whisking all the time. Taste to see if you need to add more. Add salt and pepper as you like; my mother used white pepper, so she didn't end up with black specks.

SAUCE VERTE

If you want a sharper more vinegary taste you can add ½–1 teaspoon Dijon mustard to the egg yolks in the beginning. A touch of mustard is fabulous in a sauce verte, or green mayonnaise, which is made by adding 2 tablespoons or so of chopped herbs – sorrel, tarragon, parsley, whatever – and, classically, a handful of spinach, blanched (dunked for a few seconds in boiling water), super-efficiently drained, then minutely chopped into the mayonnaise at the end. I've never actually tried using those frozen spheres of spinach purée I mention in the children's food chapter (page 459), but it occurs to me that you could try one here. Otherwise a little watercress or rocket, chopped with the unblanched herbs, in place of the spinach, is fine. And if you're in the mood, you can add some chopped capers and gherkins (about 2 teaspoons of each) as well. In other words, treat this as what it is in Italian – salsa verde (page 200) – only hanging in an egg and oil emulsion rather than just bound in the oil; this gives you the go ahead to stir in some minced anchovy if you like too.

EGG MAYONNAISE

I love sauce verte especially with cold pork, but I have to say that every time I eat real mayonnaise, in its bleached-yolk yellow and unmodified state, I am freshly surprised how good it is. And egg mayonnaise – hard-boiled eggs, sliced and masked with light mayonnaise, with or without a criss-crossing of anchovies on top – has to be one of the most fashionably underrated of dishes.

HOLLANDAISE

Hollandaise is really a kind of hot mayonnaise. As children we all took turns standing on the chair pushed up against the stove, to stir the butter we'd conscientiously cut into cubes before starting into the swell of eggs in the pudding basin which was suspended above a pan of boiling water. It wasn't until relatively recently that I came across a made-for-the-purpose *bain-marie*; previously, I had no idea they existed. So you needn't worry: a bowl and an ordinary saucepan is all you need. I prefer, now, not to use a pudding basin but a wider-curved, round-bottomed stainless-steel bowl (for which you can get a stand as well) and which is useful for whisking egg whites, off or on the heat, melting chocolate, reheating custards, whatever. But I'm glad for my early training in making hollandaise (and béarnaise, see below) because it pre-empted any fear about how difficult saucemaking might be. Even my brother, who scarcely cooks anything other than pasta, can make hollandaise.

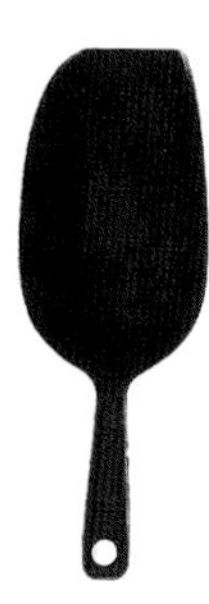

It's true, we didn't make it according to the classical canon. Most French textbooks would instruct you to make a fierce reduction to whisk into the yolks at the beginning. I think – and, since my pared-down attitude is one also sanctioned by Carême, there's no need to apologise for it – that a simple, gentler hollandaise, just eggs and butter emulsified and spruced with lemon juice, is best. If you want to try the ur-recipe, then boil down 2 tablespoons of white wine vinegar, 1 of water, a good grating of fresh pepper and the smallest pinch of salt until the liquid is reduced to about 1 tablespoon, then whisk that into the yolks at the very beginning, before you get on to adding any of the butter.

3 egg yolks

200g unsalted butter, soft, cut into 1cm cubes

juice of ½–1 lemon

Put the yolks in a bowl and suspend this bowl over a pan of cold water. The base of the bowl should be above, not touching, the water. Put the pan on the heat and whisk the yolks while the water comes to the boil. When it does, reduce to a steady simmer and start whisking in the cubes of butter. As one piece of butter is absorbed, whisk in the next and, by the time they have all been added, you should have a bowlful of thick sauce. If you feel it's reached that stage before you've finished all the butter, don't worry: just stop. And throw in extra if you feel it could take it. Still whisking, squeeze in the juice of ½ a lemon – I love watching the yolk-yellow goo suddenly lighten – and add salt, pepper (grinding in white pepper if you've got it) and more lemon juice to taste.

When the sauce is ready, you can fill another pan with tepid water and suspend the bowl on top of that (this time with the base of the bowl submerged) to keep it warm for about 20 minutes, but beat it firmly again before serving. If, when making it, the sauce looks as if it might curdle you can quickly whisk in an ice cube (to bring the temperature down) or stand the bowl in a pan of cold water and whisk well.

Hollandaise is not an essential accompaniment for asparagus, but a pretty divine one, and it is miraculous with sprouting broccoli (see page 49). I love it, too, with saffron threads – a large pinch or ¼ teaspoon, however you prefer to measure it – softened in and added with the lemon juice.

SAUCE MALTAISE

You should know that sauce maltaise is a hollandaise with blood orange juice. I don't rate it; I prefer, if I want that particular realm of flavour, to substitute Seville orange juice for the lemon juice. This means (if you don't freeze your Seville oranges) you can make it only in January or February (see food in season, page 48). As a once-a-year accompaniment to plain, baked or grilled white fish and broccoli, it might be a treat, but proceed – as with all deviations from the classical – with caution.

BÉARNAISE

for Dominic

I grew up believing erroneously that sauce béarnaise was just a hollandaise with chopped tarragon in it. Up to a point it is. And if you want to make a quick, almost-béarnaise, use my mother's method, which is to say follow the recipe for hollandaise above, adding 1 teaspoon dried tarragon to the egg yolks and then stirring in some freshly chopped tarragon at the end. Use a little lemon only, and lots of pepper. Be careful: too much tarragon can evoke that manure-underfoot, farmhouse scent, although I don't know why. When I was a child, and dried herbs weren't considered as ignominious as they are today, we made béarnaise without any fresh tarragon, though with a drip of tarragon vinegar along with the squeeze of lemon juice. Unless you are trying to create the great classic in its purest form, be kind to yourself. If you can't get chervil, be assured that the sauce will still taste fabulous with just tarragon.

This is my desert island sauce; there's little better in the world to eat than steak béarnaise. (It's also very good with salmon.) If you substitute mint for the tarragon, you have a sauce that goes very well with lamb, especially steaks cut off the leg and plain grilled.

1–2 shallots, chopped finely (to yield 1 tablespoon)
2 tablespoons fresh tarragon leaves, chopped, and their stalks chopped roughly and bruised
1 tablespoon chervil, chopped
2 tablespoons wine or tarragon vinegar
2 tablespoons white wine
1 teaspoon peppercorns (preferably white), crushed or bruised
3 egg yolks
1 tablespoon water
200g unsalted butter, soft, cut into 1cm dice
juice of 1/4–1/2 lemon

Put the shallot, tarragon stalks, 1 tablespoon each of the chopped tarragon and chervil leaves, the vinegar, wine and peppercorns in a heavy-based saucepan and boil until reduced to about 1 tablespoon. Don't move from the stove: this doesn't take long. Equally you can use 4 tablespoons of vinegar and omit the wine.

Press the reduced liquid through a sieve or tea strainer and leave to cool. Put egg yolks and water in a bowl. Set over a pan of water which has come to a simmer. Add the reduced and strained liquid and whisk well. Keep whisking, as you add the butter, cube by cube, until it is all absorbed. Taste, season as you wish and add lemon juice as you wish. Treat it as the hollandaise to keep it warm and avert curdling. Stir in the remaining tablespoon of fresh chopped tarragon as you're about to serve it.

SEPARATING EGGS

For each of the three sauces above, you need to separate the egg yolks from the albumen. Everyone always tells you that the best way to do this is by cracking open the egg and, using the broken half-shells to cup the yolk, passing it from one to the other and back again until all the white has dropped in the bowl or cup you've placed beneath and the perfect, naked round of yolk remains in the shell. I don't think so. All you need is for a little sharp bit of the cracked-open shell to pierce the yolk and the deal's off. It is easier and less fiddly altogether just to crack the egg over a bowl and slip the insides from their shell into the palm of your hand near the bottoms of your fingers. Then splay your fingers a fraction. The egg white will run out and drip through the cracks between your fingers into the bowl, and the yolk will remain in the palm of your hand ready to be slipped into a different bowl.

I cannot bring myself to throw away the whites. Occasionally, when things threaten to get seriously out of hand, I just separate the eggs over the sink, not even giving myself the agony of choice. But otherwise I freeze the rejected whites, either singly or in multiples, marking clearly how many are in each freezer bag. Just in case you forget to label them or the bag's gone wrinkly and you can't read what's written on it, you should know that a frozen large egg white weighs about 40g. From that, you can work out how many you've got stashed away in any particular unmarked bag just by weighing it.

MERINGUES

The obvious thing to make with egg white is meringue. For each egg white you need 60g sugar, and the whites should be at room temperature before you start. I use caster sugar, but you can substitute soft brown sugar to make beautiful ivory-coloured almost toffee-ish meringues, golden caster sugar if you want the ivory colour but not such a pronounced taste, and, if you're ever in Canada or Vermont or don't mind spending the fortune it costs to buy it in Harrods, you can get some maple sugar and use that for the most fabulous, smoky, gleaming, elegant meringue of all time, the colour of expensive oyster-satin underwear. The brown or maple sugar variants are worth bearing in mind to go with ice-cream or fruit compôtes of any sort or just with coffee after dinner. I wouldn't necessarily squidge them together with whipped cream, but a bowl of raspberries, another of thick cream, and a plate of sugary, creamy, soft-centred, buff-coloured meringues is easy to get together and pretty damn fabulous with it; children's tea-party food with an edge.

To make about 20 meringues 3–4cm in diameter, or 10 of 6cm, you need:

2 egg whites

120g sugar

Preheat the oven to a very low heat: gas mark 1/140°C. Whisk the egg whites until stiff. For this, I always use my free-standing mixer with the wire whip attached, but an electric beater or balloon whisk will do. When you lift the beaters or whisk out of the mixture and firm peaks retain their shape, it's stiff enough. Gradually whisk in half the sugar. The meringue will take on a wonderful satiny gleam. Then fold in the remaining sugar with a metal spoon.

Line 1 or 2 baking trays with parchment or greaseproof paper or, better still, a fabulous creation called, just as fabulously, Bake-o-Glide. This is some sort of silicon non-stick lining paper which you can re-use, more or less indefinitely (until you lose it, in my case), to line cake tins and roasting trays. Mail-order kitchen gadget places and some specialist shops stock it (see Gazetteer, page 506, for details).

I am not dextrous, but I enjoy a bit of squeezing through piping bags. It makes me feel brisk and accomplished without having to be either. Remember to fold back the hem end of the piping bag by about half its whole length as you fill it. I stand the piping bags in a straight glass to do this. Once the piping bag is half full of the meringue mixture you can unfold the bag's skirt and twist the ends together to put pressure on the meringue within, keeping one hand near the (plain) nozzle. Splodge out individual meringues to your desired size on the lined trays. Refill the piping bag, and continue until all the mixture is used up. Don't worry if you haven't got a piping bag: just use teaspoons, or tablespoons if you're making the larger size, to deposit and shape them into neat piles, one by one.

Put the trays of meringues in the oven for about 40 minutes for the smaller size, 70 minutes for the larger. When they feel firm (and you can lift one up to check that the underside's cooked) turn the oven off, but keep the meringues in there until completely cold. If you take them out too soon, the abrupt change in temperature will make them hard and dry or even crack, and they're best with a hint of chewiness within. Once they are cold you can keep them for a long time in an airtight tin.

And here are a couple of other recipes for which I use my egg whites (neither require whisking).

MACAROONS

Mix 150g ground almonds with 200g caster sugar and stir in 2 egg whites. Combine well into a thick cream, then add a scant tablespoon of flour (preferably Italian 00) and 1 teaspoon of almond extract. Pipe – through a plain nozzle – into rounds about 5cm in diameter, leaving space between each, onto baking trays lined with rice paper or Bake-o-Glide. Traditionally you should press a split almond into the centre of each, but I don't always bother. Cook in a preheated gas mark 3/160°C oven for about 20 minutes. The biscuits will harden slightly as they cool, so be careful to time them to be softish in the centre, and chewy. Don't panic at their cracked surface: macaroons are meant to look like that.

This amount should make a good dozen.

LANGUE DE CHAT

Langue de chat are the sort of biscuits that are wonderful with any pudding you eat with a small spoon. You take 60g each of butter and vanilla sugar (see page 82) or caster sugar and cream them until light and fluffy. To cream, simply put the ingredients in a large bowl and beat with a wooden spoon until soft and pale. (It helps if you beat the butter first, till it's really soft, and then beat in the sugar gradually, handful by sprinkled-in handful.) Add 2 egg whites, stirring until you have a curdy mass, add half a teaspoon of vanilla extract and then 60g flour, preferably Italian 00, and beat or stir till you have a stiffish cream. Pipe through a plain small-sized nozzle to form small strips like squeezed-out toothpaste, on a lined – or greased and then floured – baking sheet. These spread enormously, so leave a clear 5cm between each. Bake in a preheated gas mark 6/200°C oven for about 8 minutes, until they're pale gold in the centre, darker gold at the edges. These quantities make about 30.

For other ways to use up egg whites, see the hazelnut cake recipe on page 359 (substituting other nuts if you prefer), the pavlova on page 373 and the potato pancakes on page 242.

BÉCHAMEL

Béarnaise may be my favourite sauce, but béchamel is unquestionably the most useful.

All it is is a roux, which is to say a mixture of equal amounts of butter and flour (although I sometimes use a little more butter), cooked for a few minutes, to which you add, gradually, milk and then cook until thickened.

I always use Italian 00 flour, which is relatively easy to come by now, at supermarkets as well as delicatessens. The difference lies in the milling; these flours are finer-milled than our plain flour and they cook faster, so the flouriness cooks out more quickly. Undeniably, this is useful, but ordinary plain flour has been used perfectly well to make béchamel for aeons, so don't agonise over it. I find, though, that I keep no ordinary plain flour in the house: just Italian 00 (superior for pastry, too, see page 41) and English self-raising (preferably organic, from somewhere like Dove's Farm), which cuts down on clutter and lots of half-used packets in the store cupboard. I give the quantities in tablespoons first, since that really is how one is most likely to add them to the pan.

1 tablespoon butter (about 15g)
1 1/2 tablespoons flour, preferably Italian 00 (also about 15g)
300ml full-fat milk
fresh nutmeg

Melt the butter in a heavy-based pan and then stir in the flour, cooking for 2–3 minutes until you have a walnut (sized and coloured) paste. Meanwhile, heat the milk (I do this in a measuring jug in the microwave: very *moderne*) and take the pan with the roux off the heat. Gradually, using a whisk, beat the warm milk into it. Proceed slowly and cautiously to avoid lumps. Keep stirring and adding, adding and stirring and when all the milk is smoothly incorporated, add salt, pepper and a grating of fresh nutmeg. If it does go lumpy, blitz it in your blender or with a hand-held equivalent.

Return to the heat, and cook, at a lowish simmer, stirring all the time, for about 5 minutes (at least twice that if you're using ordinary plain flour) until it has thickened and has no taste of flouriness. Add some more fresh nutmeg before using. And if you want to make your béchamel in advance, you can stop a skin forming by pouring a thin layer of milk or melted butter on top.

If you want a more intensely flavoured sauce, heat 300ml of milk first with 1 onion, ½ leek or some spring onions, 2 bay leaves or some mace (or whatever flavour it is you wish to intensify) and let it infuse, lid on, off the heat for 20 minutes or so before proceeding with the sauce.

CHEESE SAUCE

To make cheese sauce, add a pinch of English mustard powder or cayenne along with the flour and about 50–100g (depending on how you want to use your cheese sauce) grated cheddar or gruyère, or half gruyère, half parmesan at the end.

PARSLEY SAUCE

For parsley sauce – heavenly with cooked ham or to blanket broad beans – just infuse the milk with the stalks from a decent bunch of parsley. Then blanch the parsley leaves (although I have to say I don't always bother), dry them thoroughly, chop them finely and add them when stirring in the milk, sprinkling over a little more parsley at the end. And you can chop up leftover ham and mix it with the cold sauce, together with some dry mashed potatoes and possibly chopped gherkins or capers, to make parsley and ham patties. I sometimes add 1 egg yolk and 2–3 tablespoons double cream to make a more voluptuous parsley sauce – especially good with poached smoked fish and mashed potato. (And you can make patties out of these, too.)

PARSLEY AND HAM PATTIES

MY MOTHER'S WHITE SAUCE

This is the way I make béchamel sauce most of the time. My mother's method was the same as above, except she put a little nut of a chicken stock cube – about ¼–⅓ of a cube – in the pan along with the butter and flour and made roux of them all together. This makes a good savoury sauce; the stock isn't very pronounced, it just gives a more flavourful saltiness. So make really sure you don't season without thinking.

I use this method to make a white sauce to coat leeks or onions, using half milk and half the water the onions or leeks have been cooking in.

Sometimes, even better, I use half single cream and half the vegetable-cooking water. If no cream's available, I beat in an extra nut of butter at the end.

VEGETABLE SOUP

A vegetable soup doesn't require a recipe, and I certainly don't want to suggest you get out your scales to make it with mechanical accuracy. But it's helpful to have a working model for a plain but infinitely variable soup. This one is not exactly the mix of carrot, parsnip and turnip my mother used to make, and which we knew as nip soup, but is based on its memory.

I use my beloved Marigold vegetable bouillon powder most of the time, but if I've got some good organic vegetables that taste properly and vigorously of themselves, I use water. A friend of mine swears that if you use Evian or other bottled still water it makes all the difference, but I haven't quite got round to that yet.

Although my hand is pretty well permanently stuck, culinarily speaking, around the neck of a bottle of Marsala, I admit that there isn't a vegetable soup in the land that doesn't benefit from the addition of a little dry sherry.

1 onion
2 carrots
1 turnip
1 parsnip
1 maincrop potato
1 stalk celery
1 leek, white part only
3 tablespoons olive oil, or 45g butter and a drop of oil
1 litre vegetable stock
1 bouquet garni
nutmeg
1–2 tablespoons dry sherry
fresh parsley, chives or chervil to sprinkle over when eating

Peel and roughly chop the onion, carrots, turnip, parsnip and potato. Roughly chop the celery and thickly slice the leek. I now put the whole lot in the processor and blitz it briefly until chopped medium-fine. Obviously you needn't use the machine, I've just got into this lazy habit.

Heat the oil, or butter with its drop of oil, in a large wide pan (one which has a lid, preferably) and then add the chopped vegetables to it, turning them over a few times so they all have a slight slick of fat. Sprinkle with salt, cover, and on a low heat let them half-fry, half-braise until softened, about 10–15 minutes, shaking the pan from time to time and occasionally opening the lid to stir (making sure nothing's sticking or burning at the bottom) before putting the lid back on again. Pour in the stock, adding the bouquet garni and a good grind of pepper, and bring, uncovered, to a simmer, then cook for about 20–40 minutes (exactly how long depends on the age of the vegetables, the size you've chopped them, the dimensions of the pan and the material of which the pan's made).

When the soup's cooked, blend or process it, or push it through a mouli. Alternatively, if you've got one of those stick blenders, you can do an agreeably rough purée in the pot. Sometimes, I take out a couple of ladlefuls, blend or process them, and put them back into the soup to thicken it, without turning it all to mush. Season to taste (I like a bit of grated nutmeg at the end) and stir in the sherry before serving, sprinkling over fresh herbs as you wish.

BREADCRUMBS

These are a regular and very ordinary kitchen requirement, but because we are all out of the habit of using up leftovers, few of us are clear how to go about making that misnomer, fresh breadcrumbs. I say misnomer, because you really want them stale.

I don't bother with drying out bread in the oven. I just take the crusts off some slices of stale-ish (but not bone dry) good white bread, cut the bread into chunks and lacerate into crumbs in the processor. I then leave the crumbs in a shallow bowl or spread them out on a plate to dry and get staler naturally. If you want to make the sort of breadcrumbs that you can buy, those very dry, very small crumbs that could coat, say, a *scaloppina Milanese*, then just leave the bread till it's utterly dried out and cardboardy beyond belief before blitzing it in the processor. You can keep breadcrumbs in a freezer bag in the freezer and use them straight from frozen. I reckon an average slice of good bread, without crusts, weighs 25g; this in turn yields approximately 6 tablespoons of breadcrumbs.

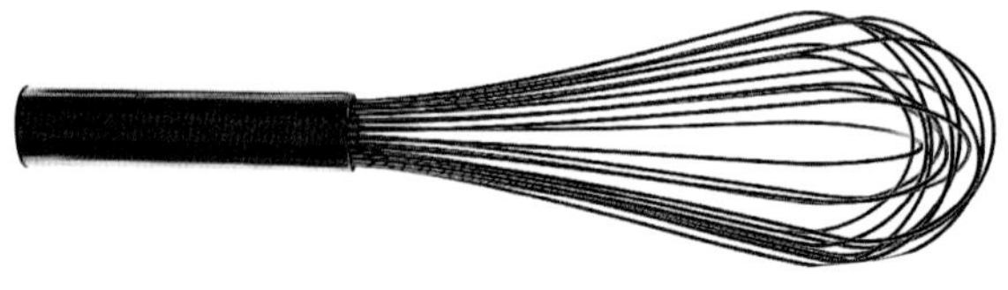

VINAIGRETTE

One of the hangovers of the hostess-trolley age is the idea that the clever cook has a secret vinaigrette recipe which can transform the dullest lettuce into a Sensational Salad. I'm not sure I even have a regular vinaigrette recipe, let alone one with a winning, magic ingredient. But we all panic in the kitchen from time to time, so here is a useful, broad-brush reminder of desirable proportions for various dressings.

PLAIN SALAD DRESSING

I sometimes think the best way of dressing salad is to use just oil and lemon juice. The trick is to use the best possible olive oil – and as little of it as possible – and toss it far longer than you'd believe possible. Use your hands for this. Start off with 1 tablespoon of oil for a whole bowl of lettuce and keep tossing, adding more oil only when you are convinced the leaves need it. When all the leaves are barely covered with the thinnest film of oil, sprinkle over a scant ½ teaspoon sea salt. Toss again. Then squeeze over some lemon juice. Give a final fillip, then taste and adjust as necessary. Instead of lemon juice you can substitute wine vinegar (and I use red wine vinegar rather than white generally), but be sparing. Just as the perfect martini, it was always said, was made merely by tilting the vermouth bottle in the direction of the gin, so when making the perfect dressing you should merely point the cork of the vinegar bottle towards the oil.

As important is the composition of the salad itself. Keep it simple: there's a green salad, which is green; or there's a red salad, of tomatoes (and maybe onions). First-course salads may be granted a little extra leeway – the addition of something warm and sautéed – but I would never let a tomato find its way into anything leafy. For more detailed explanations (genetic as much as aesthetic) of this prejudice, please see page 217. When you're using those already-mixed packets of designer leaves, you should add one crunchy lettuce – cos or Webb – which you buy, radically and separately, as a lettuce and then tear up yourself at the last minute. Herbs – parsley, chives, chervil, lovage – are a good idea in a green salad (and you can add them either to the salad or the dressing), but, except on certain, rare, occasions, I think garlic is better left out.

BASIC FRENCH DRESSING

2 teaspoons red wine vinegar
scant 1/2 teaspoon Dijon mustard (optional)
1 teaspoon sea salt
good grinding pepper
drop or two cold water
6–8 tablespoons best olive oil

If you're using the mustard (and I sometimes use a tarragon mustard – feltily green and lightly, rather than effusively, fragrant – and sometimes none at all), mix it in a bowl with the vinegar, the salt and pepper and a drop or two of cold water, then whisk or fork in the oil (I often use Ligurian, which is sweet and mild). Or you can put all the ingredients for the dressing in an old jam jar, screw on the lid and shake.

Put most – but not all – of your salad leaves in your salad bowl and add the dressing. Toss. Taste. If you find you have sloshed on too much dressing, add the spare leaves and toss again.

If you want to change oils, use part walnut or hazelnut oil, part olive oil. Don't replace the olive oil totally. Just a tablespoon of the nut oil plus olive oil should achieve the variation in flavour that you are after. If you want to change vinegars, do so uninhibitedly, but taste first to check the level of acidity and adjust the other components correspondingly.

CAKES

We no longer live in a world where baking a cake is considered a basic skill. That, one could argue, is reason enough to include a recipe here. And I don't mean a fancy cake, but just a plain, ordinary sponge.

VICTORIA SPONGE

It was easier to keep in mind the proportions of the ingredients when we used pounds and ounces, for with a plain sponge all we'd do was use equal amounts of flour, sugar and butter with the number of eggs representing, as a figure, half the amount of ounces of each. In other words, if we were using 4oz each of flour, butter and sugar, we'd use 2 eggs, if 6oz, 3 eggs. It's less snappy, certainly not easily memorable, with grams.

For a small sponge, then, use 125g each of:

sugar
self-raising flour
unsalted butter
and 2 eggs

You can flavour the sponge with 1 teaspoon vanilla extract (or use vanilla sugar, see page 82) or you can add the zest of ½ a lemon or orange. Use milk to give the firm batter a soft, pouring consistency; about 2 tablespoons should be enough for the above quantities.

If you're making a traditional Victoria sponge, in two halves, to be sandwiched together later with jam or crushed fresh raspberries and cream (and don't forget to sprinkle the top of the cake with caster sugar later), then use 225g each flour, sugar and butter and 4 eggs.

I make this cake in the processor. Realising you can make a cake without all that creaming first is a revelation. Without the beating, however, you don't get all that air into it, so you have to add some extra baking powder. I don't always sift the flour, but I probably ought to. I have found, though, that replacing some of it with cornflour gives it an almost feathery lightness. The butter must be very, very soft or it won't all blend together. I never use eggs from battery hens; most of the time I choose Martin Pitt's eggs (see page 506), which are the nearest thing in terms of taste to staggering out each morning and plucking eggs fresh from underneath the warm hens at the bottom of the garden.

225g self-raising flour or 200g plus 25g cornflour
225g caster sugar
225g very, very soft unsalted butter
2 teaspoons baking powder
1 teaspoon pure vanilla extract
4 eggs
2–4 tablespoons full-fat milk

Preheat the oven to gas mark 4/180°C. Butter 2 sandwich tins 21cm in diameter (and just under 5cm deep).

Put all the ingredients except for the milk into the processor and blitz to mix. Check that everything has mixed all right, and then process some more while pouring 2 tablespoons of the milk through the funnel. You want a batter of a soft, dropping consistency. Add more milk if necessary. Pour into the tins and bake in the oven for about 25 minutes. When ready, the tops should spring back when pressed and a cake tester or fine skewer should come out clean.

Let stand in their tins for a minute or so and then turn onto a wire rack to cool. Sandwich together with cream, jam, raspberries or whatever you like.

Obviously, you can make the cake the old-fangled way. Cream the butter and sugar till pale and soft, then add the eggs, alternating each egg with 1 tablespoon or so of flour. When the eggs are beaten in, add the vanilla, then fold in the rest of the flour. Leave out the extra baking powder, and use only one tablespoon of milk.

BIRTHDAY CAKE

It's wise to have in your repertoire a pretty failsafe chocolate cake. I call this birthday cake because that's what it seems to get made for mostly. It's plain but good, and the chocolate ganache with which it's draped is gleamingly spectacular and ideal for bearing birthday candles. With this recipe, you don't need to be dextrous or artistic – and any other form of icing for a birthday cake requires you be both. But if you want to make the sort of cake you actually write Happy Birthday on, make a Victoria sponge and look at the children's party food on page 500 for additional ideas.

So many chocolate cakes now are luscious, rich and resolutely uncakey – rather like my chocolate pudding cake with raspberries on page 351 – that I feel nostalgically drawn to this solid offering. And – this is the best bit – it is ridiculously easy to make. No creaming or beating or whisking. Stirring is about the extent of it. I know condensed milk looks like a spooky ingredient, but trust me.

A note on the chocolate: I like to make the cake with dark chocolate (minimum 70 per cent cocoa solids) but the ganache with a mixture of dark and light. The light I use is Valrhona Lacte (which I think has about 35 per cent cocoa solids), but most supermarkets sell a good quality continental chocolate which is comparable. As to what proportions to use: that really is up to you. I change them depending on who's eating the cake, but it's likely to be half dark, half light, or sometimes two-thirds dark to one-third light.

for the cake
225g self-raising flour
30g best cocoa
200g caster sugar
100g unsalted butter
200g condensed milk
100g best quality dark chocolate
2 eggs, beaten

for the chocolate ganache

250g best quality chocolate (see above)

250 ml double cream

Preheat the oven to gas mark 4/180°C. Put the kettle on. Butter a 20cm Springform cake tin (or 2 sandwich tins) and line the base with baking parchment. This last is not crucial if you're using non-stick pans, but even so it removes all worries about turning out the cake later.

Sieve the flour, cocoa and a pinch of salt together into a large bowl and set aside.

Put the sugar, butter, condensed milk, 100ml just-boiled water and the chocolate broken into small pieces in a saucepan and heat until melted and smooth. Then, using a wooden spoon, stir this robustly but not excitably into the flour–cocoa mixture and, when all is glossily amalgamated, beat in the eggs.

Pour into the cake tin and bake for 35–45 minutes; less if you're using the shallower sandwich tins. When it's ready, the top will feel firm. Don't expect a skewer to come out clean; indeed, you wouldn't want it to. And don't worry about any cracking on the surface: the ganache will cover it later.

Leave to cool in the tin for 10 minutes and then turn out onto the rack.

When completely cool, split in half horizontally; if this sort of thing spooks you, you should certainly use 2 sandwich tins and stick the 2 cakes together; though remember, even if the cake breaks while you divide it, you can stick it together with the ganache.

To make the ganache, chop up the chocolate (I put it in the processor until reduced to rubble) and put it in a medium-sized bowl, preferably a wide shallow one rather than a pudding basin shape. Heat the cream to boiling (but do not let it boil) and pour it over the chocolate. Leave for 5 minutes and then, by choice with an electric mixer, beat until combined, coolish, thickish and glossy. You want it thin enough to pour but thick enough to stay put: at this stage, think of the ganache as somewhere between a sauce and an icing; later, it will set hard and Sachertorte-shiny. Pour some over the cut side of one half of the cake, using a palate knife to spread, and then plonk the other half on top. Pour the rest of the chocolate ganache over the top of the cake, letting it drape over, swirling this overspill with your palate knife to coat the sides. Leave for a couple of hours or till set. You can make the cake the day before and then make the ganache the next morning before you set off for work. You can then get back in the evening to your gleaming masterpiece with nothing to do save puncture its flawlessly smooth surface with candle-holders.

FANCY CAKE

Well, this is not so much a fancy cake as a plain one that looks partyish. It is just an almond sponge leavened with whisked egg whites and baked in a brioche mould. It looks wonderful, intrinsically celebratory, which is why I do it. Added to any plate of fruit – fresh or thawed frozen – you can serve it after dinner or lunch. It's no harder to make than a round cake; it's just that the fancy mould (and try to find a non-stick one) makes it, illogically, look as if you've taken about ten thousand times the effort. The brioche mould won't work for a Victoria sponge because you need the whoosh of air supplied here by the whisked egg whites.

6 eggs, separated
200g caster sugar
zest of 1 lemon
200g ground almonds

Preheat the oven to gas mark 3/160°C. Butter a brioche mould (normal size, which has about a 1½ litre capacity, and preferably non-stick).

Whisk the egg yolks and sugar until you have a pale creamy mass. It's easier to use electrical equipment for this but not impossible with an ordinary, hand-held whisk.

Fold in the ground almonds and zest. In another bowl whisk the egg whites until stiff. Add a dollop of egg white to the cake batter to lighten it and make it easier to fold the remaining whites in gently, which you should proceed to do with a metal spoon. When the whites are all folded in, pour the batter into the brioche tin and bake for 1 hour. The cake will rise and grow golden, but will deflate on cooling; that's fine. When you take it out, give it a prod. If you feel it needs another 10 minutes or so (ovens do differ so radically from one another, it's always a possibility), just put it back and don't worry about the cake sinking. Think of it as accounted for.

Let cool in the tin for about 10 minutes, then unmould onto a wire rack, immediately turn to stand the right way up, and leave to cool.

A MOORISH CAKE

I ate a cake rather like this once at Moro, a wonderful restaurant with – as the name suggests – a Moorish menu. The proportions of the cake were slightly different (250g each ground almonds and icing sugar, 8 eggs, the zest of 2½ oranges), but the method was the same. The real difference was the syrup, which was spooned over the cake as it cooled, leaving some more to be handed round on serving.

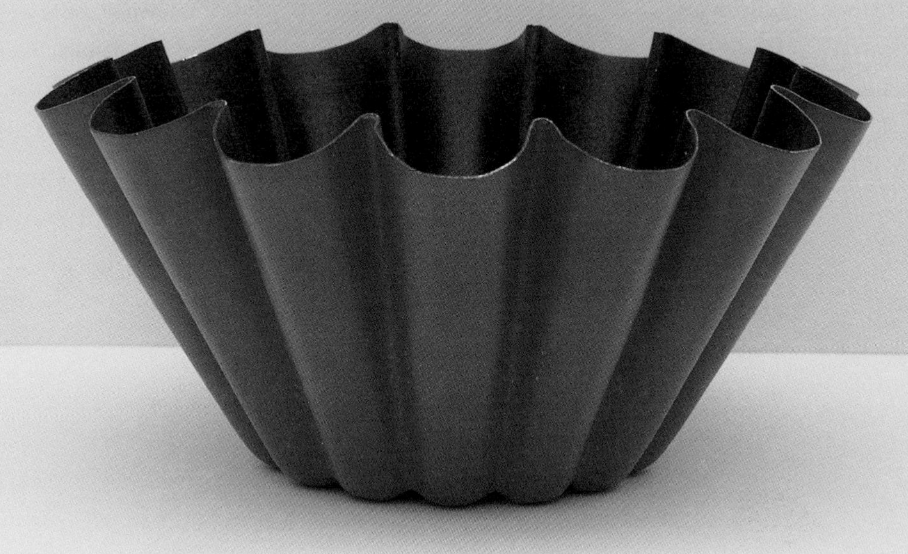

THE SYRUP

To make the syrup, combine the juice of 10 oranges, 200g sugar and a cinnamon stick in a saucepan and bring to the boil. Let it bubble away for about 10 minutes, or until the liquid is syrupy. Exactly how long this takes depends on the width of the pan and how it conducts the heat. Remove from the heat and allow to cool. If you need to cool the syrup quickly, stand the pan in a sink of cold water. And when it's cool, taste and add the juice of 1–2 lemons, depending on how sweet it is. Bear in mind that the cake will be very sweet, so it is important to keep a sour edge to the syrup for balance.

Blood oranges, available at the end of winter/beginning of spring, make a spectacular, impossibly scarlet, syrup.

BREAD

Bread is basic in the staff-of-life sense, but making it is hardly a fundamental activity for most of us. I don't get the urge that often, but every time I have, and have consulted a suitable book, I have been directed to make wholemeal bread. You may as well bake hessian. Why should it be thought that only those who want wholemeal bread are the sort to bake their own? Good wholemeal bread is very hard to make, and I suspect needs heavy machinery or enormous practice and muscularity.

Anyway, I give you this recipe for old-fashioned white bread, really good white bread, the sort you eat with unsalted butter and jam – one loaf in a sitting, no trouble. The recipe comes from Foster's Bakery in Barnsley, South Yorkshire, and found its way to me at a breadmaking workshop given at the Flour Advisory Board in London by John Foster. He was an exceptional teacher, and completely turned me, a lifelong sceptic of the breadmaking tendency, into a would-be baker.

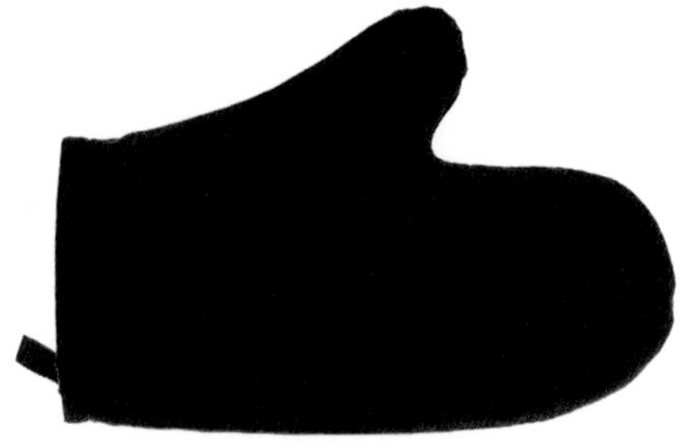

BASIC WHITE LOAF

For a good white loaf such as even I can make convincingly – a small one, so double the quantities if you want a big loaf or a couple – you need:

300g strong flour
10g fresh yeast
10g salt (1 teaspoon)
5g sugar (1/2 teaspoon)
170ml tepid water
10g fat

Buy the best flour you can (Waitrose sells some wonderful Canadian bread-making flour, and there are plenty of good mills in this country, most of which sell their flours through health stores) and use real yeast, not dried. Before you get put off, you should know two things. The first is that you can buy real yeast at any baker's, including the in-store bakeries of supermarkets; the second is that you use the real yeast here as you would easy-blend instant yeast – there's no frothing or blending or anything, you just add it to the mound of flour.

So: tip the flour onto a worktop and add the yeast, salt and sugar. Pour over the water and bring together, working with one hand, clawing at the floury mess rather as if your hand were a spider and your fingers the spider's legs. The spider analogy is apposite: you do have to be a bit 'If at first you don't suceed, try, try again' about bread-making. As the dough starts to come together, add the fat – which can be lard (my favourite here), vegetable shortening or oil – and keep squishing with your hands. When the dough has come together, begin kneading. Do this by stretching the dough away from you and working it into the worktop. Rub a little flour into your hands to remove any bits of dough that stick.

Keep kneading, pressing the heel of your hand into the dough, pushing the dough away, bringing it back and down against the work surface, for at least 10 minutes. John Foster warns that after 5 minutes you'll want to give up, and he's right. He suggests singing a song to keep yourself going; I prefer listening to the radio or talking to someone, but maybe that's just the difference between northerner and southerner.

When the dough's properly mixed – after about 10 minutes – you can tell the difference; it suddenly feels smoother and less sticky. Bring it to a ball, flour the worktop and the piece of dough lightly, and cover with a plastic bag or sheet of clingfilm and a tea-towel and leave for 30 minutes.

Then knead again for 3 minutes. Flour the worktop and dough ball again, cover as before, and leave for another 30 minutes.

Flatten the dough to expel the gas bubbles. Fold it in half, then in half again, and again, and keep folding the dough over itself until it feels as if you can fold no longer, as if the dough itself resists it (rather than you can't bear it) and then shape it into a ball again. Flour the worktop and so forth, cover the dough and leave, this time for 10 minutes.

Then shape the dough as you want: either round or oval and smooth, or you can slash the top with a knife, or put in a greased 450g loaf tin. Now, place on the baking tray (or in its tin) and put it in a warm place, under a plastic bag, for an hour, before baking for 35 minutes in a preheated gas mark 8/220°C oven. The trick is to lift the bread up and knock the base; if it sounds hollow, it's cooked. Try to let the bread cool before eating it.

IMPORTANT VARIANT

You can do the final proving in the fridge overnight (technically this is known as retarding). This doesn't cut out any work, but I find it makes things easier because I can do all the kneading when the children are in bed and before I go to bed (incidentally, it is, if not exactly calming, certainly very stress-relieving) and then bake the bread when I get up.

You do, however, need to increase the amount of yeast for this. Exactly how much you need to increase it by will depend on your fridge and the nature of your yeast. This may not be helpful, but it's true. Try doubling the yeast to 20g, then if the bread bolts when it's in the oven, you'll know to use 15g next time. When you get up in the morning preheat the oven, taking the bread out of the fridge on its baking tray as you do so. Leave it for 10 minutes or so, and then bake as above, maybe giving it an extra couple of minutes.

If you're going to start baking your own bread, what's to stop you making something to go on it?

LEMON CURD

I must admit that I don't use a double-boiler, as commonly instructed, to make lemon curd. It isn't because I'm brilliant and know how to stop it from curdling, or because I like living dangerously, but just because I'm impatient.

Fill up the sink with cold water before you start – so you can plunge the pan in it if the mixture looks like curdling – and just use a thick-bottomed saucepan (with a heat-diffuser beneath it as another safety measure if you like) and keep stirring at all times. I use an electric citrus press; if you're squeezing by hand, you'll get less juice, so use 3 eggs and 3 yolks.

4 organic or unwaxed lemons
4 eggs
4 egg yolks
300g caster sugar
200g unsalted butter

Remove the zest from the lemons. The best way of doing this is with a zester, not a grater. If you use a grater, you spend hours with a knife trying to chisel out the stuck bits later. Squeeze the juice out of the lemons after you've removed the zest.

Beat the eggs, yolks and sugar together until the sugar's dissolved. Add the butter, lemon juice and zest and heat gently in a pan on a low heat, stirring constantly, until the mixture thickens and grows smooth and looks, in fact, like lemon curd. If it's in danger of curdling, dunk the pan into the icy water in the sink, and beat like fury.

Put the lemon curd into sterilised jars – if I'm in the mood, I boil the jars in water for 10 minutes before using them, though really I think the dishwasher cleans them perfectly adequately – seal, and keep in the fridge. This makes about 2 jars, depending, obviously, on their size.

PASSION FRUIT CURD

Passion fruit curd may as well be made in half quantities (use 100g butter, 150g sugar, 2 eggs and 2 egg yolks) just because the amount of juice you get from each fruit is small, especially after you've removed the seeds. So, remove the inner pulp from 10 passion fruits and blitz it in the food processor for a minute before straining; this helps the seeds to separate from the pulp. Proceed as for lemon curd. Stir in the fresh pulp including seeds of an eleventh passion fruit, before the end.

See too the recipe for Seville orange curd on page 271.

CUSTARD

In many ways, curd is just custard made using juice in place of cream. And I mean cream: I take the view that when custard originated the milk used would have been much richer, much fattier, rather like single cream. So I use single cream or half milk, half cream.

As when making curd, I fill the sink with icy water and am prepared to plunge the pan in and start beating like mad if the custard looks like splitting.

And I don't even keep the heat all that low underneath the pan. If I do that, I lose patience, and then suddenly turn it up in a fury and then of course it does curdle.

Better to keep the heat middling and stir all the time. With the quantities below, if I'm using my widest saucepan (21cm in diameter), I find this takes 10 minutes. It's always hard to explain when exactly custard becomes custard. Like the chef Simon Hopkinson, I don't find it particularly helpful to be told that it's cooked when it coats the back of a wooden spoon, because it does that at the beginning. Think rather of aiming for it to be the texture and smooth thickness of good double cream. But you should, anyway, turn to page 377 to see my remarks about a revolutionary method for cooking pouring custard in advance in the oven, without stirring.

REAL CUSTARD

You may as well go the whole hog and use a vanilla pod. Otherwise, use vanilla sugar and/or stir in 1 teaspoon of good vanilla extract at the end. Or you can add 1 tablespoon of rum to the cream when heating it at the beginning.

It is helpful to know, when making custard, that you need 1 egg yolk for each 100ml of milk or cream. It's harder to be precise about the sugar, since that really depends on your taste, what you're eating the custard with, and whether it's going to be hot or cold, but I should say 1 heaped teaspoon of sugar per yolk should be fine.

500ml single cream or half milk, half cream
1 vanilla pod
5 egg yolks
40g sugar

Half fill the sink with cold water.

Pour the cream into your widest pan and add to it the vanilla pod split lengthways. Heat, and when it's about to come to the boil, but isn't boiling, remove from the heat and leave to infuse for 20–30 minutes.

Whisk the egg yolks with the sugar until thick and creamy and then strain the cream onto them, beating all the while, having swapped the whisk for a wooden spoon or spatula. To be frank, I find it easier just to fish out the 2 strands of vanilla; I don't lose any sleep over the speckles of vanilla finding their way into the custard. But there is something to be said (for ease of pouring alone) for straining the vanilla cream into a wide measuring jug before adding it to the yolks and sugar. Whichever way you do it, wash out the pan and dry it well, then pour in the beaten-together yolks, sugar and cream and, on a low to moderate heat, stir unceasingly for 8–10 minutes.

When the custard is cooked, even if it isn't splitting, dunk the pan quickly in the cold water in the sink and beat well with a wooden spoon. If it looks as if it is curdling, then use a whisk or, better still, an electric whisk or stick blender (or keep a blender jug in the fridge for just such eventualities) for some frenzied, violent beating here.

Pour into a bowl to cool (you can reheat it over a pan of simmering water later if you like) or serve as is.

QUICK FOOLPROOF CUSTARD

There is another way, and it's Tessa Bramley's (from *The Instinctive Cook*).

600ml double cream
1 vanilla pod
5 egg yolks
1 level teaspoon cornflour
1–2 tablespoons caster sugar

Put the double cream into a saucepan. Split the vanilla pod in half lengthways and scrape out seeds into the double cream; then bung in the pod, too. In a bowl, whisk together the yolks, cornflour and sugar. Bring the vanilla cream to boiling point. Remove pod, allow the cream to rise in the pan and then quickly pour onto the egg mixture, whisking continuously until the mixture thickens. This takes about 10 minutes with an electric mixer, so do it with a hand whisk only if you're feeling strong.

Sieve the custard and pour. That's it. You can reheat it later, and if the custard looks like curdling during the reheating, then you can save it by quickly whisking in 1 tablespoon double cream.

ICE-CREAM

Frankly, if you've made a custard, you've made (bar the freezing) your ice-cream; this asks no more of you, just of your kitchen. All that's needed is an ice-cream maker that slots into the freezer rather than a big expensive one that you plug in. Of course, you can just pour the mixture into a Tupperware and keep taking it out of the freezer to beat the mixture and break up the crystals but not only is this a bore, but the ice-cream just won't be as voluptuously smooth as if it had been churned. Though in fact, the vanilla ice-cream below is more do-able than most without special equipment; one of the reasons I include it.

BASIC VANILLA ICE-CREAM

The difference between custard and ice-cream – the temperature at which it's eaten – makes a difference to the amount of sugar you need; generally speaking, the colder you eat something, the sweeter it needs to be. All flavours, indeed, need to be intense when icy, which is why it drives me so mad when a pudding – or indeed any food – is kept in the fridge until the moment at which it's served. The cold kills the taste.

So: make the real custard above, only using 125g sugar in place of the 40g stipulated, and using single cream. And I certainly wouldn't worry here about the specks of vanilla; on the contrary, I'd welcome them. Indeed, scrape the seeds out into the cream before adding the pod strips and don't bother to strain the cream when you pour it over the egg yolks and sugar; you want maximum flavour.

When the custard's made and you've plunged the hot pan into the cold water in the sink, beating well, then you can remove the pod. Let the custard cool (if you keep it in the sinkful of water, beating every now and again, it doesn't take long) and then freeze in the ice-cream maker according to its manufacturer's instructions.

If you want to make a creamier ice-cream, you can stir 300ml double cream into the cooled custard before freezing it, in which case use about another 100g sugar. And taste for sweetness once the cream's in: if you think you need more, sieved icing sugar stirred in will dissolve easily enough.

You can flavour this ice-cream to make the flavour the Italians, who know about such matters, call *crema*. In place of the vanilla pod, infuse the cream with lemon zest, and strain as above. I like lemon custard, too, and also custard made with cream infused with the zest of an orange.

THE WORLD'S BEST CHOCOLATE ICE-CREAM

If you were only ever going to make one ice-cream, it would have to be vanilla. But once you've lost your ice-cream-making virginity, you have to allow yourself to be seduced by the world's best chocolate ice-cream. Marcella Hazan managed to procure the recipe for the Cipriani's dark and smokily voluptous chocolate ice-cream for *Marcella's Kitchen* and it is from that book that I reproduce it.

4 egg yolks
130g plus 2 tablespoons granulated sugar
500ml full-fat milk
100g dark chocolate (min. 70 per cent cocoa solids)
40g best cocoa available

Whisk the yolks and 130g of the sugar in a bowl until thick and creamy, forming pale ribbons when you lift the beaters or whisk. Bring the milk to the boil and add it to the beaten yolks, pouring slowly and beating all the while.

Melt the chocolate by breaking it up into small squares or pieces and putting it in a bowl above (but not touching) some simmering water in a pan. Then whisk this, followed by the cocoa, into the eggs and milk. Now pour the chocolate–custard mixture into a pan and cook on a low to moderate heat, stirring with a wooden spoon, until everything's smooth and amalgamated and beginning to thicken. You don't need to cook this until it is really custard-like, which makes life easier. Now for the bit that gives this ice-cream its essential smoky bitterness. Put 2 tablespoons of sugar with 2 teaspoons water into a thick-bottomed saucepan and turn the heat to high. Make a caramel: in other words, heat this until it's dark brown and molten. Live dangerously here: you are after the taste of burnt sugar. As it browns, whisk it into the chocolate custard; don't worry if it crystallises on contact as the whisking will dissolve it.

Turn into a bowl or wide jug and cool. Plunging the pan into cold water and beating, as usual, will do the trick. Then chill in the fridge for about 20 minutes (or longer if that's more convenient) before churning it in your ice-cream maker according to instructions.

PANCAKES

At some time in your life, if only on Shrove Tuesday, you might want to make pancakes. Obviously, a batter is a batter is a batter: you could easily consult the recipe for Yorkshire pudding. But it is surprising how useful it is just to know what the proportions of a regular batter are, especially since the Yorkshire pudding recipe I give (see page 281) isn't the traditional one.

125g plain flour, preferably Italian 00
1 egg
300ml milk
15–30g cooled butter, melted (optional)

The way I remember pancakes being made when I was a child is as follows.

Make a mound of the flour in a bowl, add a pinch of salt, then make a dip in the top. Crack open the egg and let it slip into this hole at the top of the hill and, with a wooden spoon, beat well, gradually incorporating the flour from the sides, and beating in the milk to make a smooth batter. Stop when the batter's creamy, change to a whisk and then whisk in the melted butter if you like (ordinary pancakes, as opposed to fancy crêpes, don't need butter). Leave the batter to stand for at least half an hour; overnight wouldn't matter. The batter might thicken in the meantime, in which case add milk or water (or possibly a little rum if you're making crêpes) to get the batter back to the right, thickish single-cream consistency.

The trick of the pancake is not so much in the batter, though, as in the frying: use very little oil and very little batter. The pan must be hot, and what I do is heat oil in it, then empty the oil down the sink before putting in the batter. Use less batter than you would imagine you need: you want just to line the pan. When bubbles come to the surface, the pancake is ready to flip. You should be prepared to throw away (and by that I mean eat yourself standing up at the cooker) the first pancake. It never works. Re-oil every 4 pancakes or so. Using a 20cm crêpe pan, you should get about 12 pancakes out of the above quantities. You don't need a special pan but you must use a well-seasoned frying pan. Non-stick pans are hopeless here as the pancakes they make are blond and pallid and rubbery; the batter seems steamed rather than seared.

There is nothing better on a pancake than a thick sprinkling of sugar (I keep only caster in the house now, but granulated is the gritty taste I remember from my childhood) and a good squeeze of lemon juice.

If you want to make American breakfast pancakes, to be eaten, preferably, with maple syrup and maybe even some crisp shards of bacon, you should alter the balance of the ingredients. Obviously you want a thicker batter, so add another egg, double the flour and to that flour add 1 teaspoon sugar and 4 teaspoons baking powder and regard the melted butter later as obligatory. Cook them, in about 8cm rounds, on a hot griddle or pan. Makes about 22.

PASTRY

On the subject of pastry, I am positively evangelical. Until fairly recently I practised heavy avoidance techniques, hastily, anxiously turning away from any recipe which included pastry, as if the cookbook's pages themselves were burning: I was hot with fear; could feel the flush rise in my panicky cheeks. I take strength from that, and so should you. Because if I can do the culinary equivalent, for me, of Learning to Love the Bomb, so can you.

It came upon me gradually. I made some plain shortcrust pastry, alone and in silence, apart from the comforting wall of voices emanating from Radio 4: it worked; I made some more. Then I tried some pâte sucrée: it worked; I made some more; it didn't. But the next time, it did; or rather, I dealt better with its difficulties.

But shortcrust, or even rich shortcrust, is really easy, and that's all you need to know. If you want something a little more exalted, you can make almond pastry (see page 292): this is as simple as the plainest shortcrust, tastes rich and rolls out like Play-Doh; the ground almonds seem to make it stretchy and extra-pliable.

SHORTCRUST

At its simplest, pastry is just a quantity of flour mixed with half its weight in fat and bound with water.

So, to make enough plain shortcrust to line and cover a 23cm pie dish (in other words for a double-crust pie), you would mix 240g flour with 120g cold, diced fat (half lard or vegetable shortening and half butter for preference), rubbing the fat in with your fingertips until you have a bowl of floury breadcrumb or oatmeal-sized flakes. Then you add iced water until the flour and fat turn into a ball of dough; a few tablespoons should do it. But as simple as that is, I can make it simpler; or rather, I can make it easier, as easy as it can be.

The first way to do this is not to use our ordinary plain flour but Italian 00 flour. This is the flour Italians at home, rather than in factories, use for pasta and it's certainly true that it seems to give pastry an almost pasta-like elasticity.

The second part of my facilitation programme is as follows.

Measure the flour into a bowl and add the cold fat, cut into 1cm dice. You then put this, as is, in the freezer for 10 minutes. Then you put it in the food processor with the double blade attached or into a food mixer with the paddle attached, and switch on (at slow to medium speed if you're using the mixer) until the mixture resembles oatmeal. Then you add, tablespoon by cautious tablespoon, the iced water, to which you've added a squeeze of lemon and a pinch of salt. I find you need a little more liquid when making pastry by this method than you do when the flour and fat haven't had that chilling burst in the deep-freeze.

When the dough looks as if it's about to come together, but just before it actually does, you turn off all machinery, remove the dough, divide into two and form each half into a ball, flatten the balls into fat discs, and cover these discs with clingfilm or put them each inside a freezer bag, and shove them in the fridge for 20 minutes. This makes pastry anyone could roll out, even if you add too much liquid by mistake.

Now, this method relies on a machine to make the pastry. To tell the truth, I culled and simplified the technique from a fascinating book, *Cookwise*, by an American food scientist called Shirley O. Corriher, and she does all sorts of strenuous things, including making the pastry by tipping out the freezer-chilled flour and fat onto a cold surface and battering it with a rolling pin until it looks like 'paint-flakes that have fallen off a wall'. She does, however, sanction the use of a mixer bowl (well-chilled) and paddle (set on slowest speed) and I have found it works well in the processor too. I know that I am not up to her hand-rolling method, or not yet at any rate.

RICH SHORTCRUST

'Rich', in terms of shortcrust, normally implies an egg to bind, and more than half fat to flour, but I find my method makes the pastry taste both more tender and more buttery anyway, so I don't change the basic shortcrust ratio. You can, of course: in which case, with 120g flour, use 80g fat. In all cases, I prefer half lard, half butter. Lard is unfashionable these days, but it is seriously underrated, both as a frying medium and, here, as a pastry shortener; it helps the crust get wonderfully flaky.

Since one of the things I learnt from *Cookwise* was that a slightly acidic liquid makes the pastry more tender (the freezing of the flour and fat, which makes for flattened crumbs rather than beady ones, contributes to its desirable flakiness), I have taken to using lemon or orange juice instead of, or as well as, an egg yolk and water to bind. And sometimes I just add a little sour cream, yoghurt or crème fraîche, whatever's to hand. For instance, when I make an onion tart (see page 392) I use some of the crème fraîche I've got in for the onion-covering custard. I always use just the yolk, not the whole egg, when making rich shortcrust.

Anyway, to make rich shortcrust to line a deep 20cm or shallow 23cm flan ring, you need:

120g flour, preferably Italian 00
60g butter, cold and cut into 1cm dice
1 egg yolk
1 teaspoon yoghurt or crème fraîche or sour cream or orange or lemon juice

Measure the flour into a bowl, add the butter and put in the freezer for 10 minutes. Beat the egg yolk with a pinch of salt and whatever acidic ingredient you choose and put it in the fridge. Keep a few tablespoons of iced water in a jug or bowl in the fridge in case you need them, too.

As above, you can make this either in a food processor or a mixer. Put the flour and butter in the processor with the double blade fitted or in a mixer with the flat paddle on slow and turn on. After barely a minute, the mixture will begin to resemble oatmeal or flattened breadcrumbs, and this is when you add the yolk mixture. Add, and process or mix. If you need more liquid, add a little iced water but go slowly and carefully; you need to stop just as the dough looks like it's about to clump, not once it has.

When it looks right, take it out and form into a fat disc, then put the dough disc into a freezer bag or cover with clingfilm and put into the fridge to rest for 20 minutes.

SWEET PASTRY

I have to say I mostly use unsweetened rich shortcrust for sweet pies and flans, in the first instance because making pâte sucrée can give me a nervous breakdown at the best of times, in the second, because I nearly always think that a plain, sugarless, neutral base is best. There are some pies or tarts though – the custard tart on page 318 for example, or any French fruit flan – which do need a crisp and sweet crust. This is it. It is as easy as the pastry recipes above, but it has the sweet, short, flan-base delicacy of far more complicated pastries. Just use it whenever you see pâte sucrée stipulated. I can't guarantee your sanity otherwise.

120g plain flour, preferably Italian 00
30g icing sugar
80g butter
1 egg yolk
½ teaspoon pure vanilla extract

Sieve the flour and icing sugar into a dish and add the cold butter, cut into small cubes (and here I do use just butter). Put this dish, just as it is, in the deep-freeze for 10 minutes. In a small bowl beat the egg yolk with the vanilla extract, a tablespoon of iced water and a pinch of salt. Put this bowl in the fridge. Then, when the 10 minutes are up, proceed with the flour and butter as above (i.e. in processor or mixer) and when you reach porridge-oats stage, add the egg mixture to bind. Be prepared to add more iced water, drop by cautious drop, until you have a nearly coherent dough. Then scoop it out, still just crumbly, push it into a fat disc, cover with clingfilm and stick in the fridge for 20 minutes.

BLIND BAKING

If you're going to fill the pastry case with anything creamy or liquid, you should blind-bake first. This simply means covering the pastry with greaseproof paper or foil, covering that with beans and baking it. The beans can be ceramic, especially bought for the purpose, or you can use any old pulses as long as you remember not to cook them later to eat by mistake. I remember reading in an American magazine that a metal dog lead (a relatively fine one) is useful here, since the metal conducts the heat well and you don't have to worry about dropping all the beads on the kitchen floor (apparently there are those who worry about just this); I'm longing to try it.

I like to bake blind at a slightly higher temperature than many people. The drawback is that the pastry sides can burn, so I keep the edges covered with foil strips for the final bit of baking.

Take the pastry disc out of the fridge and unwrap it. Flour a work surface, put the pastry on it and sprinkle the pastry and the rolling pin with flour. An ordinary wooden rolling pin will do; those beautiful stainless steel ones sold in modish kitchen shops are not a good idea except for rolling out fondant icing, which needs heavy battering.

Roll out the pastry fairly thinly. I can't see the point of giving measurements here since you are hardly going to get your ruler out to check, are you? Anyway, in all recipes I've given specific quantities for the pastry to make exactly the right amount for the stipulated flan case, so once you've rolled it in a circle to fit, the thickness should be right too.

You can lift the pastry over to the flan tin by carrying it on the rolling pin or you can fold it in quarters and carry the pastry over, placing the corner of the dough in the centre of the ring and opening it out to cover. Or just lift it up. One of the benefits of pastry made by the blitz-freezing method is that it travels, as it handles, well.

Now you have a choice. You can either line the tin with the pastry, letting it hang slightly over at the rim – use a metal flan ring with a removable bottom, not one of the ceramic flan dishes that make the soggiest pastry – and then roll the pin over the edges to cut off the pastry at the top, which looks neat and clean and smart. Or you can keep the overhang so that if it shrinks (which it can) as it cooks, you won't find you've got a truncated and filling-leaking pastry case. (I never prick the base, as I think it just makes holes for the filling to seep through later.) Whichever you decide – and I veer towards the latter – put the pastry-lined tin back in the fridge for 20 minutes or longer indeed: you can make the pastry and line the flan ring the day before you bake it; if so, keep it covered with clingfilm.

When you want to bake, preheat the oven to gas mark 6/200°C, put in a baking sheet and line the pastry case with either crumpled greaseproof paper or tinfoil. Then fill with the beans of your choice and bake on the hot sheet for 15 minutes. Take out of the oven and remove beans and greaseproof paper or foil. Cut out a long strip or a couple of strips of foil and fold over the edges so they don't burn. Put the foil-rimmed but bare-bottomed pastry case back in the oven and give it another 10–12 minutes or until it is beginning to colour lightly. Sweet pastry burns more easily, so turn down the oven to gas mark 4/180°C for the second bout in the oven.

I used to bake blind and then fill the flan as soon as it cooled a little; but my friend Tracey Scoffield, one of the best cooks I know and the daughter of a wonderful pastry-maker, has taught me that you can bake blind a day in advance as long as, when the case is cool, you slip it into a freezer bag and seal and keep it in the fridge. It must be wrapped airtight – clingfilm would do – or it will go soggy. The advantage of staggering the work, making the pastry, rolling it out and blind-baking it on 3 different days if you really want to, is that you never need to spend more than a few minutes on it each evening. But even in one go, this method is relatively painless.

CRUMBLE

I can't say I don't ever use machinery to make crumble, but there is something peculiarly relaxing about rubbing the cool, smooth butter through the cool, smooth flour with your fingers: it also makes for a more gratifyingly nubbly crumble; the processor can make the crumbs so fine you end up, when cooked, with a cakey rather than crumbly texture. So just remember, if you aren't making this by hand, to go cautiously.

In either case, the texture is improved by a quick blast in the deep-freeze: but rather than freezing the flour and butter mixture before working on it, as with the pastry recipes above, I plonk it in for 10 minutes or so after it's been rubbed together. And if you want you can just leave it in the deep-freeze, in an airtight container, on standby for when you get home from work and want to make something sweet and comforting quickly.

PLAIN APPLE CRUMBLE

I find this mixture makes enough to cover 750g fruit in a 1-litre pie dish, which should easily be enough to feed 4–6 people. To make plain apple crumble (though see also the recipe on page 174), peel, core and segment the apples and toss them for a minute or so in a pan, on the heat, with 1 tablespoon of butter, 3–4 tablespoons of sugar (to taste) and a good squeeze of orange juice, before transferring to the pie dish and topping with the crumble. In fact I use orange with most fruits: it seems to bring out their flavour rather than striking an intrusive note of its own. Make a blueberry or blackberry crumble by tossing the fruit in a buttered pie dish with 1 tablespoon each of flour and sugar for the blueberries, 2 each for the blackberries, and the juice of ½ orange. For rhubarb crumble, trim 1kg of the fruit, cut it into 5cm lengths and toss, again in a buttered dish, with a couple of tablespoons each of caster and light muscovado sugar (or more to taste), the zest of 1 orange and the merest spritz of the juice.

BLUEBERRY, BLACKBERRY OR RHUBARB

Add spices – ground ginger, cinnamon, nutmeg, even a pinch of ground cardamom – as you like to the crumble recipe below; treat it merely as a blueprint.

120g self-raising flour (though see below)
90g butter, cold and diced into about 1cm cubes
3 tablespoons light muscovado sugar
3 tablespoons vanilla sugar (and see below)

Put the flour in a bowl with a pinch of salt. I tend to use self-raising flour for crumbles simply because (to save on cupboard space) the only plain flour I keep in the house is Italian 00 and its qualities are just not required here. Add the cold cubes of butter and, using the tips of your fingers – index and middle flutteringly stroking the fleshy pads of your thumbs – rub it into the flour. Stop when you have a mixture that resembles porridge oats. Stir in the sugar. I love the combination of muscovado and vanilla sugars, but if you haven't got round to making vanilla sugar yet (and see page 82) then don't worry about what white sugar you use: any will do.

Keep the mixture in the fridge until you need it or put the bowl, as is, in the freezer for 10 minutes. Preheat the oven to gas mark 5/190°C and when ready to cook sprinkle the crumble over the prepared fruit in the pie dish and cook for 25–35 minutes.

FOODS IN SEASON

Don't believe everything you're told about the greater good of eating foods only when they are in season. The purists may be right, but being right isn't everything. If you live in the Tuscan hills, you may find different lovely things to eat every month of the year, but for us it would mean having to subsist half the time on a diet of tubers and cabbage, so why shouldn't we be grateful that we live in the age of jet transport and extensive culinary imports? More smug guff is spoken on this subject than almost anything else.

There is no doubt that there are concomitant drawbacks: the food is out of kilter with the climate in which it is eaten; it's picked underripe and transported in the wrong conditions; the intense pleasure of eating something when it comes into its own season is lost; the relative merits, the particular properties of individual fruits and vegetables are submerged in the greedy zeal of the tantrumming adult who must Have It Now. There's no point in eating flown-in asparagus which tastes of nothing (though not all of it does), or peaches in December, ripe-looking but jade-fleshed. But my life is improved considerably by the fact that I can go to my greengrocer's and routinely buy stuff I used to have to go to Italy to find.

I love fresh peas, but they aren't the high point of our culinary year for me. Once they get to the shops, all that pearly sugariness has pretty well turned to starch anyway. As far as I'm concerned, the foods whose short season it would be criminal to ignore are:

rhubarb, the forced, best and pinkest: January–February
Seville oranges: January–February
purple-sprouting broccoli: February–March
home-grown asparagus: May–June
elderflowers: June
grouse: 12 August–10 December
damsons: August–September
quinces: November–December
white truffles: November–January

RHUBARB

Rhubarb is amply covered in this book. I know many people are put off because of vile experiences in childhood. I have faith, however, or rather passionate hope, that I can overcome this prejudice. And since my own childhood contained little traditional nursery food, it takes on, for me, something of the exotic. My adult love affair with rhubarb is heady illustration of this (see Index).

SEVILLE ORANGES

You can now buy Seville oranges in supermarkets, but they are regarded almost exclusively as for making marmalade. This is such a waste. Seville oranges have the fragrance and taste of oranges but the sourness of lemons. Try them, then, wherever you'd use lemons – to squirt over fish, to squeeze into salad dressings, to use in a buttery hollandaise-like sauce or in mayonnaise to eat with cold duck. A squeeze of Seville orange is pretty divine in black tea, too. And although you can only buy them in January or early February, they freeze well. See, also, the recipe for Seville orange curd tart on page 271.

CANARD À L'ORANGE

Traditionally, oranges go with duck: real canard à l'orange should be made with bitter and not sweet oranges; you shouldn't end up with jam. Put half a Seville orange up the bottom of a mallard and squeeze the other half, mixed with 1 teaspoon honey or sesame oil, as you wish, over the breast before you cook it. Roast in a hot gas mark 7/210°C oven for 40 minutes. You won't even need to deglaze the pan to make a sauce to go with the mallard: the juices there will be good enough just as they are, though if you wish you can add more Seville orange juice, sweetened with honey to taste or left sharp. If you want something more saucelike, thicken with 1 teaspoon cornflour, made first into a paste with some of the juice.

SCALLOPS WITH BITTER ORANGES

Scallops have been cooked with bitter oranges since the eighteenth century. You can do a modern turn on the same theme simply by sautéing each glorious white disc (remove the coral for the time being) in bacon fat, butter or olive oil, 1 minute or so each side, before removing and deglazing the pan with a good squirt of Seville orange juice. Make sure you've also got enough juices in the pan to make a dressing for the watercress with which you're going to line the plate.

If they make up supper in its entirety, I'd get about 5 scallops per head. If you want to eat the corals with the scallops, then fry them for about thirty seconds after you've removed the fleshy rounds, or freeze them to fry up later with a lot of minced garlic to eat, alone and greedily, spread on toast.

SEVILLE ORANGE MARMALADE

I confess I have never made marmalade. The nearest I've got is buying a box of oranges which then, reproachfully, went mouldy in my larder. I have since never even pretended to myself that I'm the sort of person who's about to turn into a bottler and canner and storer of good things, though I live in hope. A friend, however, swears it's easy – you cook the fruit whole – and it doesn't produce so much that you feel like you're starting a marmalade-making factory.

700g Seville oranges
1.2 litres water
juice of 2 lemons
1.4kg sugar

Put the oranges in a pan with the water, bring to the boil and then simmer robustly until soft: about 2 hours. Remove the oranges, keeping the water in the pan, and cut up, pulp and all, into whatever size peel you prefer.

Remove pips and put them in a small pan, with a small amount of water to cover, and boil for 5 minutes. In the meantime, put the chopped oranges and the lemon juice into a bowl. Strain out the pips, and add the water to the lemon juice and chopped oranges.

Return to the pan and over a low heat add sugar and stir until dissolved. Then bring to boil and cook till set. To establish this, put a small amount, 1 scant teaspoon, on a cold saucer. Let it cool and then prod or stroke it with a fingertip. The marmalade's set if the surface wrinkles. You should remove the pan of marmalade from the heat while you test just in case setting point has been reached. About 15 minutes is usually fine for a softish set.

Take off the heat and pot, after removing any scum and stirring to make sure the peel is mixed through. This should fill a couple of warm, cleaned jam jars. Leave to cool a little more before screwing on the lids.

PURPLE-SPROUTING BROCCOLI

Purple-sprouting broccoli is avoided by those who think that good food has to be fancy. Clearly they don't deserve it.

Steam or lightly boil it and eat as you would asparagus, dipped into hollandaise, into plain melted butter (with or without breadcrumbs fried with it) or into a sharp, semi-emulsified sauce made by warming through some finely chopped anchovy fillets in wonderful olive oil. There can't be a wrong way to eat broccoli; just with soy sauce is fine enough.

I like a plate of sprouting broccoli mixed with asparagus (imported – it has to be). They make a good couple.

ASPARAGUS

English asparagus is expensive in restaurants and easy to cook well at home. Don't worry about special asparagus pans, just cook the asparagus in abundant boiling salted water in a pan or couple of pans which are wide and big enough for the whole spears, stem, tip and all, to be submerged. Cook for 3–5 minutes (test and taste regularly – it's better to waste some spears than for them to be either woody or soggy) and drain thoroughly, first in the colander and then lying flat on the draining board, but do it gently, too: you want the spears to stay beautiful and remain intact.

The usual accompaniment, and always a successful one, is hollandaise (see page 16), but often I like to do something more homey and give each person a boiled egg in an eggcup for them to dip their asparagus into, like bread-and-butter soldiers. The eggs have to be perfectly soft-boiled; there is no room whatsoever for error. I don't wish to frighten you, but it's the truth. Provide 2 per person and smash or cut the tops off each as soon as they're cooked.

If you feel safer with a non-traditional method, then roll the asparagus in a little olive oil, then roast it, laid out on a tray, in a seriously preheated gas mark 8/220°C oven for 15–20 minutes. When cooked, the spears should be wilted and turning sweet and brown at the tips. Sprinkle over some coarse salt, arrange on a big plate and line another big plate with thin slices of prosciutto (San Daniele or Parma). Let people pick up the hot, soft, blistered spears using the ham to wrap around the asparagus like the finest rosy silk-damask napkins.

ELDERFLOWERS

You don't need to have a vast estate with elderflowers springing lacily to flower from that avenue of trees lining the drive; just pick them roadside whenever you see them.

ELDERFLOWER CREAM

I don't normally go in for individual puddings, each precious darling to be ceremoniously unmoulded from its ramekin. But I make an exception here, would have to. This is, in effect, *panna cotta*, and as with the Italian pudding, this very English-tasting cream needs to be set with as little gelatine as possible. I've tried with big moulds and just can't set it enough without turning it halfway into rubber. These are perfection as they are, and anyway, I use a mixture of teacups, sticky-toffee-pudding moulds and ramekins, feeling that the pleasurable lack of uniformity makes up for any potential dinkiness. Line the moulds, cups and so on with clingfilm, pushing it well against the corners and over the rim so you've got a tuggable edge; it may make for the odd wrinkle or crease on the surface of the set cream, but that doesn't matter; what does is that you will be able to unmould them easily.

900ml double cream
18 heads of elderflower
6 tablespoons caster sugar
3 leaves gelatine

Heat cream over low heat in saucepan with the elderflowers. When it comes bubbling to a simmering near-boil, turn it off, remove from the heat and cover. Leave for up to a couple of hours, but not less than 1/2 hour, to infuse. Then stir in the sugar and bring back to boiling point. Taste to see if more sugar is needed and then sieve into a jug. While the last of the headily aromatic cream is dripping off the elderflowers, soak the leaves of gelatine in cold water. In 5 minutes or so, when the gelatine is softened, squeeze the leaves out and then beat into the warm cream in the jug. Make sure they are dissolved and dispersed and pour into the clingfilm-lined moulds. Cool and then put in the fridge overnight.

GOOSEBERRIES

With these serve a contrastingly lumpy bowl of gooseberries: the Victorians knew well, and invoked often, the muscatty aptness of the combination of elderflower and gooseberry; about many things they were wrong; about this they were right. Put 750g gooseberries in a pan with 350ml water and 6 tablespoons of sugar. Bring it all to the boil and simmer for a couple of minutes. Drain, reserving syrup, then put the fruit in a bowl and return the lightly syrupy juices to the pan. Bring it to the boil again and let boil for 5 minutes. Pour it into a bowl or jug to cool, while the fruit cools separately in its bowl, then when you're about it eat, put the gooseberries in a shallow dish and cover with the syrup.

GROUSE

Grouse should either be roasted plain, first smeared thickly with butter, in a gas mark 6/200°C oven for 30–45 minutes (the size of the birds varies, but you want the flesh to be rubied and juicy, but not underdone to the point of tough quiveriness) and eaten with bread sauce (see page 66), or stuffed with thyme and mascarpone (yes, really), as on page 169.

DAMSONS

Damsons are a glorious fruit. They can't be eaten raw and are a chore to prepare and cook, but it's only once a year ...

DAMSON FOOL

I sometimes make damson ice-cream, but damson fool is the recipe for which I wait most greedily. This fool is not difficult to make, but it is stunning, utterly distinctive: you can taste in it both the almost metallic depth of the sour fruit and billowy sweetness of the bulky cream. And it's wonderful after grouse.

500g damsons
2 teaspoons each dark muscovado, light muscovado and caster sugar
¼ teaspoon mixed ground spice
300ml double cream, whipped with 2 tablespoons icing sugar

Put the whole damsons (try to stone them now and you'll go really mad) in a pan with 125ml water and the sugars, bring to the boil and cook till soft. Push through a sieve or food mill to get rid of the stones and add the spice and more sugar to taste if you think they need it.

When cool, stir into the sugar-whipped cream and pour either into individual pots or into a bowl. This will fill 6 glasses of the sort you'd eat pudding from, but if you're putting the fool in a bowl then count on feeding only 4.

QUINCES

Quince, the apple which Paris presented to Helen and maybe even the one which grew in the garden of Eden (although there is, it's argued, a more convincing academic case to be made for the pomegranate here) is a ravishing mixture of *One Thousand and One Nights* exotic and Victorian kitchen homeliness. It looks like a mixture between apple and pear, but tastes like neither. And actually the taste is not the point: what this fruit is all about is heady, perfect fragrance. I have something of an obsession for quinces, although they are in the shops only for a scant eight weeks, aren't at all easy to deal with and can't be eaten raw. In the old days, quinces were kept in airing cupboards to perfume the linen, pervading the house with their honeyed but sharp aroma, so you needn't feel bad if you buy a bowlful and then just watch them rot in a kitchen or wherever.

You should add a quince, peeled, cored and sliced or chunked to apple pie or crumble. Poach them as you might pears (only for longer, and see the recipe for quinces in muscat on page 366) or make mostarda. Although I am not someone who goes in for preserve-making, I do make mostarda.

MOSTARDA DI VENEZIA

There's mostarda di Cremona, which has become modishly familiar over here, those stained-glass-window-coloured gleaming pots of fruits glossily preserved in mustard oil: no one, even in Italy apparently, makes their own. But mostarda di Venezia is different. You can't buy it and it's easy to make. It's just quinces boiled up with white wine, with the addition of sugar, candied peel and mustard powder. It's wonderful with any cold meat (which makes it very useful for Christmas and, since you have to leave it a month or so before eating, rather well timed for it, too). I risk a culinary culture-clash by eating it alongside couscous and curries and to pad out the sort of low-fat, highly-flavoured food on pages 404–27. Or you can eat it with a dollop of mascarpone, sweetened (and perhaps bolstered with egg, as on page 122) and flavoured with rum, as pudding.

This recipe is adapted from the one in Anna del Conte's *Classic Food of Northern Italy* which, as these things do, has a mixed parentage of its own. I have changed it a little. I simplify the procedure (see below) and also make it hotter and with almost double the amount of candied peel. Now, I loathe and detest commercial candied peel, but it's different here, not least because you must not use the ready-diced, bitter and oversweet at the same time, vile stuff in tubs. Seach out the good candied peel, whole, in large jars.

The second time I made mostarda di Venezia I didn't peel and core the quinces. It's such hard work. Instead I just roughly chopped the fruit and then pushed the lot through a fine food mill. Laziness prompted this modification, but since the peel and core help the set and intensify the flavour, you should have no qualms. If you don't own a mouli-légumes I suppose you could just push the fruit through a sieve, but that's strenuous too. So if you don't own this cheap and useful piece of equipment, it would be easier to peel, quarter and core to start with.

1.8 kg quinces
1 bottle (750 ml) white wine
grated rind and juice of 1 unwaxed lemon
sugar (1–1.2kg, see below)
8 tablespoons English mustard powder
250g candied peel (see above), cut into small cubes

Roughly chop the quinces, put them in a pan and cover them with the wine. Add the lemon rind and juice and cook until soft, about 40 minutes. Purée the mixture by pushing it through a food mill, weigh and add the same weight in sugar. Return to the pan. Dissolve the mustard powder in a little hot water and add to the purée with 1 teaspoon salt and the candied peel. Cook gently until the liquid is reduced and the mostarda becomes dense and, normally, deeper-coloured, about 20–30 minutes.

Sterilise some jars (I find the dishwasher's performance adequate) and fill with the mostarda. When it is cool, cover, seal and store away. Keep for about a month before you use it.

What you should also know about quinces is that for all their hardness, they bruise very easily. Whenever I have got a batch of quinces, at least a third of them have been riddled within with speckles, or worse, of what looks like rust. I just ignore it, unless of course it's obviously rotten. Anyway, quinces darken as they cook, going from glassy-yellow to coral to deepest, burnt terracotta; the odd bit of bruising really won't show.

WHITE TRUFFLES

No greedy person's mention of foods in season could ignore the white truffle. I don't really understand the fuss about black truffles, but a white truffle – called by Rossini the Mozart of funghi – is something else. And you don't do anything to it. You just shave it. And if you're buying a truffle you may as well go the whole hog and buy the thing with which to shave it over a plate of buttery egg pasta or into an equally rich risotto made with good broth. It is instant culinary nirvana. And although expensive, so much less so, unbelievably less so, than eating it in a restaurant.

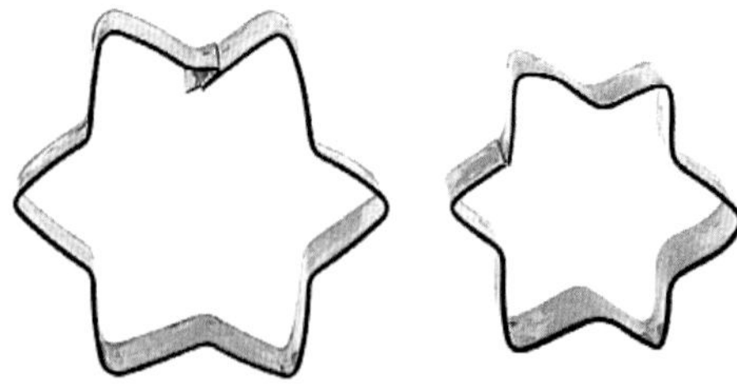

CHRISTMAS

Seasonal food doesn't come much more seasonal than at Christmas; this is not exactly to do with what's in season, but with what's expected of it – and you. Christmas is every cook's nightmare. Maybe it isn't helpful to say that it doesn't have to be a nightmare because if anything will increase your dread it is the sense that other people somehow find it a complete breeze. They don't. All the problems of cooking are intensified at Christmas: too many people to cook for; too many meals to cook; and too many people hanging around you all the time you're cooking.

If you are going to be cooking two meals a day – or even just one, with leftovers for the other – for upwards of six people for a week, you will need to be organised. It is hard not to feel swamped by food and food preparation, and even if you like cooking, Christmas can induce panic and depression. And all this food can also begin to instil a sense of unease: so much excess is unsettling, and it feels decadent to be the creator of it in the first place.

This isn't, of course, purely a moral distaste – after all, food is celebratory and it's perfectly respectable to choose to appreciate its plentifulness – but, rather, a narcissistic anxiety. We feel uncomfortable with the prospect of over-eating. But just as we fear it, we court it, because the truth is that we don't have to plough our way through seasonal cakes and chocolates and nuts and pies. We feel we have an excuse, and so we plunge into an orgy of over-indulgence which is utterly unnecessary, and which makes us feel both guilty and resentful at the same time.

For me, an urban person, Christmas is rather like the country: not much to do apart from eat and drink. I end up suffering from boredom-induced bloat. But cooking itself can make a difference. It's the amount of packaged and processed food around at Christmas that makes us feel truly bad. Not all Christmas food has to be the sort that leaves us stultified and slumped over the table for hours after we've eaten it.

Christmas Day itself is, in my view, non-negotiable. It's fashionable to decry the traditional lunch as boring and turkey as dry, but I love it all, and on 26 December start longing for next year's lunch. My great-grandmother was so keen on Christmas lunch, and felt it was such a waste to eat it only once a year, that she had a second one each Midsummer's Day.

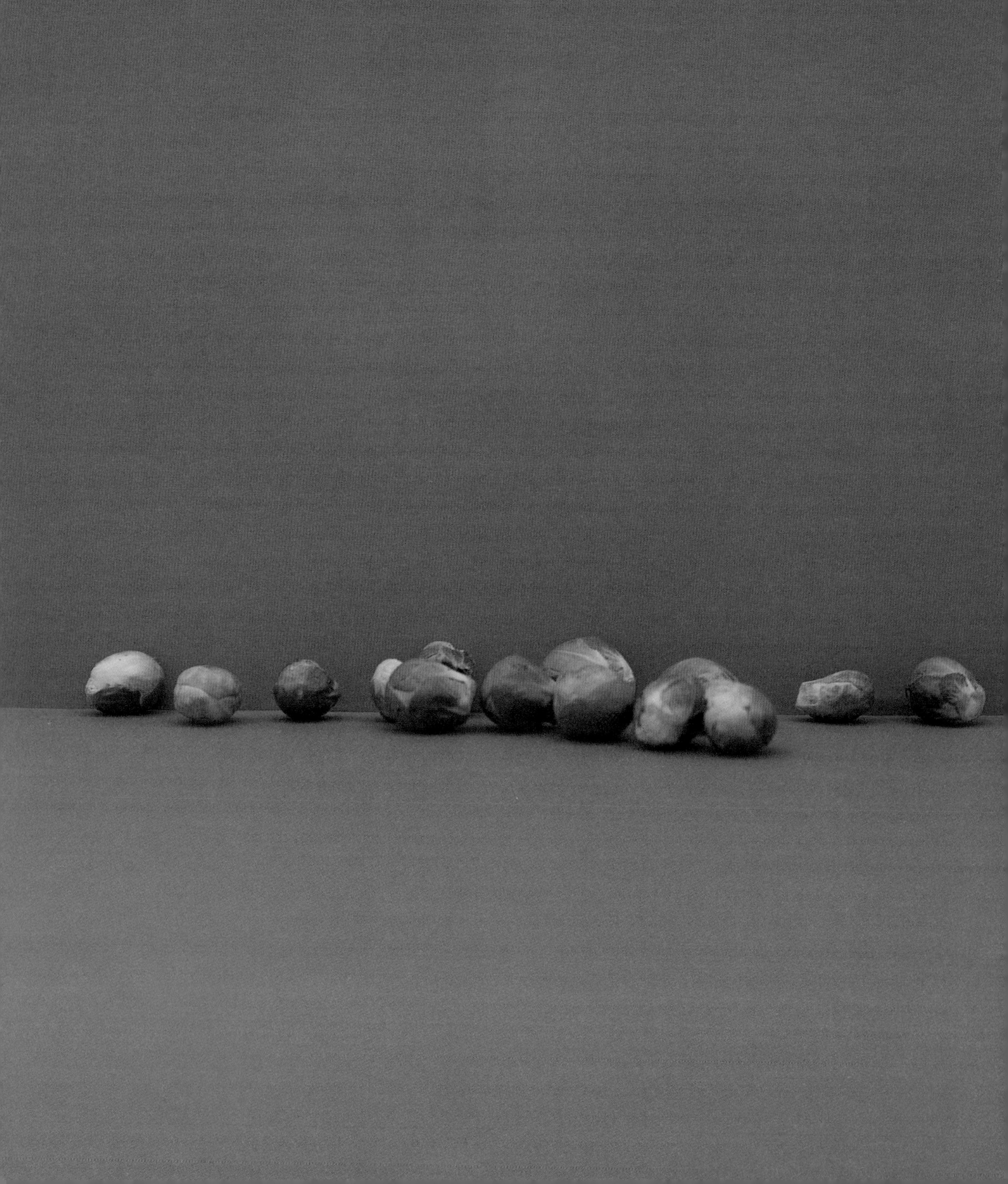

I have heard the arguments for goose, and eaten it, and have no fierce objections, but I don't think I would like to see my turkey ousted by it. Cooking a goose for Christmas Eve dinner seems to me the best idea, since one can then make sure at least of getting some leftovers to go with the cold turkey. Goose is anyway much better cold than hot.

What I really object to are the bright, magazine alternatives to Christmas lunch – medallions of pheasant in Armagnac sauce, guinea fowl with grapes and sweet-potato galettes, rolled breast of turkey with chestnut and pine-nut stuffing and celeriac rösti. I do see that if you're a vegetarian an alternative is required. But, frankly, I would still avoid the nut-roast route. Either forget the whole thing and eat as normal on Christmas Day, or just do Christmas lunch without the turkey. Not being vegetarian, I would miss turkey and, perhaps even more, its stuffings (I am not convinced chipolatas are necessary and I feel bacon rolls, a late innovation surely, are not), but, if I were prepared to make the sacrifice, I would be happier with a plate of roast potatoes, darkly golden and resonant, some brussels sprouts with chestnuts and sweetly aromatic bread sauce – along with other vegetables – than with some jaunty ersatz number.

At least you know what you're doing for Christmas lunch, the choice is made for you. But even if Christmas Day itself is sorted, there are still the other days to think of. I think it helps if you divide up, in your head, the pre-25 December meals from those eaten afterwards. The reason is that anything you cook before your Christmas turkey can be devised to go with it after. I am a huge fan of cold leftovers. Resist, please, the tendency to camouflage, to go in for makeovers. Cold turkey, as long as it hasn't been overcooked, is wonderful, and better still if you have some cold ham, cold duck, maybe even some cold lamb to go with it, too.

The best sorts of leftover meals are those which are glorified picnics. Alongside the cold meats, you need a good butcher's pork pie. Also put on the table a plate of tomatoes – best left whole, so people can take and cut them as they like – and some other salad and bread. I sometimes add cheese to this board, sometimes serve the cheese after the meat has been eaten and cleared away. And at Christmas, I have to hand some good English cheeses – an excellent stilton naturally, but some cheddar and possibly some Appleby Cheshire, too.

You need some sort of mayonnaise, if only for sandwiches (see recipe on page 13). And sandwiches, especially for eating television-side, are an essential part of Christmas food.

But other sauces are important for cold turkey, too. Cranberry sauce is an obvious one (see page 66), but I also have to have mustard (as I do with hot turkey: I have a painful Christmas memory of lunch at a friend's house where everything was perfect, only there was no English mustard). Mustard is especially good with cold stuffing as well. Mango chutney is fundamental to a good turkey – or for that matter chicken – sandwich, and if you are eating cold goose you should make sure you have some horseradish. You should try here, too, that Jewish mix of horseradish and beetroot called chrain. And while we're on this particular culture clash, potato latkes (see page 70) are wonderful with cold turkey.

I think it's all right to give people leftovers if they're coming for dinner around Christmas, but in that case make a hot pudding. It needn't be complicated, but it looks as if you've made some effort. Soup, too, not out of a carton, gives a hospitable uplift to the inevitable leftover offerings.

However much you like cold cuts and leftovers, you can't eat them for every meal. Christmas food divides into food that is seasonal and food that is deliberately not. By this latter category I don't mean you should be serving strawberries flown in from distant hemispheres, but that it can be a relief to eat food which is innocent of any seasonal connotation. So much Christmas food, too, is so palate-stickingly luxy: every magazine, every food programme is pushing smoked salmon rolls and salmon mousse roulades. At home avoid all that prinking and puréeing and packaging. Keep it simple, make it fresh. Avoid the slavish overprovision of rich food that turns eating into a burdensome duty rather than a pleasure and turns cooking into an entirely out-of-character exercise.

CHRISTMAS EVE GOOSE

Years ago, I cut out this recipe for goose stuffed with mashed potato from one of Simon Hopkinson's columns in the *Independent*. The recipe comes via Peter Langan, and was his Grandmother Callinan's. It must represent a curious axis, where Irish and Polish culinary practices meet, for I've only come across something similar in a book on Polish-Jewish cooking.

Simon Hopkinson, no namby-pamby when it comes to food, says this recipe feeds 6 and I believe him (normally I treat printed portion sizes with distrust), so if you're having more than 6 guests, cook a couple of geese, eat all the unctuous stuffing, and have the cold meat later on in the week. Because you need to dry out the skin well before you start, you have to get cracking early.

1 goose, dressed weight about 4½kg or so, with giblets
2 tablespoons oil
1.4kg potatoes, peeled, cut into large chunks and rinsed thoroughly
50g butter or goose fat (and see below)
4 onions, peeled and chopped coarsely
2 cloves of garlic, peeled and chopped finely
1 heaped tablespoon fresh sage leaves, chopped
grated rind of 2 lemons

for the gravy
4 rashers streaky bacon, chopped
25g goose fat
1 goose neck bone, chopped coarsely
1 goose gizzard, cleaned (ask your butcher) and chopped coarsely
1 onion, peeled and chopped
1 carrot, peeled and chopped
2 sticks of celery, chopped
2 tablespoons Calvados
150ml Madeira
300ml strong chicken stock
1 scant tablespoon redcurrant jelly
1 heaped teaspoon arrowroot, slaked with a little water

First prepare the goose, and render some lovely goose fat. Remove all the gobbets of pale fat that lie just inside the goose's cavity, attached to the skin. Put them in a pan with 2 tablespoons oil and place on a very low heat and let melt. Render it all down, pour into a bowl or tin and add to this, later, the great glorious amounts of fat that drips off the goose into the pan as it roasts. The goose fat will be wonderful for roast potatoes on Christmas Day – or any day.

Now, get to work on the goose's skin, so that it crisps up in the oven like Chinese duck. Put the goose on a rack in a tin, puncture the skin several times with the point of a thin skewer or very sharp knife, then pour over boiling water. Tip all the water out of the tin and let the goose dry. You can do this by placing it by an open window – at this time of year I think you can reckon on a fair breeze – and leave for hours, preferably overnight. Even better, direct an electric fan towards the bird for a few hours. Remember to turn it regularly so that all sides get dried. You are often advised to hang the bird up, but this is hard enough to do with a duck and a coathanger, and a duck is very much lighter than a goose. But if you've got a butcher's hook handy, and somewhere to hang it, why not give it a try?

Your goose is prepared: now preheat the oven to gas mark 7/210°C. Boil the potatoes in salted water until tender, drain well and mash coarsely; just use an old-fashioned masher or fork. Fry the onions in the recently rendered goose fat until golden brown. Add the garlic and stir them both into the mashed potato, along with the sage, lemon rind and pepper. Rub a generous amount of salt over the goose and put a good grinding of pepper inside the cavity. Then pack the mashed-potato mixture into the cavity and put the goose back on its wire rack over the largest possible roasting tin and place in the oven.

Roast for 30 minutes and then turn the temperature down to gas mark 4/180°C. Cook the goose for a further 2½ hours or so. Don't baste: you want the fat to run off the goose, the more the better; but do remember to remove fat regularly during the goose's cooking or you might have a messy and dangerous accident.

Make the gravy while the goose is cooking. Fry the bacon in goose fat in a heavy-bottomed pan, until crisp and brown. Add the neck bone and cook until well coloured, then do the same with the vegetables. Pour off any excess fat and add the Calvados and Madeira (I'd be happy using my usual Marsala here). Bring to the boil and reduce until syrupy. Pour in the chicken stock and redcurrant jelly and simmer for 30 minutes. Strain through a fine sieve into a clean pan. Allow to settle and with some kitchen paper lift off any fat that is floating on the surface. Whisk in the arrowroot and bring the gravy back to a simmer until clear and slightly thickened. Make sure you don't let it boil or the arrowroot can break down and thin the gravy. Keep warm. Just putting the lid on a good saucepan should do this, or use a heat-diffuser and keep the flame low.

When your goose is cooked, remove it from the oven and let it rest for 15 minutes or so before carving. Simon Hopkinson suggests serving some extra potatoes (in addition to the potato stuffing – now you see why I trust him on portion size), fried with garlic in some of the goose fat you've collected, and sprinkled with parsley, and some big bunches of watercress. You certainly don't need sophisticated vegetables: frozen petits pois, good and buttery, with some blanched and buttered mangetouts stirred in would be good.

After eating the goose, I'd just make sure there were big bowls of lychees, clementines and some nuts on the table.

CHRISTMAS LUNCH

I think for Christmas lunch it has to be turkey; furthermore, this turkey has to be a Bronze (see Gazetteer, page 506). A good turkey, reared well, is what makes the difference. My mother did a splendid job, though, with a less illustrious bird, by soaking some J-cloths in melted butter, then bandaging the turkey's breast with them for the first part of the roasting, first on one side, then on the other. But a good turkey removes instantly all association with dryness for ever.

I have never gone in for starters at Christmas lunch. I can't see the point of blunting your appetite before you even get to the main event.

THE TURKEY

The turkey needs to be stuffed, and I should in all honesty own up that I get my butcher, Mr Lidgate, to do that for me. I couldn't improve on his recipes, and so I've got them for you, one for chestnut stuffing, the other for cranberry and orange. This is the perfect pair: the one sweet and mealy, the other sharp and fruited; the quantities in both are enough to stuff, one at each end, a 5½–6½kg bird, with some stuffing left over to cook in a separate dish. If you don't make extra stuffing, you can run out before second helpings, which is a grave error.

LIDGATE'S CHESTNUT STUFFING

175g shallots, peeled and chopped finely
75g butter
75g smoked streaky bacon, chopped
2 eggs
1 435g tin unsweetened chestnut purée
1 200g tin or vacuum-pack whole chestnuts
200g so-called fresh breadcrumbs (see page 24)
bunch parsley (approx. 40g), chopped
fresh nutmeg

Cook the shallots in the butter, melted in a heavy-bottomed pan, with the bacon (keeping the rinds for the gravy, see page 63) for about 10 minutes on a lowish heat or until soft and beginning to colour. Beat the eggs and add to the chestnut purée to help slacken it, or it will be hard to mix everything together later (unless you've got one of those sturdy free-standing mixers). Roughly chop the chestnuts and add them to the eggy purée, along with the breadcrumbs, parsley and buttery shallots and bacon. Add salt and pepper and a good grating of fresh nutmeg.

LIDGATE'S CRANBERRY AND ORANGE STUFFING

zest and juice of 1 large orange
500g fresh or thawed cranberries
125g butter
500g fresh breadcrumbs (see page 24)
2 eggs
fresh nutmeg

Zest and juice the orange. Put the cranberries into a heavy-based saucepan with the orange juice and zest. Bring to simmering point on a moderate to high flame, then cover, turn down the heat slightly, and simmer for about 5 minutes. Add the butter in slices and stir, off the heat, until it melts, then add the breadcrumbs and the eggs, beaten. Season with salt and pepper and a good grating of fresh nutmeg.

NB: Remember to weigh the stuffings before adding them to the turkey because you'll need to count them in the total cooking time.

Neither stuffing here uses sausagemeat; if you think you'll miss it, just get a pile of sausages or chipolatas to cook alongside.

Right, to cook the turkey, proceed as follows.

Remove the giblets (though you should have done this when you first got the bird home). Reserve them for the gravy. Wash the inside of the bird with cold running water. Drain well and blot dry with a few kitchen towels.

Fill the neck end with the chestnut stuffing: you want to fill it firmly but don't pack it in; cover the stuffing with the neck skin when you've done. Use the wing tips rather like pincers – or paper clips – to keep the neck skin in place while it's cooking. Now, fill the body cavity with the cranberry and orange stuffing. Melt some goose fat (if you've got any) or some butter (if you haven't) and brush over the turkey breast.

I don't understand why people make such a song and dance about the length of time a turkey needs to be cooked. My mother made a great point of getting up at the crack of dawn to put the turkey in the oven. But one of the things that I discovered the first time I actually cooked Christmas lunch myself is that turkey doesn't need that much cooking.

I have always followed the instructions given to me by my butcher, and the turkey's been cooked perfectly. So don't be alarmed by the shortness of the cooking times, below. And *do* remember to take the turkey out of the fridge in good time: it should be at room temperature when it goes in the oven.

Put the turkey breast down in the roasting tray: the only fat deposits in a turkey are in the back and this allows them to percolate through the breast meat as it cooks; this makes for the tenderest possible, succulent meat.

Preheat the oven to gas mark 6/200°C and keep it at this temperature for the first 30 minutes. Then turn it down to gas mark 4/180°C.

For the following weights of turkey (stuffing included, remember) you need to cook it for these times:

Weight	*Time*
2¼kg	**1½ hours**
4½kg	**2 hours**
6¾kg	**2¾ hours**
9kg	**3½ hours**
11½kg	**4½ hours**

It is not possible to give one serve-all timing based on minutes per kg; this time decreases as the weight of the bird increases. But if you are buying a true Bronze turkey as recommended (and the times are given for this superior bird) you can consult those who are selling it to you. The turkey will weigh too much for kitchen scales to cope with, so you'll need to confer as it is.

Baste regularly throughout the cooking time, and turn the bird the right way up for the last half hour of cooking to brown. I use no foil without, but if you want to use foil, add an hour onto cooking time; and still remove it for the last, breast-burnishing half-hour.

To see for yourself that the turkey is ready, poke a skewer or fork where the meat is thickest – behind the knee joint of the thigh – and if it is cooked the juices will run clear.

GRAVY

Now for the gravy. I am not one of life's gravy-makers – I make disgusting coffee, too: obviously brown liquids are not my thing. This one works, though.

Make the giblet stock well in advance. Keep the liver covered with milk in a dish in the fridge till you need it.

giblets from the turkey
1 bouquet garni
4 peppercorns
1 onion, peeled and halved
1 carrot, peeled and quartered
1 stick of celery, roughly chopped
bacon rinds left over from chestnut stuffing
1 tablespoon plain flour, preferably Italian 00
1 tablespoon butter
1 tablespoon Marsala

Put all the giblets except for the liver in a pan (that's to say the heart, neck and gizzard), add the bouquet garni, the peppercorns, onion, carrot and celery and bacon rind, and cover with 1 litre water, sprinkling over 1 teaspoon salt. Bring to the boil, cover, lower the heat and simmer for a couple of hours. Strain into a measuring jug. Set it aside if you're doing this stage in advance, or else get on with the next stage, which takes place when the turkey's cooked and sitting, resting, on its carving board.

Pour off most of the fat from the roasting tin, leaving behind about 2 tablespoons plus all the usual sticky and burnt bits. Put it back on the hob at a low heat, and in a separate little bowl mix together the flour with, gradually, 3–4 tablespoons of the liquid from the pan. When you have a smooth, runny paste, stir it back into the pan. Cook for a couple of minutes, scraping up any bits from the bottom and incorporating them, but make sure the pan's not so hot it burns. Still stirring, gradually pour in 500ml of the giblet stock, or more if it seems too thick, bearing in mind you're adding the liver later.

While the gravy's cooking gently, leave it for a moment (though keep stirring every now and again) to fry the liver. Melt the butter in a small pan and toss the liver in it for 1–2 minutes, then remove to a board and chop finely.

Add the liver to the gravy. Add the Marsala, and stir well, cooking for another few minutes, before pouring into a couple of gravy boats. Since first making this gravy I have bought a blender and would now add a little more of the giblet stock, say 600ml, and blend the gravy after the liver has been chopped and added.

POTATOES

You should parboil and roast the potatoes as instructed in the Weekend Lunch chapter on page 281, and use goose fat if you have any (it can now be bought from supermarkets, especially at Christmas). The oven the turkey is in is not hot enough for the potatoes. If you don't have a double oven, you can leave the turkey to sit while you're blasting the potatoes.

BRUSSELS SPROUTS AND CHESTNUTS

I know there are chestnuts in the stuffing, but I'd put still more of them in with the brussels sprouts. I don't suggest you peel your own: buy them vacuum-packed. Using prepared sprouts (though never frozen) isn't the end of the world, either. What does make a difference is the butter you add after cooking: there should be lots of it. And season well with pepper and fresh nutmeg.

For 10 people, buy about 1½kg sprouts and 200g vacuum-sealed chestnuts. Roughly chop the chestnuts so that some are cut in 2, some in 3; that's to say, you don't need them whole, but nor do you want mealy rubble. After you've cooked the sprouts – lightly – drain them and melt about 100g unsalted butter in a large pan. Toss the chestnuts in the butter and then add the sprouts. Add salt, pepper and fresh nutmeg and coat well with the butter in the pan before turning into a couple of warmed bowls.

You need other vegetables too, but if you're a large group of people it cuts down the possibilities of what can be done easily. Delicious though a sharp-edged bowl of shredded cabbage would be (see page 372) you hardly want to stir-fry a large amount at the last minute. But you do want crunch. Barely blanch a bowl of sugar-snap peas. Or buy some already-prepared broccoli florets and toss them, just cooked, in butter to which you've added a little sesame oil. And I know it's unseasonal, but green beans, imported from Kenya or wherever, are not a bad idea. I wouldn't mind one puréed vegetable as well, though it's not crucial. You can do this much earlier, even the day before, so it doesn't add too much horror. Puréed Jerusalem artichokes would be my choice.

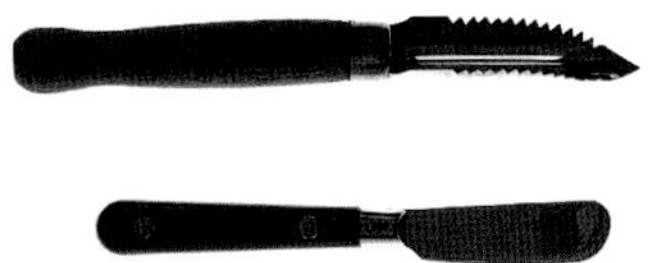

BREAD SAUCE

This is essential: of course it is. For 10 people you need:

2 small onions, peeled and each stuck with 3 cloves
1 bay leaf
4 peppercorns
blade of mace or 1/4 teaspoon ground mace
800ml full-fat milk
150g fresh breadcrumbs (see page 24)
30g butter
2 tablespoons double cream
fresh nutmeg

Put the clove-stuck onions, bay leaf, peppercorns and the blade of mace (or sprinkle the ground mace over) into a pan with the milk. Add a good pinch of salt and bring to the boil, but do not actually let boil. Remove from the heat, cover the pan and infuse. I tend to do this first thing in the morning when I get up, but if you forget or can't, then just make sure you get the infusion done about an hour before eating.

Back on a very low heat, sprinkle over and stir in the breadcrumbs and cook for about 15 minutes, by which time the sauce should be thick and warm. I have to say I don't bother with removing any of the bits, the onions, the peppercorns and so on, but you can strain the milk before adding the breadcrumbs if you want to. Just before serving, melt the butter and heat up the cream together in another pan, grate over quite a bit of nutmeg, and stir into the bread sauce. Taste to see if it needs any more salt or, indeed, anything else.

CRANBERRY SAUCE

We always had cranberry sauce out of a jar at home, which is why I'm fond of it, as I am of horseradish sauce out of a bottle, too. But both, truly, are better freshly made. Cranberry sauce is so easy as not to be worth even hesitating about.

500g cranberries
225g sugar – or to taste
30g butter
zest and juice of 1 orange
1 tablespoon Grand Marnier, optional

Put the cranberries, sugar, butter, juice and zest of the orange, and Grand Marnier if using, in a pan. Add 100ml water and bring to the boil. After a minute or so's fierce bubbling, lower to a simmer and cook for about 10 minutes, until the berries have popped and you have a thick, fruity sauce. Don't panic if it's still fairly runny, though, as it solidifies on cooling. Taste to see if you want more sugar, then decant to a bowl and let cool before serving.

I have to say I have never yet made my own Christmas pudding. I will, I will. One day. And so, I'm sure, will you. But buying one seems an entirely sensible thing to do. The best I've found so far, and it's the best by a long way, is Anton Mosimann's (see page 506). And I pass on a tip of Fanny and Johnny Craddock's (from their *Coping with Christmas*) which is to use vodka in place of the brandy for flaming the pudding. Apparently it burns for much longer: Fanny boasts of keeping the flame alive for 11 minutes at her spectacular at the Albert Hall.

But I do make my own brandy butter to go with my unashamedly bought pudding, the brandy butter of my childhood, and I have recently taken to making an odd sort of semi-frozen rum sauce, too, which is a variant of the eggy, brandy-spiked cream a friend of mine makes.

BRANDY BUTTER

This is what was always traditionally called Hard Sauce, but somehow it looks affected and twee to call it that now. We all know it as brandy butter these days. I add ground almonds – because my mother did, so it's the taste I know, and because they give it a glorious marzipanny depth and velvetiness.

You need the butter to be as soft as possible before you start, but not at all oily. Obviously it makes life easier if you can make this in a machine, either a mixer or processor; I prefer the former.

150g unsalted butter, soft
225g icing sugar
50g ground almonds
3 tablespoons brandy or to taste

Beat the butter until soft, then add the sifted icing sugar and beat them together till pale and creamy. Mix in the ground almonds and, when all is smooth, add the brandy. Add a tablespoon at first, then taste, then another and see if you want more. You may find that the suggested 3 tablespoons is far from enough: it is a question of taste and what is lethally strong for one person seems insipid to another; you must please yourself since you can't please everyone.

ICED RUM SAUCE

This is a sort of rum-sodden and syrupy egg-nog with cream that's kept in the freezer until about an hour before eating. You put it on the searing hot pudding and it melts on impact. It's odd, but it works.

300ml double cream
2 egg yolks
2 tablespoons golden syrup
2 tablespoons dark rum

Beat the cream until stiff. In another bowl, beat the yolks until extremely frothy. Add golden syrup and rum to eggs, still beating. Then fold this egg mixture into the cream. You could serve straightaway, as it is, un-iced; the plan, though, is to put it in the deep-freeze to set hard and then take it out and let it ripen for about an hour in its tub in the fridge so that it's frozen but beginning to flop by the time you add it to the hot pudding.

MINCEMEAT

Mince pies, I feel, are a bit like Christmas pudding: you may as well buy in. I once made my own mincemeat – adding quince in place of the more usual apple, and eau de vie de Coings instead of the brandy – but it was years ago and I've still got most of it lying about. I am not, therefore, inspired to repeat the experience just yet.

What you can always do, if you want to go one step further than getting shop pies, is buy a 400–500g jar of the best mincemeat you can find and, a couple of weeks before Christmas, grate in a cooking apple or a quince, stir in 3 tablespoons of rum, Grand Marnier or eau de vie de Coings, add some chopped flaked almonds (about 60g) and the juice of ½ lemon and ½ an orange each, and a bit of the grated zest of both. Then you'll almost feel you have made your own mincemeat.

There are two ways of approaching the making of the pastry for your mince pies: either make tiny pies (which I think I like best) and use a plain shortcrust (see page 41), binding the dough with iced, salted orange juice in place of water, or make them the usual size but out of almond pastry (see page 292). For the small pies, cut out circles of dough, put in tartlet tins, add a scant 1 teaspoon of mincemeat to each, and top, not with a round lid, but with a star stamped out with a specially shaped cutter. About quarter of an hour in a gas mark 6/200°C oven should be fine. For the bigger pies, use an almond pastry base and top with a dollop of frangipane. Cook at gas mark 6/200°C for about 10 minutes, then at gas mark 4/180°C for about another 15–20 minutes.

LEFTOVERS

BUBBLE AND SQUEAK

Cold brussels sprouts have become something of a byword for the culinary awfulness of Christmas. But my absolute favourite Christmas Day or Boxing Day supper is a bubble and squeak made by frying the leftover and roughly chopped sprouts with an onion and some mashed potato in a pan, then topping it with a fried or poached egg, and maybe some crisp, salty bacon.

And I know I said that cold turkey must be left to eat cold, not reformulated in any way, but here is the exception.

ED VICTOR'S TURKEY HASH

Obviously, one can't be specific about amounts: who knows how much you've got left or how many people you are trying to feed? I give you this recipe, then, just as my literary agent, Ed Victor, gave it to me. Use whatever quantities and proportions feel right, taste good, to you.

'Sauté chopped onions and green peppers in a mixture of butter and olive oil in a large pan. Add diced turkey (white and dark meat) plus any leftover stuffing to the cooked onion and peppers mixture, and cook till warmed through. You can season it at this stage with salt and pepper.

Then stir in pitted ripe black olives and toasted almonds. Finally drizzle over the top some beaten eggs mixed with double cream, and stir till set.

Optionally, you can finish the hash off with some grated parmesan on top and brown it under the grill.

Voila! It's usually much, much better than the turkey itself. In fact, it's the only reason to eat turkey on Christmas Day!'

I don't concede that last point, but we should allow a man his prejudices.

POTATOES

You don't need to do very much to make cold cuts interesting, as long as the meat's good to start off with. I suggest serving alongside potatoes, cut small, and roasted till crisp. Cut them into about 1cm dice, toss in a freezer bag with garlic-infused oil and dried thyme, and then turn into an oven tray, or just sprinkle with the thyme and drop in a pan of hot goose fat, and roast for about an hour at gas mark 6/200°C. When the potatoes are done, remove to a plate and sprinkle with coarse sea salt. Work on rations of about 150g potato, weighed raw, per person. And serve with salad: one green, another of tomatoes.

ROASTED WHOLE GARLIC CLOVES AND SHALLOTS

My other regular standby is a plate, a huge plate, of roasted whole garlic cloves and shallots. When I'm eating hot meat alongside (as with the chicken on page 9) I don't peel them; but with cold cuts I do. This is made easier if you blanch them first. So, preheat the oven to gas mark 3/160°C. And, reckoning on half a head of garlic and 125g of shallots per person, peel the shallots and put them in a tray in the oven with some olive oil. They'll need about 45 minutes, and the garlic will need about 25, so give the shallots a 20-minute head start. Meanwhile, separate the cloves of garlic, put them in a pan of cold water, bring to the boil and let boil for 2 minutes. Drain and peel the garlic: the blanching will have made it very easy; just exert pressure on one end of the clove and it will pop out of its skin at the other. Put the garlic in its tray, with some olive oil, too, and roast.

When both garlic and shallots are cooked, mix on a large plate and sprinkle salt and parsley over them. I know half a head of garlic each and all those shallots sounds a lot, but people always seem to eat incredible amounts of this. You can also eat them cold, with a little more olive oil and a drop or two of balsamic vinegar poured over them, along with a load of fresh parsley and maybe some toasted pine nuts. They reheat well, too, if you stir them over a low heat in a heavy-bottomed pan on the hob, so don't skimp.

LATKES

If you want to make latkes to eat with the cold meats, then – for 6 or so people – push about 2kg of potatoes, peeled, through the grater disc of the food processor. Remove and drain in a sieve, pushing well to remove all excess liquid. Then fit the double-bladed knife and put a peeled medium-sized onion, coarsely chopped, 3 eggs, 1 teaspoon salt, some pepper and 4 tablespoons self-raising flour or fine matzo meal in the bowl and process briefly. Add the grated potatoes and give a quick pulse till the mixture is pulpy but not totally puréed. You should have a thick mess; add more flour if it's at all runny.

Fry the latkes in lumps of about 1 tablespoon each in a heavy-based frying pan with hot oil bubbling away in it to a depth of about 2cm. About 5 minutes a side should do it, maybe even less. These are not great if they are left lying around to cool off, but you can fry them earlier, then reheat in a very hot, about gas mark 8/220°C, oven for about 5–10 minutes. You can even fry them, freeze them, defrost and reheat them – or so I'm told – but I am not the freeze-ahead type.

And while we're mixing culinary cultures, I should mention that Sameen Rushdie's potatoes with whole spices are wonderful with the Christmas cold cuts. I don't include the recipe here just because it includes nigella seeds; but I admit that I was inspired to cook this for the first time by just such embarrassingly egomaniac promptings. You might need to go to a specialist store for them: you should know, then, that their Indian name is *kalonji*; or you can buy the particular spices below – panchphoran – ready mixed.

PANCHPHORAN ALOO
(POTATOES IN WHOLE SPICES)

900g potatoes, peeled
vegetable oil
1/2 teaspoon turmeric
1/2 teaspoon red chilli powder
1/2 teaspoon fenugreek seeds
1/2 teaspoon nigella seeds
1/2 teaspoon black mustard seeds
1/2 teaspoon white cumin seeds
1/2 teaspoon fennel seeds
3–4 tablespoons freshly chopped coriander

Slice the potatoes into 1/2–1cm rounds, then dice these further into small, evenly-sized cubes. Using a wok or other non-stick pan, take the minimum amount of oil needed and fry these cubed potatoes over a high heat to start with and then turn the heat down and cover. When the potatoes are a little more than half done, add the turmeric, red chilli powder and some salt, closely followed by the whole spices, mixed together. Stir to combine and put the lid back on once again. When the potatoes are nearly ready (and you will have to be vigilant to ensure they don't get too soft), take the lid off, turn the heat up and stir-fry to enable any excess liquid to evaporate.

Garnish with fresh coriander and serve.

LENTIL AND CHESTNUT SOUP

Another way of adding zip to cold leftovers is to serve hot soup first.

I first had this aromatic, velvety, manilla-coloured soup at Le Caprice about ten years ago, and still hanker after it. This is, with some help from the restaurant, my interpretation of it.

I have specified vegetable stock, and I tend to use Marigold vegetable bouillon powder, but obviously you can use chicken stock if you prefer.

Peeling chestnuts gives me a nervous breakdown, so for this, I use the Clément Faugier cans of chestnuts (and so, I have since found out, does Le Caprice). Their slightly candied taste adds a honeyed oomph to the soup.

1 small onion
1/2 leek
1 carrot
1 stick celery
2 tablespoons olive oil/goosefat/butter
225g red lentils
1 1/2 litres vegetable stock
225g cooked chestnuts
parsley and double cream to serve

Finely chop the onion, leek, carrot and celery. Heat the oil in the pan, add the chopped vegetables and let sweat and soften in the fat. Add the lentils and stir, then add the stock. Bring to the boil and simmer until the lentils are very soft (about 40 minutes). Add the chestnuts and simmer for a further 20 minutes or so. Liquidise until smooth, adding water as you need. When you want to serve it, reheat and, at the table, sprinkle each full bowl of soup with parsley and lace with cream. Serves 4–6.

You can otherwise make any old supper, whether of cold meats or whatever's lying around, seem a little more effortful (and indeed it will be a little more effortful) by making a pudding to have after. A hot pudding, I mean. And my favourite for this time of year is one of the recipes I did for my first piece as foodwriter for *Vogue*. It's a version of the rightly named queen of puddings, which has mystifyingly never come into fashionable focus like bread and butter pudding, to which it is grandly, indubitably, superior.

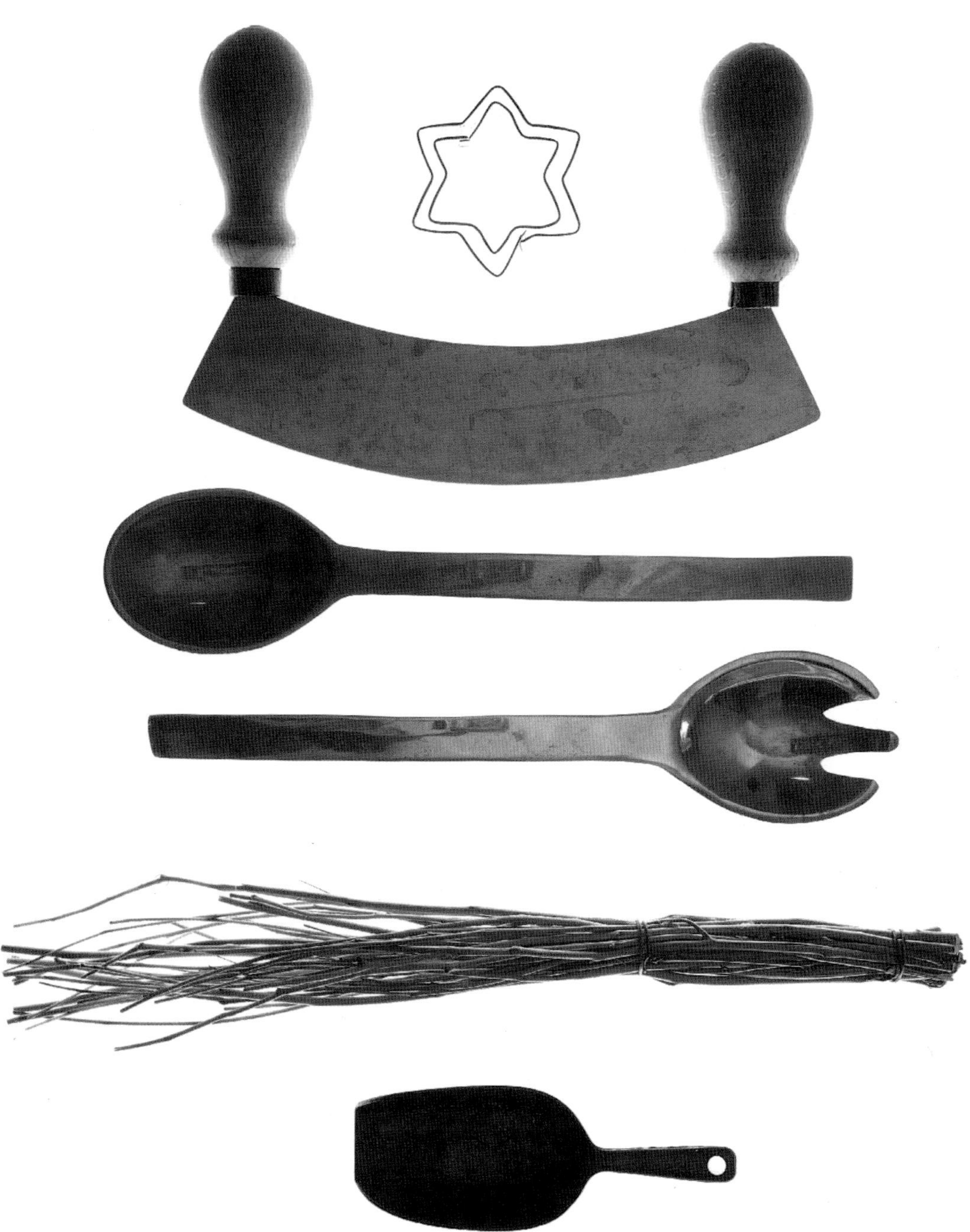

CHRISTMAS QUEEN OF PUDDINGS

The only things that are remotely Christmassy about this are that I use marmalade (sweetened with golden syrup) in place of the more usual jam, replace the lemon zest with orange zest (the smell of oranges, see also clementine cake below, always feels Christmassy to me) and I make the crumbs (in the processor as normal) not out of bread but out of pandoro, one of those yeasty cakes (this one's unfruited) which Italians eat in significant numbers, as we do too these days, at this time of year. You don't need to get pandoro, you could just as easily use brioche, or indeed the normal white breadcrumbs.

And since Christmas is very much the season for declassé liqueurs, I would serve this with double cream with a hint of Grand Marnier or Cointreau whipped up into it.

150g pandoro breadcrumbs (see above)
1½ teaspoons caster sugar
zest of 1 orange, preferably organic
orange-flower water, optional
575ml breakfast milk for preference, or else full-fat
40g unsalted butter, plus butter for greasing dish
5 eggs
3–5 tablespoons good quality fine-cut marmalade
1–2 teaspoons golden syrup
125g caster sugar, plus extra for sprinkling

Put the pandoro crumbs, caster sugar and the zest of the orange with 1–2 drops orange-flower water, if you have it, in a bowl. Heat the milk and butter in a pan until hot but just not boiling and then stir into the bowl of flavoured crumbs. Leave to steep for about 10 minutes and then thoroughly beat in the egg yolks.

Grease a shallow dish (I use a round dish about 10cm deep, 25cm in diameter because that's what I've got, but an oval dish is traditional) with butter and pour in the crumb custard. Bake at gas mark 3/160°C for about 20–30 minutes depending on depth of dish.

When it's ready the custard should be set on top, but may still be runny underneath. Let it stand out of the oven for a few minutes so that the top of the custard gets a bit harder while you turn your attention to the marmalade and egg whites. Heat the marmalade in a pan. Add 1–2 teaspoons golden syrup to the hot marmalade and then pour over surface of custard. Meanwhile whisk the egg whites until stiff and then whisk in half the sugar. In a few seconds the egg whites will become smooth and gleaming, and then fold in the remaining sugar with a metal spoon.

Cover your pudding with meringue mixture, sprinkle with sugar and then put it back in the oven for about 20 minutes or until meringue is browned and crispish. Serves 4–6.

CLEMENTINE CAKE

Another fixed item in my Christmas repertoire is my clementine cake. This is suitable for any number of reasons. First, it's made of the clementines which are seasonal. Then there's the fact that you need to cook them for 2 hours: you're more likely to be hanging around the house and to feel in the mood for this sort of thing during the Christmas period. It's incredibly easy to make; even if you're stressed out, it won't topple you over into nervous collapse. And, finally, it's such an accommodating kind of cake: it keeps well, indeed it gets better after a few days, and it is perfect either as a pudding, with some crème fraîche, or as cake to be eaten with seasonally sociable visitors in the mid-morning or afternoon. What more do you want?

It was only after I did this a few times – the route it took to get to me was circuitous, as these things can be – that I realised it was more or less Claudia Roden's orange and almond cake.

It is a wonderfully damp, dense and aromatic flourless cake: it tastes like one of those sponges you drench, while cooling, with syrup, only you don't have to. This is the easiest cake I know.

4–5 clementines (about 375g total weight)
6 eggs
225g sugar
250g ground almonds
1 heaped teaspoon baking powder

Put the clementines in a pan with some cold water, bring to the boil and cook for 2 hours. Drain and, when cool, cut each clementine in half and remove the pips. Then pulp everything – skins, pith, fruit – in the processor (or by hand, of course). Preheat the oven to gas mark 5/190°C. Butter and line a 21cm Springform tin.

Beat the eggs. Add the sugar, almonds and baking powder. Mix well, adding the pulped oranges. I don't like using the processor for this, and frankly, you can't baulk at a little light stirring.

Pour the cake mixture into the prepared tin and bake for an hour, when a skewer will come out clean; you'll probably have to cover with foil or greaseproof after about

40 minutes to stop the top burning. Remove from the oven and leave to cool, on a rack, but in the tin. When the cake's cold, you can take it out of the tin. I think this is better a day after it's made, but I don't complain about eating it any time.

I've also made this with an equal weight of oranges, and with lemons, in which case I increase the sugar to 250g and slightly anglicise it, too, by adding a glaze made of icing sugar mixed to a paste with lemon juice and a little water.

FREEZER

I lived for years without a freezer without ever minding very much. Certainly this allowed me the luxury of dreaming of all the goods things I would cook and put by should I ever have one: I imagined with pleasure the efficient domestic angel I would then become. Now that I do have a freezer, and a big American one to boot, it is indeed full. And, yet, I feel faintly resentful of its fullness.

The difficulty I find with stuffing a freezer full of food to eat at some future date is that when that future date comes I probably won't want to eat it. This is not because the food will spoil or disappoint, but because every time I open my freezer I see the same efficiently-stowed-away packets of coq au vin or beef stew or whatever it may be, and I get bored with them. I begin to feel as if I've eaten them as many times as I've opened the freezer door.

The freezer can easily become a culinary graveyard, a place where good food goes to die.

If you're someone who is meticulous about cooking, freezing, filing and then thawing in an orderly fashion, you need no advice from me as to how best to use your freezer. But you must be honest with yourself. There is no point in stowing away stews and soups if you are going to let them linger so long in its depths that finally all you can do is chuck them out. You'll probably find you stand more chance of eating the food you cook in advance if – when you put it in the freezer – you do so with some particular occasion in mind rather than just stashing it away for some unspecified future time. Obviously, if you know people are coming for dinner on Friday but the only time you can get any cooking done is on the weekend before, then the freezer will be useful (see Cooking in Advance). But unless you have an astonishingly capacious freezer and a mania for planning in advance, I wouldn't advise stocking up for more than one or two such occasions at any one time. However, there are two areas in which even I am ruthlessly efficient about freezing and then using food: cooking for children and dieting are both unimaginably easier if you create a form of culinary database in the deep freeze (see Feeding Babies and Small Children, and Low Fat).

Leftovers are obviously better put away in the freezer if the alternative destination is several days lingering in the fridge and then the bin. On the other hand, beware against using the freezer as a less guilt-inducing way of binning food you know you don't want. If no one, including you, liked the soup the first time round (and that's why you've got so much left over) there is no point in freezing it for some hopeful future date when, miraculously, it will taste delicious. But bagging leftovers – say stews – in single portions can be useful for those evenings when you're eating alone. Take the little packet out of the deep-freeze before you go to work in the morning and heat it up for supper when you get back at night. Immensely cheering.

The freezer really comes into its own not so much when you don't have time for cooking as when you don't have time for shopping. In other words, the best use for the freezer is as a store cupboard.

As with a store cupboard, you must be on your guard against overstocking. In fact having far too much in the freezer can be very much worse than a mouldering store cupboard, because food so easily gets buried and really forgotten about rather than simply ignored. But a solid supply of ingredients with which to cook, rather than just wholly prepared dishes, can really help you make good simple things to eat without exhausting last-minute trawls around the supermarket.

TIGER PRAWNS

You should always have in your freezer some raw tiger prawns. Cooking with raw prawns rather than cooked ones makes such a difference, and the raw ones anyway seem to be sold only in their frozen state, so you just transplant them from the fishmonger's freezer to yours. You can cook them from frozen (which means you don't need to think about defrosting in advance) by plunging them, unthawed, into boiling water, salted and maybe spiked with a little vinegar. Peel them and pile them on top of garlicky puy lentils or mix them, cooled, into a fennel salad. When I was in Los Angeles some years back, I ate at Joachim Splichal's Patina the most wonderful starter of mashed potatoes and truffles with warm Santa Barbara shrimp on top. The combination works. Purée some potatoes (they need to be whipped as well as

MASHED POTATOES, TRUFFLE OIL AND WARM SANTA BARBARA SHRIMP

mashed) with butter and white pepper, put a small, or maybe not so small, mound on a plate, add some barely cooked prawns, then drizzle over some truffle oil if you have some, or some Liguarian olive oil if you haven't.

BACON

Bacon is another ingredient any cook should keep in store. (And I like to keep some pancetta there too.) I always freeze bacon in pairs of rashers, so that they defrost in minutes. The point about bacon is that everywhere, even the corner shop, sells it, but the good stuff is hard to find. I get my bacon from my butcher, and I know when I cook it that 1) white froth won't seep out of it, and 2) it will taste of bacon. If your butcher doesn't have excellent bacon (and very few do), I really wouldn't turn to the supermarket, however upmarket its reputation: find instead a mail-order supplier (see Gazetteer or consult Henrietta Green's *Food Lovers' Guide to Great Britain*) and get some sent to you.

Nothing is as good as a bacon sandwich made with white bread. There are times when you just need to have that salty-sweet curl of seared flesh pressed between fat-softened, rind-stained spongy slices. My guiding rule is that I always have the wherewithal for a bacon sandwich in the house. I aim to keep all the ingredients for spaghetti carbonara to hand, too.

BREAD

Bread is worth keeping in the freezer. It freezes well, and I keep good bread in loaves and plastic white bread (such as is needed for bacon sandwiches) in pairs of slices. It's when I have to go shopping for basics such as bread and milk that I come back having spent far too much on absolute

MILK

unnecessities. Many varieties of milk now freeze all right, too: just check the labels first. For various reasons, all of them good ones, I try to keep visits to a supermarket to a minimum: I use my freezer to help keep me away.

STOCK

You must keep stock in your freezer, and also the bones you have saved up to make it. Turn your freezer into your very own Golgotha, by throwing in lamb bones, chicken carcasses and any other bones that, these days, you are allowed to boil up. I have been known to take home the carcasses with me after a dinner party once I've found out that a) they have come from my butcher and b) they were going to be thrown away. Keep ham bones or leftover trimmings from gammon joints, too, to flavour pea and bean soups at some later date. It may make your freezer look like Dennis Nilsen's, but that is a small price to pay.

Freeze your own, consequent, home-made stock in manageable portions (see page 11). I also keep a couple of tubs of Joubère stock (see Gazetteer) in my freezer. Certainly, Joubère fish stock is very useful to have on hand: making a good fish fumet is rather more serious work than making a chicken stock, and I feel guiltless about having someone else do it for me, especially if it's done better than I would myself.

PARMESAN

Parmesan rinds can be stowed away for future use. Every time you come to the end of a wedge of parmesan, or if you've left it out unwrapped for so long that it has become rebarbatively hard, don't throw the piece away, but chuck it in the freezer (preferably in a marked bag) to use whenever you make a minestrone or other soup which would benefit from that smoky, salty depth of flavouring.

SUMMER FRUITS

As for puddings, other than the obvious ones that are meant to be frozen, such as ice-cream, you don't need to do more than keep a packet or so of frozen summer fruits, which can be made to serve in most eventualities. Remember that defrosted strawberries take on the texture of soft, cold slugs. Remove them from the packets of mixed fruits, and chuck them out.

WINE

EGG WHITES

If, like me, you're not much of a drinker, then you can stop yourself from wasting leftover wine after dinner parties by measuring out glassfuls and freezing them, well labelled (or you'll mistake white wine for egg whites, and see below), to use for cooking later on. And as for egg whites: I've got so many frozen my freezer is beginning to look like a sperm bank.

STORE CUPBOARD

Unless you want to spend your every waking free hour buying food, you need to have at home basic ingredients that you can use to make something good when you haven't had time to shop or plan for a particular meal. But don't believe what you are told about essentials: all it means is that you'll have a larder full of lost bottles of Indonesian soy sauce with a use-by date of November 1994. There is a compromise. Buy those few ingredients which really do provide a meal quickly and easily, and don't weigh yourself down with various tempting bits and pieces that you think you may get round to using one day.

I don't want to be too dictatorial, though. Apart from anything else, so much depends on the amount of space you've got. I am the Imelda Marcos – she who had a cushion with Nouveau Riche is Better than No Riche At All embroidered on it – of the foodshop world. I am not safe in delicatessens. No wonder I can't move for food I've bankrupted myself to buy. You have to avoid finding yourself in the same position. For there is no such thing as having food to cover most eventualities which doesn't also involve regularly throwing away food that goes off before you eat it.

It's not easy to hold back. Nothing is as good as buying food. Buying store-cupboard food is highly seductive, because it doesn't go off and you don't have the stress of actual, imminent here-and-now cooking. It's fantasy shopping – and that's why it gets out of hand. Food bought on these expeditions lingers on for years, untouched. Partly this is because items you buy to store away are so often expensive, rarefied delicacies which, having bought, you then feel you have to save for something special. If you can get out of that frame of mind – which is the same mind-set that leads you to buy an extremely expensive piece of clothing which you then leave hanging in the wardrobe rather than allow it to be sullied by being worn around the house – then food shopping isn't quite such a dangerous pastime.

But it isn't the pattern of extravagance followed by austerity, nor the habit of saving things for best, which argues against intensive stockpiling. There is a hard-headed practical reason for being modest in your supplies: the food that people buy packets and packets of – flour, spices, rice, lentils – doesn't actually keep for ever. The chances are that you will end up with a larder full of stale pulses. It's not that this food goes off, necessarily, but it becomes less good to eat. It's comforting to know that you've got a bag of chick peas, but you must be strict with yourself and use it, not just keep it there for some rainy day when you fondly think you'll stay in and cook *pasta e ceci*. After a few years, they won't be dried, they'll be fossilised – and tasteless.

Anyway, unless you live in a very remote part of the country, the chances are that it won't be too difficult to go shopping for any special items you need for a specific recipe. A store cupboard is much more useful for keeping stuff in that you know you'll want regularly. This sort of food is likely to be the food you eat alone, or with your family. You want to be able to cook something in the evening after work without having to go shopping, and you don't want to have to start thinking about it before you get home. (I always want to think about what I'm going to eat, not in any elaborate organisational way, but because the speculation gives me pleasure. But there are many times when idly, greedily speculating is indeed the most energetic thing I can manage to do in advance. So what I need to know is that I have some food at home that won't take long to cook and won't demand too much of me.)

PASTA

The most important ingredient to keep in your larder, or food cupboard, or whatever it might be, is pasta. Stick to a few different shapes only: if you try and cover too many bases, you will simply end up with about 10 opened, almost finished, packets and you will never be able to make a decent plateful of any of them. It's useful to have rather a lot of spaghetti, so that you can suddenly cook a huge plateful of something for a kitchen-load of people if need be. Linguine are sufficiently different to be worth having as well. Short pasta is quick and easier to cook for chidren; choose fusilli or penne, for example. Some kinds of eggy pasta need little cooking, and are therefore wonderful for when you feel like Elizabeth Taylor shouting 'Hurry!' to the microwave, as Joan Rivers' cruel joke had it.

GOOD TOMATO SAUCE

If a store cupboard is there so that you know you can always cook yourself something good with what you've got at home, then you need some pasta sauces in it too. A good tomato sauce is indispensable. What you want to avoid is having your fridge full of large opened jars and bottles which have been half used up. I buy a whole tray of smallish bottles at a time, so that I know there's always some on hand. With jars and cans, it is worth getting as much as you have room for, since anything heavy is a nightmare to buy: better to get it over and done with in one exhausting go. (For this reason, I also buy baked beans, the 220g size, in bulk.) I would never be without two jars of pesto, one on the go, the other in the cupboard. If you can have pasta with tomato sauce or pasta with pesto in an everyday emergency, then you have all you need in your larder.

PESTO

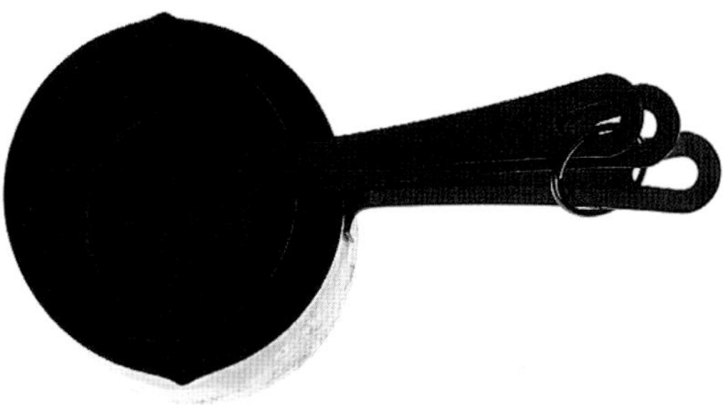

I do keep, though, a mixture of canned foods (soup, baked beans) so that there's something there for when I don't want to cook at all.

I know I said that flour and so forth doesn't keep for ever, but I do keep a modest and restrained selection, including flours, especially Italian 00, sugars, salt, spices, oil, vinegar, tinned tomatoes, vanilla extract, stock cubes and Marigold vegetable bouillon powders. I also make up a jar of vanilla sugar – simply by filling a Kilner jar with caster sugar and chopping a couple of vanilla pods into about 5cm lengths to go in it. This takes very little effort, makes one feel positively holy and also gives one gloriously scented sugar to use in cakes, puddings, custards and so forth whenever needed. The pods give out their sweet and fleshy scent for ages; just pour over fresh sugar as you use it.

VANILLA SUGAR

Naturally, what I want to keep in my kitchen cupboards might not be what you want to have in yours. But I couldn't live without Marsala, Noilly Prat (or Chambéry), dry sherry and sake pretty close to hand. I don't drink much, and so don't tend to have bottles of wine open; so if I need alcohol for cooking, I need to have it in the sort of bottles that come with a screw-top. Most often, I use Marsala in recipes which specify red wine, vermouth where white's required. Other drinks have their part to play: as ever, follow your own impulses; go with your own palate.

MARSALA, NOILLY PRAT

CHAMBÉRY, DRY SHERRY AND SAKE

Any time I let myself run out of garlic or onions, I curse. The base-note ingredients should be a given in your kitchen, or you always feel you're scrabbling around before you can make *anything*. And for me, fresh nutmeg is crucial, too. You don't have to get a special little nutmeg grater (you could just shave off bits with a sharp knife) but it's not expensive, and it is useful.

GARLIC

ONIONS

FRESH NUTMEG

FRIDGE

I keep a modest but restrained selection in my fridge, including butter, eggs, milk, salad leaves, some herbs and blocks of parmesan cheese. That's in theory; in reality it's a constant culinary clutter. I have either too much or not enough. But that's life.

ORGANIC FOOD

Not everything in my kitchen is organic, but it seems to be going that way. Eggs, I've already mentioned: though make sure the box says organic and free-range – or better still, Martin Pitt, see page 506 – as free-range alone doesn't signify anything very edifying. I can't buy meat any longer from a supermarket. I want it free-range, traceable – the buzzword in organic farming – and not pumped full of revolting things: so I go to the butcher. And now that supermarkets have got wise to the ever-more-widespread lure of organic produce it's easier to find vegetables from organic farms that aren't utterly covered in mud just to show their virtuous credentials. I worry about the chemicals in non-organic reared fruit and vegetables, but to tell the truth it's the improved taste of the organic stuff that's the clincher. If you can't muster the energy or interest to go wholly organic, just buy organic carrots. A few years back the government advised us to peel carrots because of the potentially harmful residues of chemicals which had been used in their cultivation. This is enough to make me feel that the real truth must be very much worse. Besides, organically grown carrots taste so much better. You should know that the difference in taste between organically and non-organically farmed potatoes is also pronounced. And it's worth buying organic oranges and lemons just because they're unwaxed and therefore better for zesting. But without the wax, they don't keep as long – there is a trade-off here – so just store them in the fridge if your turnover's slow.

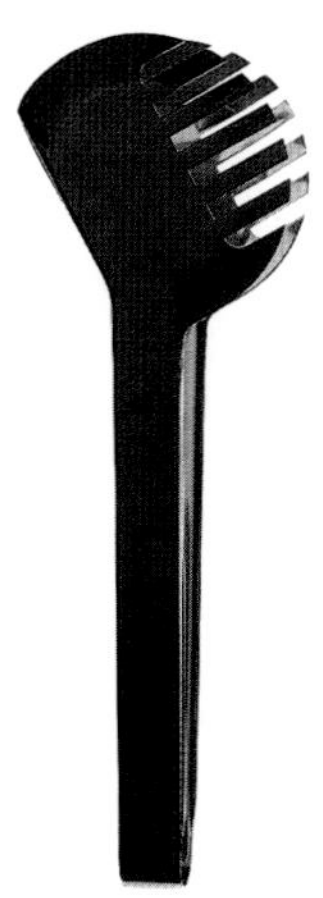

cooking in advance

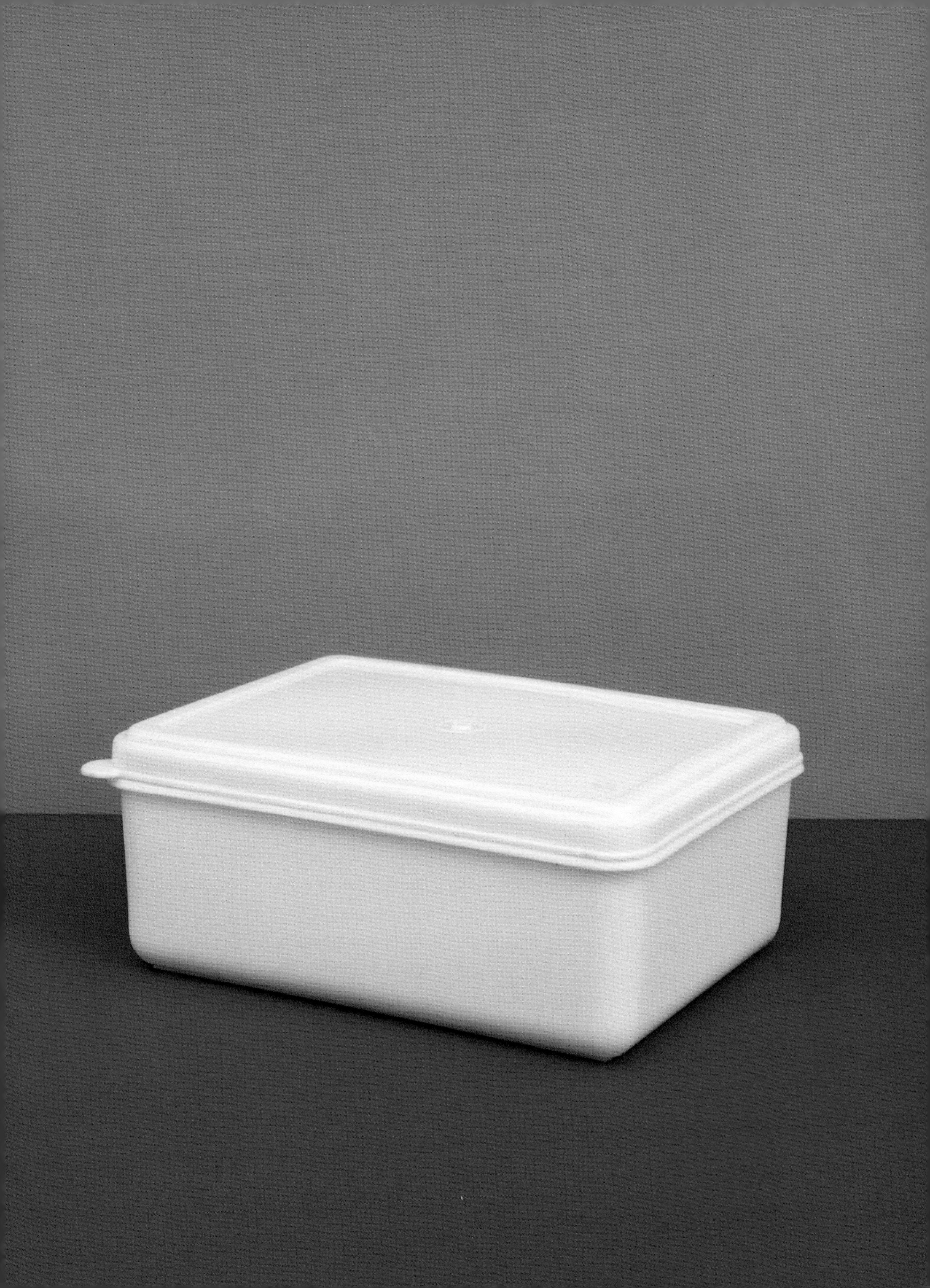

Quick cooking has become so implanted in people's minds as the way to eat well without having a nervous breakdown that everyone ignores the real way to make life easier for yourself: cooking in advance. Knocking up a meal in fifteen minutes is good for everyday cooking, when there's just one or two of you, or if you're one of those people who feels uncomfortable with too much planning. But when you're having people to dinner, life is made so much simpler if you don't have to do everything at the last minute. If you feel flustered at the very idea of cooking, indeed hate it, doing it in advance takes away some of the stress: if you enjoy it, you'll enjoy it more if you don't put yourself under pressure; that's for the professionals, who thrive on it. I love the feeling of pottering about the kitchen, cooking slowly, stirring and chopping and getting everything done when I'm feeling well-disposed and not utterly exhausted. When I cook with too much of an audience I immediately worry about what'll happen if something goes wrong, and then, of course, something does.

Cook in advance and, if the worst comes to the worst, you can ditch it. No one but you will know that it tasted disgusting, or failed to set, or curdled or whatever. That may sound a rather negative approach, but in fact it's liberating; moreover, because you're not stressed out or desperately working against the clock, there's less chance of disaster. And if something does go wrong, you have the time calmly to find a way of rectifying it.

And things do go wrong in cooking. Indeed, it's one of the ways you learn and eventually find your own style. Some of the best food I've cooked has been as a result of trying to make up for some fault, some blip. It's when you're exploring and trying out, not simply following a recipe, that you feel what the food needs, what will make it taste how you want it to taste. Without the pressure of having to perform, you can concentrate on the food. This is not to say that cooking has to be a solitary pursuit. In a way, there's nothing better than cooking with someone to talk to while you do it. But I am someone who panics if there's too much commotion or if I've got too little time to think.

cooking in advance

Perhaps this is a temperamental thing, but cooking is about temperament, and so, I think, is eating. You have to find a way of cooking that suits you, and that isn't just about your life, your working hours, your environment, though these, of course, matter. But what counts, too, is whether you're the sort of person who's soothed or cramped by list-making, whether you're impatient or tidy, whether spontaneity makes you feel creative or panic-stricken. Most of us like eating, but many people feel flustered and a sense of panic and, frankly, boredom when it comes to cooking. It's difficult to be good at something you aren't really interested in. But some people don't like cooking simply because they've never given themselves the chance to do it calmly and quietly and in the right mood. Obligation can be a useful prompt to activity, but it can be a terrible blight, too. Cooking in advance is a good way to learn confidence, to learn what works and why and how, and from that you can then teach yourself to trust your intuition, to be spontaneous: in short, to cook.

Cooking is about working towards a goal, towards something you have decided upon in advance. But any creative work (however cringe-makingly pretentious it sounds, cooking *is* creative, has to be) needs to liberate itself from the end product during the act of producing. This can be very difficult. There are practical constraints, which are what make the form, in cooking as in poetry. You have to learn to use these constraints to your advantage. Get over economic constraints by buying ingredients you can afford rather than making do with inferior versions of expensive produce. Make the best of the equipment you happen to have in your kitchen. Be ready to adapt to what you've got. But some other constraints – such as lack of time – merely add to your obstacles, and to the risk that if your dinner is inedible you and your guests will just have to live with it.

Some food actually benefits from being cooked in advance. Stews, for example, are always best cooked, left to get cold and hang around for a while, and then reheated. Puddings can need time to set or for their flavours to settle and deepen. Soups mellow. That's why I love this sort of cooking: the rhythms are so reassuring; I no longer feel I'm snatching at food, at life. It's not exactly that I'm constructing a domestic idyll, but as I work in the kitchen at night, or at the weekend, filling the house with the smells of baking and roasting and filling the fridge with good things to eat, it feels, corny as it sounds, as if I'm making a home.

SOUP

Soups are the obvious place to start for those thus in domestic goddess mode. Soups, of course, are some of the quickest meals that you can make. Somehow the home-made soup, lovingly prepared in advance, is no longer popular. I think it comes down to stock: our disinclination to make it from scratch, together with our disdain for cubes. It is important to stress that even though the better a stock the better a soup, it does not follow that no good soup, no superlatively good soup, can be made with stock cubes. Naturally, it depends on the kind of soup: no consommé or delicate broth should be made with anything but home-made stock; but a hearty vegetable soup can, frankly, be made with water; and in between these two extremes, use stock cubes. I am keen on the Knorr Italian ones or bouillon powder (the ones made by a company disconcertingly called Marigold. See page 10 for making your own stock and Gazetteer for cube stockists.)

If you haven't already got a supply of home-made stock in the freezer, you'll need a good day's grace: time to make the stock, to cool it, to skim the fat off it. A ham stock (just the liquid in which a gammon's been cooked) makes all the difference to a pea soup; a chicken stock, light though it may be, gives instant depth and velvety swell to a very basic parsnip soup. Grate fresh parmesan over the pea soup; drop chilli oil into the pale sweetness of the parsnip to add a probing fierceness. To both you could add some bacon, fried, grilled or baked in a hot oven, and crumbled into salty shards; marjoram, too, would work equally well with either.

Both these soups can be made in advance and kept in the fridge for reheating throughout the week, whether on the hob or in the microwave.

The soups that you really have to cook in advance are the ones made from pulses. Most legumes need a good day's soaking. I tend to put beans into soak as I go to bed even if I won't actually be cooking with them until the next evening. Chick peas need 24 hours, and I don't mind if I give them 36. And they need a lot of cooking, much longer than you are usually told. There seems to be a conspiracy to misinform you about chick peas: I cannot believe the number of times I've read that 45 minutes will do, when it takes double that time to cook them. Anna del Conte is realistic about this, admitting that some chick peas can take as long as 4 hours. I use her technique for preparing chick peas. Put them in a bowl and cover them with cold water. Then mix together

CHICK PEAS

1 teaspoon bicarbonate of soda and 1 tablespoon each of salt and flour – or those ingredients in that ratio: a very large quantity of peas will need more of this tenderising mixture – add water to form a runny paste and stir this paste into the soaking chick peas. Leave for a good 24 hours. Then, when cooking the chick peas (drained and rinsed), don't lift the lid off the pan for the first hour or so or the peas will harden. (Curiosity often gets the better of me.) Broad beans similarly need longer soaking than, say, cannellini or borlotti (both of which are fine with 12 hours), and all are better if you leave the salting till the last moments of the cooking time. If you're cooking in advance, it doesn't matter how long it all takes: and good though canned chick peas are, dried, soaked and cooked ones are so much better. You can taste the full, grainy, chestnutty roundness of them.

Chick pea and pasta soup is my favourite soup of all. You can cook it days before you actually want to eat it. Obviously it can't all be done in advance because the pasta must be cooked at the last minute, but since you have to reheat the soup anyway, what does it matter to you if, when reheating, you keep it simmering for 20 minutes or so extra while the ditalini swell and soften.

I cook this soup so often – just for us, at home, for supper, in great big greedy bowlfuls; for a first course when I've got people coming for dinner; or, if they're coming for a Saturday lunch, for a main course, with a salad and cheese after – that I don't follow a recipe any more. But this is the recipe that started me off. It is Anna del Conte's, adapted from her *Entertaining All'Italiana*. I have several copies of this book: one in the kitchen, where, eccentrically perhaps, I tend not to keep my cookery books; one in my study, where all books on food notionally live (in practice they are dotted on floors, in lavatories, throughout the house); and one in the bedroom, for late-night soothing reading and midnight-feast fantasising.

ANNA'S CHICK PEA AND PASTA SOUP

This will make enough soup for 8. I sometimes add a glass of white wine or any stock to hand, from whatever animal it emanates, but the soup has quite enough taste with simply water. If you want a vegetable stock, choose the low-salt Marigold bouillon powder. You can make the soup (bar the pasta) up to 3 days in advance, or longer if you want to freeze it.

400g dried chick peas
2 teaspoons bicarbonate of soda
2 tablespoons flour
2 tablespoons salt
3 litres vegetable stock (or meat stock or white wine and water)
3 sprigs rosemary
8 cloves garlic, peeled and bruised
120ml extra virgin olive oil
400g fresh tomatoes, skinned and seeded
270g small tubular pasta such as ditalini
parmesan for grating over
chilli oil and flat-leaf parsley if you want

Put the chick peas in a bowl and cover with plenty of water. Mix together the bicarbonate of soda, flour and salt and add enough water to make a thin paste. Stir this mixture into the bowl with the chick peas and leave to soak for at least 12 hours and preferably 24.

When the chick peas have doubled their size (you don't have to get your ruler out: trust your eyes) they are ready to be cooked. Drain and then rinse them. Put them in a large pot and add the vegetable stock, meat stock or white wine and water or the same quantity of water.

Tie the rosemary sprigs in a muslin bag and add to the pot. This will make it possible to remove the rosemary without leaving any needles to float in the soup. This might sound pernickety, but when I ignored the advice I found the sharp and, by now, bitter needles an unpleasant intrusion. If you feel intimidated by the idea of muslin then use, disgusting though it sounds, a popsock or stocking and tie a knot at the open end, or a tea-infuser. Frankly, it doesn't matter what you use providing it does the job, although I imagine untreated muslin is better. You can get muslin or cheesecloth in any kitchen shop or haberdashery department and, come to think of it, in a baby department selling muslin napkins, one of those posset-catching squares you wear over your shoulder to catch infant regurgitations would do.

Add the garlic and pour in half the oil. Cover the pan tightly and bring to the boil. You will have to gauge this by ear without peeping in. Lower the heat and cook over the lowest simmer until the chick peas are tender, which can take 2–4 hours. Take a look after 1½ hours. Do not add any salt until the chick peas are nearly ready. If you put it in too soon, they'll harden.

When the chick peas are tender, remove the garlic and the rosemary bundle, which should be floating on the surface. Purée the tomatoes through a food mill or in a food processor and add to the soup with their juice. Stir well, add salt and pepper to taste and cook for a further 10 minutes or so. This is the point at which you should stop when you're cooking the soup in advance.

When you want to eat it, put it back on the hob and reheat it, so that you can proceed to the final step, which is to cook the pasta. Before you add the pasta, check that there is enough liquid in the pan. You may have to add some boiling water. Now, to the boiling soup, add the pasta and cook till al dente. I like to add some freshly chopped flat-leaf parsley, but the glory of this soup will be undiminished if you prefer not to. But do pour some of the remaining oil into the pot of soup, and drizzle some more into each bowl after you've ladled the soup in. Or just pour some into the big pot and let people add what they want as they eat. I would put good extra virgin olive oil on the table as well as a bottle of chilli oil for those who like some heat: and it does work. Serve, too, the parmesan, put on a plate with a grater, so people can add their own.

SPLIT PEA SOUPS

Split pea soups don't need to be cooked in advance, since the pulses don't need soaking, but it is a rare soup – or stew, for that matter – which doesn't improve with a few days' hanging around. The only thing to remember is that you will need to add more liquid when you reheat it, as pulses seem to carry on drinking up their cooking liquid for ages. I love all split pea soups, and remember wonderful grainy, tobacco-tinted purées eaten in Amsterdam – thick, puddingy soups, smelling of sausage. But green split peas are the ones I tend to cook the most. Whenever I've boiled a ham, I save the salty stock. Into this I throw some green split peas and sliced leeks, maybe a potato or two, for a near-enough instant supper. When the weather is relentlessly, intrusively windy and cold, then a thick, pale green sludge of split peas is perfect. Recently, though, I've begun to think that the ham stock is even better used as a base for a pea soup with fresh (or frozen) peas on a spring or summer's day.

Cooking ahead is the only way to keep sane when you're cooking for a lot of people. Thick soups will do, as you don't need to add too much to fill people up: good bread, good cheese, good wine. I was never particularly keen on black bean soup till I had a bowlful in a small Cuban place in South Beach, Miami: I loved its spice-fuggy muddiness. The recipe that follows attempts to evoke it. It serves about 8 people, but obviously the quantities can be boosted without requiring a doctorate in higher mathematics on the part of the cook.

SOUTH BEACH BLACK BEAN SOUP

450g dried black turtle beans
2 bay leaves
200ml extra virgin olive oil
2 large red peppers, seeded and chopped
2 shallots, chopped
2 onions, chopped
8 cloves garlic, chopped
1 tablespoon ground cumin
2 tablespoons ground dried oregano
zest of 1 lime, plus more limes for serving
½ tablespoon light or dark muscovado sugar
2 tablespoons dry sherry
1 red onion, diced, to serve
coriander, chopped
250ml sour cream, to serve, optional

Place the beans in a large pan and cover with 2 litres water. There is no need to soak. Add the bay leaves and bring to the boil. Reduce the heat and simmer the beans for 1½–2 hours till soft but not squishy, stirring frequently and adding more water if necessary to keep them well covered.

Meanwhile, heat the olive oil in a large, deep frying pan and sauté the peppers, shallots and onions over medium heat until the onions are translucent (about 15 minutes). Add the garlic, cumin, oregano and lime zest, and sauté for an additional 5 minutes. Transfer to a blender and purée until smooth.

When the beans are almost tender, add the puréed mixture, sugar and 1 tablespoon salt (or to taste) to the beans and cook until just tender (20–30 minutes). Adjust the seasonings and add the sherry if you're serving straight away, but otherwise season and sherry the soup when you're reheating it later, and you will also need to add water as the soup thickens on cooling. Put the coriander, chopped red onion, quartered limes and sour cream on the table in separate bowls so that people can add their own as they want. I'd add a bottle of tabasco while I was about it, too.

But *the* soup you have to make in advance, and a soup unjustifiably ignored today, is consommé. There is, for most people, a ring of bon viveur – the Frenchified works of Fanny and Johnnie – about the word consommé: it conjures up a world of napkin-arranged gentility and brisk effortfulness. Well, then, call it *brodo*. A beautiful, clear, flavour-infused liquid is unsurpassable. And it's strange that, in our gush and lust for all things Italian, that amber broth, which is such an ordinary and integral part of the Italian diet, gets routinely ignored.

I've come to the conclusion that our disdain is twofold: it is fuelled in the first part by fear and the second by insecurity. The fear is culinary, the insecurity social. There are certain words which immediately make people feel the recipe they are reading is not for them. Stock, pestle and mortar, double-boiler are just some such. And stock is, I think, the most terror-laden. But more than that, people are afraid that a plain consommé will be boring. For all our modern talk about valuing simplicity, we baulk when faced with something truly, perfectly simple. We want the vibrant, the robust, the instant, the *simplified*: that's different. A consommé strikes us – correctly – as a dish that belongs to a formal dinner. We are afraid that borrowing from the earlier canon of the elaborately arranged dinner party will mark us out as infra dig, out of touch or just plain suburban.

A clear soup, made properly, is not at all without personality. It is uplifting, delicately but insistently flavoured. But even chefs, with their splendid stockpots, are rarely sufficiently confident to serve an unadorned broth. Too often these days it comes fashionably spiked with lemongrass or pebbled with beans. I love all variations – and I do willingly admit that the point of a good broth is that it is a wonderfully deep-toned base for the bits you can float in it – and am happy with just about any innovation that has integrity, but an ordinary, straightforward consommé or *brodo*, golden poolfuls of the stuff, is a joy and a restorative: bracingly elegant.

It is time-consuming to make but not difficult, and a wonderfully mood-enhancing way of putskying around in a kitchen. You need to get started a good day before you're planning to eat it – in order to let it cool and skim off the fat – but you can leave it in the fridge for 3 or so days and not worry.

The recipe here is from a book which should never have been allowed to go out of print: Arabella Boxer's *Book of English Food* – subtitled *A Rediscovery of British Food from Before the War* – which was published in 1991. You don't read cookery books just for culinary instruction – I don't – but also for comment, for history, for talk. And it is for all these that I want Arabella Boxer's literary company. Here she is on the fashionable emergence of the consommé in the 1920s:

> Roughly speaking, the more elegant the occasion, the smoother, or clearer, the soup. A consommé was considered the ultimate test of a good cook, and the ideal start to an exquisite meal. It might be served quite plain, or

with some small garnish floating in it: small vegetable dice, a few grains of rice, or minuscule soup pasta. In a less conventional household a more elaborate garnish might be served separately: round croûtons piled high with whipped cream, or a bowl of saffron-flavoured rice, or even a jug of beetroot juice for adding, with cream, to a consommé made with duck and beef stock. This practice of handing round a number of elaborate garnishes separately amused the English. Part of its appeal was that by enabling the guests to assemble their own dishes it pandered to their distrust of what they described as 'mucky food'.

CONSOMMÉ

Arabella Boxer adapted this recipe from June Platt's *Vogue* column in the 1930s and prefaces it with the remark – pertinent here – that it is best made over 2 days, adding that 'the original recipe calls for 12 pints (6.8 l) of water, but few of us have pans that large. I use half that amount, filling up the pan from time to time with more cold water'. Boiling fowls are difficult to come by, but not impossible. Halal butchers sell them, or you may find frozen boiling chickens. I don't want to be too prissy, but I like to feel confident about the origin of the birds. I don't want to eat some miserable fowl raised on fish pellets in squalor somewhere. The French free-range corn-fed birds can provide wonderful stock, as, I've found, can poussins (see page 11).

The idea of cooking anything for 7 hours seems incredible these days. Consider using a heat-diffuser: you want a gentle simmer, the odd bubble rising up. Avoid at all costs all the precious liquid's ungovernable evaporation.

1 large chicken, preferably a boiling fowl
1.15kg shin of beef, cubed
2 large carrots, sliced thickly
2 onions, sliced thickly
2 leeks, sliced thickly
3 stalks parsley
3 sprigs thyme
1 large clove garlic, peeled
2 cloves

Wash the chicken and put it in a large soup pot, add the shin of beef and cover well with 3.6 litres cold water. Let stand for ½ hour, then put on the fire and bring slowly to the boil. Remove the scum, add 120ml cold water and bring to the boil again. Repeat this process twice. Simmer very slowly for 1 hour, then add the carrots, onions, leeks, parsley stalks, thyme, garlic, salt and pepper and the cloves. Let simmer for 7 hours.

Strain through a fine sieve, then through a wet cheesecloth. You can use muslin for this or even a clean J-cloth or a paper funnel-shaped coffee filter. Kitchen paper lining a sieve doesn't work: it's too absorbent and ends up not sieving anything.

Chill overnight and when cold carefully remove grease. Makes 2.75–3.6 litres, serves 12.

A basic *brodo* of an Italian sort provides a fragrant liquid base for tortellini or gnocchetti di semolino (see below) or any other manner of culinary punctuation. This broth is cooked for less time than the one above and so one would expect it to be lighter, more delicate and less suited to being served just as it is. It is also, pre-eminently, designed to make divine risotti.

ITALIAN BROTH

1 piece of beef flank, approx. 500g
2 ossobuchi
approx. 500g chicken wings or a chicken carcass or a poussin
1 onion, cut in half, each half stuck with a clove
2 carrots, sliced chunkily
2 celery stalks, sliced chunkily
2 leeks, white part only, sliced
1 ripe tomato, halved or 1 tinned plum tomato, drained of juice
1 clove garlic, peeled
1 bay leaf
6 parsley stalks
6 black peppercorns
1 teaspoon salt

Put all the ingredients into a stockpot or large saucepan and cover with water, to which you've added a teaspoon of salt, by about 6cm. Bring to the boil slowly – over a medium flame – and then turn down the heat so that it simmers gently. Skim the scum from the surface and keep an eye on it so that you can see when more scum rises to the surface and needs to be skimmed off again. Do this about 3 times in quick succession, then every hour. Let simmer – always very gently, and you may well need a heat diffuser if even at the lowest heat on the hob the broth bubbles over-exuberantly – for 3 hours.

Remove the large pieces of meat and vegetable with a slotted spoon and then pour the broth into a large bowl (a wide one makes it easier to remove the fat later) through a sieve lined with muslin or a clean, single-thickness J-cloth. When cool, put in the fridge. When it's set (overnight or after about 8 hours), skim the fat off the surface. I find wiping the top, firmly but not so brutally you break into the jelly below, with a few pieces of kitchen towel the easiest way of degreasing it. It keeps in the fridge for up to 3 days.

GNOCCHETTI DI SEMOLINO

Somehow these sound rather better in Italian than they do in English: semolina dumplings have a heavy, puddingy ring to them; and these are light, puffy things.

250ml full-fat milk
100g semolina
45g butter, softened
1 egg, separated
4 tablespoons grated parmesan (about 20g)
fresh nutmeg

Bring the milk to the boil but do not let it actually boil. Off the heat, add the semolina to the milk: whisking constantly, hold the semolina in your fist and letting a light rain of grain fall into the pan as you beat. Keep beating till you have a thick paste and then let cool.

Mix the butter with the egg yolk, the cheese and a good grating of fresh nutmeg and a pinch of salt. Mash the egg–cheese–butter mixture into the semolina paste to combine. Whisk the egg white with a good pinch of salt till stiff, and then fold in; you may find this easiest if you stir in a tablespoonful of whites quite briskly first to loosen the semolina. If it helps, too, do everything a few hours in advance up to the whisking and incorporating of the egg white, but don't keep in the fridge.

When the broth's boiling, form little oval balls by scooping out bits with a teaspoon, and drop them in. They'll take about 10 minutes to cook, when they'll swell and rise to the surface.

ROAST POTATOES

Some food won't suffer if allowed a little resting time. By all means parboil potatoes before you need to roast them. I have eaten for Sunday lunch roast potatoes which were parboiled on Friday evening. My one proviso here is that they shouldn't be put in the fridge in the interim. I find potatoes go slightly powdery and heavy after they've been put in the fridge, even leftover mashed potato. Just leave them out somewhere cold, like a larder.

If you are parboiling in advance, before roasting, rub over the surfaces of the potatoes, though gently – you're not trying to make rosti – with the coarse side of a grater, just to rough them up before putting them in the hot fat. Cook in a hot oven.

SKINNING PEPPERS

Skinning peppers a day or so before you want to eat them is sensible even when you're not planning anything elaborate. They're better the longer they sit in their oily juices. So: blister them under the grill or in the oven and while they are still very hot, put them either in a plastic bag which you tie tightly at the neck or in a bowl which you seal quickly with clingfilm. The peppers then steam, and this enables the skins to be removed more easily. Skin them, seed them and cut them into strips, being sure to catch the juice to add to the dressing. Make them glisten with some peppery glass-green olive oil. You can pound some anchovies into a paste and mix that with the olive oil now, or, just before you want to eat the peppers, arrange them on a plate, criss-cross them with the best anchovy fillets you can find and dot here and there (not too neatly) with some stoned black olives, halved to form shiny little squished black rounds, like a teddy bear's nose. Pour over some fresh olive oil and eat. I like the anchovies striating the glossy, flat mass of peppers rather than being actually part of the dressing, just because that can make the whole look rather muddy. Garlic and rosemary, added at any and all stages, are also to be welcomed. With food like this, you should just relax and do what tastes best to you. Peppers and anchovies are an incomparable mix and, pertinently, one that has consistently found favour, regardless of fashion, from the age of the hors d'oeuvres trolley to the balsamic-soused present.

Some sauces can be cooked a day ahead and left in the fridge until you need them. If you don't want a skin to form, then cover with a disc of buttered greaseproof paper or a thin film of full-fat milk, if it's a milk-based sauce. Obviously those egg–butter liaisons – hollandaise, béarnaise and so on – need to be done at the lastish minute but a white sauce, béchamel, anything with a roux base, can be cooked and then forgotten for a while. Just reheat slowly and be prepared to add more liquid.

Pasta sauces can be made up to 3 days before you need them. At least, those pasta sauces which are not predominantly cream or butter can. Any vegetable-based sauce, even if it does contain cream, can be made when it suits you, which may well not be at the same time as cooking the pasta. Pasta itself obviously needs to be cooked at the last moment, unless, that is, it's baked pasta. This is incredibly useful if you've invited quite a lot of people for lunch or supper when you're not going to be at home very long before you want to eat. You can cook the pasta, the sauces, assemble everything a couple of days or so in advance, and then give the whole thing about 40 minutes in a hottish oven when you want to eat it.

This is the only baked pasta dish I go in for much: it's mellow, comforting but resonantly flavoured as well; you're not swamped in puddingy béchamel, as you can be. My children love it, incidentally, and since you can feed a good 8 people (more if children are included in the numbers) this makes it a good filler for one of those low-key mixed generation meals, when you're too busy with everything else you have to do to be absolutely full-on in the kitchen before you eat.

BAKED VEAL AND HAM PASTA

The name I give it evokes, and is meant to, the old-fashioned flavours of those hot-water-crust pies: picnic food to be eaten on scratchy rugs; this is the winter, indoors variety. But it's very garlicky, too, so it's not a complete transposition of that mild, sausagey taste. If you boil the garlic, it not only makes it easier to peel, but it reduces any latent acridness, producing, later, warmth rather than smoky heat. The ham in question is pancetta (or chopped bacon if you prefer) but if you've got some cold cooked ham in the fridge, do use that: cut it into small cubes and stir it into the quantity of béchamel the pasta is coated in later.

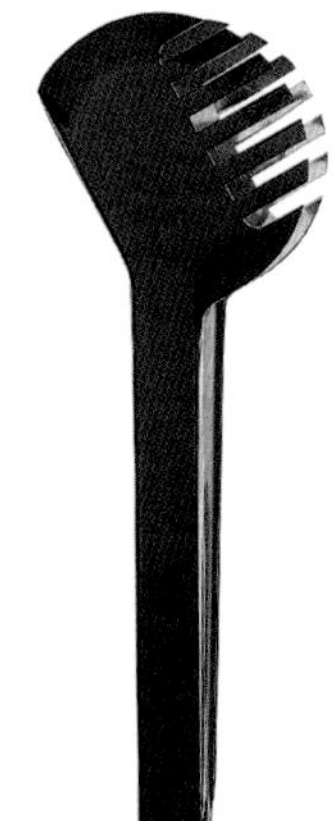

6 cloves garlic
75g pancetta
2 sticks celery
1 onion
1 carrot
good handful fresh parsley
2 heaped tablespoons lard or 2 tablespoons olive oil
1/4 teaspoon paprika
1/4 teaspoon ground mace
3 tablespoons Marsala
325g veal, minced
95g butter, plus more for greasing and dotting (see below)
95g flour, preferably Italian 00
pinch mace, plus one further 1/4 teaspoon
1.4 litres full-fat milk
5 bay leaves
fresh nutmeg
110g parmesan, freshly grated, plus more for grating over later
500g penne or rigatoni

Put the cloves of garlic in a small pan, cover with cold water, bring to the boil and boil for 7 minutes. Drain. Derind the pancetta, chop roughly and put into the bowl of the food processor, fitted with the double-bladed knife. Roughly chop the celery, peel the cloves of garlic (just press them and they will pop out of their skins), peel and quarter the onion, peel and roughly chunk the carrot and throw them all in too, along with the parsley, and process until finely chopped. Melt the lard or oil in a heavy-based shallow pan (I use the lid of my Le Creuset Marmitout, using the bottom bit for the assembled dish later) and then, when hot, add the vegetable and pancetta mixture. Stir well over highish heat for a minute or so, adding Marsala, mace and paprika, then turn the heat down to low and cook, stirring regularly to make sure it doesn't stick, for 15 minutes.

While this is happening, put copious water on to boil for the pasta.

When the 15 minutes are up, briefly turn the heat back to high, add the minced veal and turn well for a minute or so before, again, turning down to low for 15 minutes. While this is cooking, get on with the béchamel. Melt the butter in a large saucepan, stir in the flour and pinch of mace, and cook for a couple of minutes, still stirring, adding a fat pinch of salt and some pepper. Off the heat, slowly stir in the milk. I don't bother to heat the milk up; there's too much of it.

When all the milk's smoothly amalgamated, add the bay leaves and put back on a medium heat, stirring, until the sauce cooks and thickens. Although you want to cook this for a good long time – about 20 minutes – so it's velvety, bear in mind that this is meant to be a thin, runny sauce. Towards the end of cooking time, taste for salt (though remember you will be adding quite a bit of salty parmesan later) and pepper and add, too, the remaining mace and grate in some nutmeg. When the sauce is cooked and the flouriness gone – taste after 12 minutes if you're using 00 flour – turn off the heat and stir in the parmesan, beating well with your wooden spoon to make sure all is smoothly incorporated. You should by now have started cooking the pasta. You want it slightly undercooked, since it will be cooked again in the oven. On the packets of penne I have at home, the instructions are to cook for 13 minutes; for this, I drain them after 10.

Butter the pan, or whatever the pasta's to be baked in (a lasagne dish or any form of shallowish casserole would be fine) and pour in about a third of the béchamel; don't bother to measure, just make a rough estimate by eye. Add the drained pasta and turn well to coat. Add the veal and toss well again, then another third of the béchamel and give a good final mix, tasting for salt and pepper. Level the pasta in the pan and pour over the last third of béchamel. Let cool then put, covered, in the fridge for a couple of days or so before baking, though of course you can put it straight away in the oven to bake if you want (in which case it will need less time than otherwise mentioned).

If you've fridged it, take it out and make sure it's at room temperature before you bake it. Sprinkle with more parmesan and dot with butter and bake in a preheated gas mark 5/190°C oven for about 40 minutes.

KAFKA-ESQUE OR SOFT AND CRISPY DUCK

You'd think, wouldn't you, that a roast could never ever be done in advance. Yes, we all know that any joint needs to rest after it's come out of the oven and before it goes on the table, but I now do a roast duck – the best roast duck I have ever eaten, let alone cooked – that can be started a good few days before you want to eat it. This is semi-cooking in advance and I'm blazingly evangelical about it. A method of doing the perfect roast duck which leaves you with just three-quarters of an hour's cooking on the night – and all in the oven, no basting, no faffing, nothing – has to be a good thing. I let the duck sit around in the fridge in a state of semi-cookedness for up to 3 days; but if you feel at all nervous about this, don't leave it as long. But actually, before we get on to it, it isn't that new an idea: Apicius – he of the first cookery book – likewise instructed his readers: 'lavas, ornas et in olla elixabis cum acqua, sale et aneto dimidia coctura'. Admittedly, even if he suggested boiling the duck in water (with dill as well as salt) until half-cooked, the second half's cooking would not be exactly by roasting; it would have been more like pot-roasting. Nevertheless, it reminds us pointedly that there is nothing new in cooking. That's if it's to taste good.

But this is the story: when I was last in New York I bought a copy of Barbara Kafka's *Roasting*, the premise of which is that roasting at very high temperatures makes for the most succulent, fleshily yielding and crispy skinned birds and joints. The drawback is that you need a clean oven, otherwise all that roasting at very high temperatures gives you a smoky kitchen, burning eyes and an acrid glaze on the putative pièce de résistance. I noticed that there was a recipe for roast duck which involved poaching the bird first in stock for about three-quarters of an hour and then blitzing it in the oven for half an hour. The result: tender flesh and crisp skin. And it's true, if you're not careful when you roast a duck in the more usual way you often find that the desirably crunchy carapace comes at the cost of overcooked and thus stringy meat. Everyone has an answer to this one: covering the bird with boiling water, hanging it up on a clothes line on a blustery (but dry) day, suspending it on high by means of a clothes hanger then getting a stiff wrist by aiming a hair-dryer, at full though icy blast, at it for hours.

The *echt* Kafka-esque technique involves poaching the duck, upright, in a thin, tall pot in duck stock. I couldn't quite see why you needed to poach the bird in stock, since the flesh is rich itself. More to the point, I had none. So the first time I tried it, I put the water into the requisite tall thin pot (the bottom half of my couscoussier), added the giblets, brought it to the boil, added salt, and lowered in the duck. Then, as directed, I made sure the bird was submerged for the whole 40 minutes. I did this in the morning, let the duck get cool, put it in the fridge and then brought it out in the evening, letting it get to room temperature before roasting it for the 30 minutes as recommended.

The next time I tried it, I made some changes. For one thing, duck doesn't yield much flesh, and cooking a single, lone, duck is no use unless there are only 2 or 3 of you eating. But I couldn't get 2 ducks into my couscoussier, and getting even one out, from an upright position, tore its skin. So I decided to be even more disobedient. Figuring that the ducks would stay moist if they were steamed, not necessarily submerged, I put one duck, breast down, in a large, oblong casserole and the other in a large, deep, all-purpose frying pan. Both pans were filled with boiling salted water. The casserole had its own lid, and for the frying pan I made a tent of tin foil. I wasn't sure it would work, but there's only ever one way of finding out.

I had decided anyway – on the evidence produced by my first stab – to swap around cooking times: that's to say, poach the birds for the ½ hour and roast them for ¾ hour. The ducks weren't exactly the same size (one was about 1½kg, the other perhaps 300g heavier) but I didn't alter the poaching times to suit: I merely took the lighter one out of its water first. And it is very much easier taking the ducks out when they are flat rather than upright. Use wooden paddle-spoons or rubber spatulas to make sure you don't rip the flesh. It would be even easier to steam the birds breast up, and frankly I doubt it matters which way up they are. I noticed some slight scalding to a patch on both ducks where the breast had come into contact with the hot base of the pan, but this didn't seem to make any difference either.

Boiling ducks produces a rather pongy fug which can linger in the kitchen, so open a window; but I was going away for the weekend and had promised to cook something. I knew I wouldn't have time to poach the birds on the Friday so did them on Thursday at about six in the evening, let them cool on a baking tray with a wire-mesh grill arrangement set over it, and then put them in the fridge before going to bed.

For travelling on Friday evening I just put them in a plastic bag and put that plastic bag in a picnic coolbag. On arrival, I put the ducks, uncovered, on a large plate in my friends' fridge. When I got around to cooking them – which turned out to be Sunday lunch – it transpired that the Aga had died. I put the birds, anyway, into the supposedly hot oven, which turned out to be a rapidly cooling sooty box, and left them there for a hopeless 20 minutes. The ducks just got greasy, not even hot, and I got more teary and mutinous by the minute. But someone living in a neighbouring farm set her oven to high for me (she was doubtful about having ducks at top whack so we compromised on gas mark 8/220°C): the ducks were driven over to her, roasted for 45 minutes and came back, after the brief car journey, bronze and crisp and perfect.

I don't think it is possible to try out a recipe more conclusively than that.

I love having someone in the kitchen just to talk to as I chop, and weigh, and stir, and generally get things ready. I love cooking with other people, too. I do it rarely, though used to often with my sister Thomasina. There's something about that industrious intimacy that is both cushioning and comforting, but also hugely confidence-building. I love that sense of companionable bustle, of linked activity and joint enterprise. It makes it easier to attempt food that normally you would shrink from, not because you rely on another's superior capabilities or experience necessarily, but because you aren't isolated in the attempt. Everything doesn't feel geared towards the end product because it is a shared activity – and that itself is pleasurable. You feel a sense of satisfaction about the process. It isn't drudgery.

Claudia Roden, writing about her memories of childhood in Egypt, recollected kitchenfuls of women kneading and pummelling pastries, stuffing them, wrapping them, baking them together. But I suppose those Middle-Eastern delicacies, meticulous confections with their elaborate *farces*, could have sprung only from a culture in which the cooking was carried out by posses, by armies, of sisters and female relatives. It doesn't do to get too lyrical about this culinary companionship, though: which of us now would want our lives to be spent in such service, companionable though it might have been?

Still, it's a pity to lose all of it, never to become immersed in that female kitchen bustle. For me, so much of cooking in advance is tied up with that image, that idea: that's when cooking feels like the making of provisions, the bolstering up of a life. I don't see it as a form of subjection (unless the position is a forced one) and I don't see it as a secondary role, either. Some people hate domesticity, I know. I'm glad I don't: I love the absorbing satisfactions of the kitchen. For me, the pleasure to be got from cooking, from food – in the shop, on the chopping board, on the plate or in the pan – is aesthetic. I think it's that I find food beautiful, intensely so.

Not that I need to be tackling hideously complicated recipes. I feel just as caught up with the domestic spirit when I'm making a very basic stew. I love the reminder that good food is simple food. It's as if there's a sort of alchemy about a stew: what do you put in it? Onions, carrots, meat, wine or beer, stock or water. And you don't even do anything to it: it just cooks, slowly, and turns, untouched, into something restorative, comforting, toothsome and wonderful.

STEWS

I love oxtail, but at the moment this is an illicit desire, since at the time of writing beef on the bone is an illegal substance. It's in a spirit of optimism, then, that I give you a recipe.

Oxtail has to be cooked at least a day ahead because you'll need to let the stew get cold so that you can degrease it properly. To tell the truth, I'm happy with the fat left in: I love the artery-thickening deep and unctuous sauce it provides. But oxtail always makes for a good gravy, always gratifyingly thickens the liquid in which it cooks. What I don't like is oxtail which has been boned, chopped, piled into darioles or ramekins and then unmoulded artistically on the plate, surrounded by its sauce-soused vegetables. In a restaurant, that's fine. In the home, I like food to be less messed around with. Sprinkling with parsley is one thing, sculpture is quite another. My grandfather – and mother after him – used to speak disparagingly about landscape cookery.

I have a rather wonderful book, published by W.H. Allen in 1960 at the cost of 25 shillings, that I picked up in a second-hand bookshop. It is Rupert Croft-Cooke's deliciously camp, charmingly authoritative *English Cooking, a New Approach*, dedicated to Noël Coward who, one hopes, appreciated it. Regarding oxtail, Mr Croft-Cooke advises, 'if you like producing meat moulds with subtle decorations, an oxtail is a splendid thing to work on for the stock from it will set hard and firm. You boil till you can remove the meat from the bones and putting this aside with fresh seasoning, herbs and spices, you boil the bones for another hour or two then mix the stock and meat and pour into a mould. It looks', he concludes devastatingly, 'what cook used to call "a picture".'

Oxtail can be cooked in any beer or wine. I love to use Mackeson, which is sweeter than Guinness and has a creamy roundness that suits the fatly honeyed flesh from the oxtails, or Sam Smith's Imperial Stout, which isn't as sweet as Mackeson but has a smoky licoriceness. Of course you can use red wine if you prefer, in which case just substitute it for the beer, below.

OXTAIL WITH MACKESON AND MARJORAM

I would buy oxtail only from a butcher, and what's more, a butcher I knew and trusted, in which case you can get him to joint it for you. What you want are rounds of oxtail that are nice and chunky (not little and scrawny, though these you can profitably use for soup) and as near to the same size as is possible. As for the stock: if you can, use any home-made you may have stowed away in the freezer or else use a tub of Joubère beef stock (see page 506); otherwise, to be frank, you could use water.

65g fat or oil
4 onions, sliced finely
2 cloves garlic, chopped finely
1 teaspoon dried marjoram
65g plain flour
1 teaspoon mustard powder
small bunch flat-leaf parsley
½ teaspoon powdered mace
½ teaspoon ground cloves
2½kg oxtail, jointed
2 celery sticks, whole
1 400g tin plum tomatoes
4 carrots, cut into slim batons about 4cm long
2 bay leaves
400ml Mackeson (see above)
300ml beef stock or water
flat-leaf parsley for serving

Preheat the oven to gas mark 2/150°C.

Melt half the fat in a large casserole (I use a big cast-iron rectangular one measuring 37cm by 25cm, which goes across 2 burners on the hob and in the oven) and fry the onions over a gentle heat until they are translucent (not brown), which will take about 15 minutes. About 2–3 minutes before you think they're done, add the garlic, marjoram and 1 tablespoon chopped parsley. Remove to a plate.

Spread the flour out on a large plate or, better still, a chopping board and mix in the mustard powder, ground mace and cloves and some salt and pepper. Dredge the oxtail in this, melt the remaining fat in the casserole and brown the meat well on both sides. Top with the already softened, garlicky and marjoram-flecked onions, then pile on the carrots, the tinned tomatoes (not their juice, but don't throw it away, you may need it later), the celery sticks and the bay leaves. Pour over the stout and stock or water and

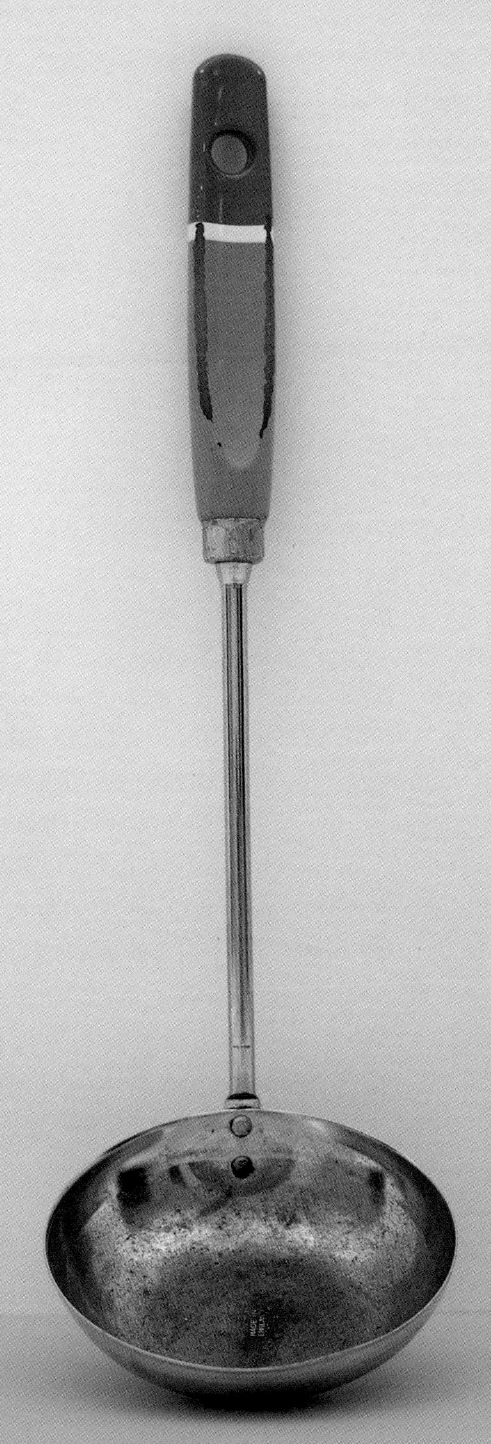

bring to the boil. If the liquid looks too sparse – you want to have a decent amount covering the oxtail – throw in the juice from the tinned tomatoes. Put the lid on the casserole and transfer to the oven.

Cook for 3–4 hours, or until unctuous and tender. Remove the celery sticks and cool before putting in the fridge. The next day, remove the fat that has risen to the surface. And when you want to eat it, taste for seasoning (you may well need to add a pinch or so of salt) and then reheat, either on a gentle flame on the hob for about 1 hour or at gas mark 4/180°C for about 3/4 hour. Before serving, sprinkle with flat-leaf parsley. And I think the parsley necessary, not a poncy optional extra: without the bright, jewel-vivid flecks of green the meat can look rather sludgy. This final touch somehow brings it to life, seems to give it the gloss of a seventeenth-century Dutch painting.

Mashed potato is traditional with oxtail stew, and I wouldn't offer a dissenting voice. But rice (I like basmati) works as well.

The rediscovery of British cooking over the past few years has tended to overlook the Welsh contribution. Part of this is perhaps due to the fact that if you're not Welsh, your experience of Welsh food will probably have been in pubs or restaurants. In other words, you'll have eaten badly – and probably little that is specifically Welsh. I felt much the same way in Spain. After a week of eating indifferent food in public places, I had to be stopped from ringing the doorbells of private houses and begging, pleading, to be allowed to go in for supper and to eat some real Spanish food cooked at home.

Good peasant cooking needs a rural society, and it is true that Wales is not quite that any more. Good bourgeois cooking needs a large and successful middle class, and Wales doesn't seem to have that either. But I feel affectionately drawn towards Welsh food. I first had cawl (pronounced 'cowl') when I was staying with my sister Thomasina, who lived in Wales. Her neighbour, Dai, would make it and bring pots of it over.

There is no one set of rules for making cawl any more than there is for pot au feu, or any of those other soupy stews – cockaleekie, Scotch broth, Irish stew – which change from region to region, from household to household. Cawl just means stew, and it is made with beef just as often as with lamb. That's in theory: in practice it has always been lamb, as is the one that follows.

CAWL

Obviously the quantities are variable, but the amounts given will be enough for about 6 people. It's not necessary to finish it all at one sitting. Traditionally in Wales cawl was always eaten over a couple of days: the broth and vegetables on the first day, the meat the next; both with a great deal of bread and butter. Now people eat it all together, but it is still important to have lots of bread and butter.

750g scrag end or middle neck of lamb or best end of neck chops
2 large onions
6 medium or 3 large potatoes
2 parsnips
1 swede
3 large carrots
2 leeks
parsley

Put the lamb in a large saucepan and fill with cold water to cover. Bring to the boil, add salt, and then cook gently for about 1 1/2 hours. Remove from the heat, let it get cold and leave somewhere cool overnight.

The next day, or when you want to eat, skim the fat off. Put it back on the heat, bring it back to the boil and then throw in the onions, sliced, and the potatoes, parsnips, swede and carrots, cut into chunks. Cook for about 1/2 hour, or until the vegetables are nearly tender. I would test the carrots, since they seem to take the longest, but check the potatoes, too; obviously the relative size of the vegetables will determine how long they take to cook, so use your initiative. About 10 minutes before you think everything's ready, add the leeks, sliced. Sprinkle some freshly chopped parsley on top when you serve the cawl.

Giving actual recipes for stews always sounds inappropriately bossy. All you ever need to do is fry some onions and carrots, brown (or not) the meat and add seasoning, wine or other liquid and that's it. Once you get in the habit of making stews you won't even think of measuring this or weighing that. You'll be comfortable building around what you've got in the kitchen, accommodating the odd bottle of wine left without a cork or half-empty can of anchovies. But even so, a recipe can be a prompt to action, a reminder of possibilities.

One of the advantages of cooking lamb stews in advance is that you can use shoulder rather than leg and just remove the fat when it's cold. I love the oozy, sticky juice you get from shoulder, and the extra fat keeps the meat tender.

GREEK LAMB STEW

Meats such as lamb and venison you'd presume would be best stewed with red wine. I love them cooked with white. When you cook this Greek lamb stew please don't do what I did and use retsina. It wasn't a good idea. Joubère make a good lamb stock (see page 506) but water is fine, and you can always ask the butcher for the shoulder-bone, chopped, and throw it in while the stew's cooking. Obviously, since the stew has pasta in it, it can't be cooked entirely in advance. But just add the pasta when you reheat. What is so useful about this stew is that you certainly don't need vegetables. Just make a salad to serve after.

The addition, when you eat, of crumbled feta and oregano (or basil if you like) may not be exactly authentic, but it tastes wonderful.

4 tablespoons olive oil
2½kg boned shoulder of lamb, trimmed of excess fat and cut into cubes about 6cm x 3cm
750g onions, sliced finely
4 cloves garlic, minced
2 stalks celery, chopped finely
leaves from 4 sprigs thyme
1 teaspoon dried oregano
3 bay leaves
2 carrots, cut in half lengthways and then half across
3 400g tins chopped tomatoes
300ml lamb stock or water
1 bottle dry white wine
500g pasta – ditalini or macaroni
300g feta
parsley, oregano or basil

Preheat the oven to gas mark 3/160°C.

Into the largest pan or casserole you have that will go in the oven pour about 3 tablespoons of oil. Brown the meat in batches over high heat and remove with a slotted spoon to a plate nearby. You may need to add more oil as you do this. The onions certainly need it, so pour in more, add the onions, sprinkling a little salt over them, and cook them until soft and translucent. Add the garlic, celery, thyme and oregano: these should be fairly well minced, and the easiest way to do this is just to bung them all in the processor. After a couple of minutes or so, when the smell of garlic wafts up, remove half the mixture. Then add the meat to the layer of onions and garlic mixture in the pan, cover with the remaining half, add the bay leaves, carrots, tins of tomatoes, stock and wine. I use a big but flattish casserole and this amount of liquid covers the meat, but if you find you need more liquid just top up with water: you want a lot of liquid, because you will, eventually, be cooking some pasta in it. Bring to the boil, remove scum, and let bubble for about 3 minutes and then cover, transfer to the oven and cook for about 2–2½ hours, or cook on a very low heat on the hob. The meat should be tender and yielding. Remove the carrots (and eat, cook's treat) and bay leaves, too, if you want, and season to taste.

Of course you can proceed to the final stage now, but I am presuming you're not going to. In which case, let the stew cool and keep it in the fridge until you want it. Skim the fat off the top, and do remember to take it out of the fridge a good 1–2 hours before you cook it again. You can reheat this in the oven, but since you will be putting the pasta in on the hob, I tend to start off there, too. Make sure the stew is piping hot before you add the almost-cooked pasta. Put on a large pan of water. When it boils, add salt and then the pasta. Cook this till it's nearly but not quite cooked: it should have a couple of minutes still to go.

Then drain the pasta and add quickly to the bubbling juices in the casserole, making sure first that there are enough bubbling juices. You don't want the meat to be drowned, but you want enough for the pasta to be covered. The pasta will absorb some of the liquid as it finishes cooking, of course. If you don't have a pan that will accommodate all the meat and all the pasta and is heat-proof, then you will just have to cook the pasta completely separately and find some other cavernous vessel (remember to warm it first, even if it's just by filling it with some hot water in the sink) and mix the lot together in that. You'll lose something, I know: the pasta won't suck in any of the sweet, tomatoey, winey juices, but it won't be the end of the world.

In a couple of minutes the pasta should be cooked. Crumble some feta and put in a bowl with some finely chopped oregano, parsley or basil. Stir to combine and then leave the spoon with it, so that people can sprinkle the herb-spiked cheese over as they wish. Ladle the stew into shallow soup bowls. This should be plenty for about 10.

One of the advantages of the following stew – apart from its honeyed and luscious taste – is that it can be done seriously in advance: that's to say, you can leave the venison in its marinade for 2–3 days in the fridge and then put the cooked casserole back in the fridge when it's cold, where it can stay for another 2–3 days.

I don't necessarily scale down the quantities if I'm cooking for rather fewer people (these quantities are enough for about 8) since the oniony juices, with or without the leftover meat, make the most fabulous pasta sauce the next day.

VENISON IN WHITE WINE

for the marinade
1 bottle dry white wine
2 tablespoons olive oil
2 bay leaves
2 carrots
1 large onion
2 sticks celery
2 garlic cloves, squashed with flat of knife
10 juniper berries, crushed slightly
10 black peppercorns, crushed slightly

for the rest of the stew
1½kg venison, cut into chunks about 3cm x 6cm
20g dried porcini
100g unsalted butter or goose or duck fat
1kg onions
drop olive oil
1 tablespoon sugar
3 sage leaves
½ teaspoon ground cinnamon
½ teaspoon ground cloves
½ a nutmeg, grated
300ml beef or game stock
3 tablespoons flour
300g mushrooms, preferably brown cap or chestnut mushrooms
chopped parsley

Put the venison into a bowl and cover with the marinade ingredients. Give a good stir and cover with clingfilm and leave overnight somewhere cool. If the weather's warm (though you are unlikely to be wanting to eat this in summer) or you just want to stow this away for a few days, then put it to marinate in the fridge, but make sure you take it out and get it back to room temperature before you want to cook it.

When you do, preheat the oven to gas mark 2/150°C and, at the same time, cover the porcini with hot water. Then put 75g of the butter and a drop of oil in a large casserole and when it's melted add the onions, very finely sliced (I use the processor), and cook for about 10–15 minutes or until the onions are soft and translucent. Strain the dried mushrooms, reserving the water, and then chop them very small. Add these to the onion and give a good stir. Cook gently for another minute or so, stir again, then sprinkle with the sugar. Turn up the heat and caramelise slightly and then add the spices and sage. Tear a piece of kitchen foil about the same measurements as the casserole and place it just above the onions. Turn the heat to low – you may need to use a heat diffuser – and cook for 30–40 minutes, lifting up the foil every now and again to give a gentle prod and stir. You want a brown, sweet mess under there.

Pour the venison into a colander or sieve placed over a pan. Then pick out the marinade ingredients or meat (whichever is easier). Remove half the onions and cover the half still in the pan with the venison. Season with salt and pepper, sprinkle with the flour, and cover with the rest of the onions. Heat up the marinade liquid in its pan, add the stock and reserved, strained mushroom-soaking liquid, and pour over the venison. If the meat isn't covered you can add some more wine (though heat it up first) or stock (ditto). Put in the preheated oven, and cook for about 2½ hours or until very tender indeed.

You can now let this cool and keep it in the fridge for 2–3 days. Forty minutes at gas mark 4/180°C, or on the hob, should be enough to reheat it, but do remember it should be brought back to room temperature first. About 15 minutes before the stew is hot again, wipe the mushrooms, cut them into quarters, melt the remaining 25g butter in a small frying pan and cook the mushrooms in it, sprinkling with salt and pepper. After about 5 minutes, add them to the stew in the oven. Leave it there to cook for another 10 minutes.

Sprinkle the stew with parsley when you serve it. I always have this with mashed potato and I like sliced green beans with it, too.

Cooking chicken in white wine is hardly revolutionary, but then the point of cooking is not to surprise but, gratifyingly, to satisfy. Chicken doesn't benefit from sitting around in its cooking juices for as long as meat does – you want the meat to be tender rather than sodden – but a day or two definitely helps with brown meat.

CHICKEN AND CHICK PEA TAGINE

I have done this stew with dried, soaked and cooked chick peas and with canned, and it is, I have to tell you, better with dried. I cook them till more or less tender first. If you want to substitute tinned ones, add 2 or 3 cans of them, drained, on reheating.

You can choose whether or not you want to keep the skin on your chicken thighs, but make certain they have not been boned.

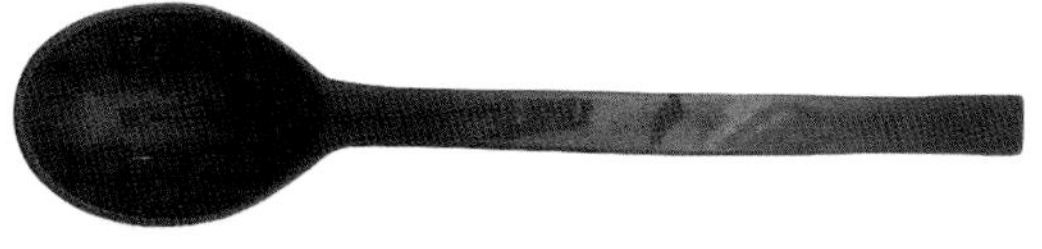

175g dried chick peas
1 large onion
5 cloves garlic
1 stick celery
3 tablespoons olive oil
10 chicken thighs
2 carrots, cut into small batons
1 tablespoon flour, preferably 00
½ teaspoon ground cinnamon
1 teaspoon each ground cumin and turmeric
400ml white wine
300ml light chicken stock
fresh coriander to serve

Soak and cook the chick peas, following instructions on page 88 but removing them from the pot slightly before they're soft. Drain and reserve.

Put the onion, garlic and celery in the processor and blitz till chopped. Put the oil in a casserole or tagine on the hob and, when hot, brown the chicken thighs; remove to a plate. Now add the onion mixture to the casserole and cook till soft – about 5 minutes – then add the carrots and cook for another 5 minutes. Mix the flour with the spices and stir in, cooking for a couple of minutes. Put the chicken pieces back in, add the chick peas and pour over the wine and stock. Season and cook on a low heat, covered, for about 1 hour. Let cool and then stick in the fridge for up to 3 days.

I love eating this with fresh chopped coriander on top. And a pile of pine-nut-sprinkled couscous to the side.

Serves 4–5.

This next stew resolutely uses red wine, and makes the most of it, too. I think it is a waste, almost, if you don't cook it in advance as the anchovies seem to get mellower after a day or two's soaking. It's delicious straight off, too, but you get its full, deep-bellied roundness when it's given time to rest and wallow between cooking and reheating. I don't think you should necessarily tell people about the anchovies. In my experience, many people who claim not to be able to stomach them love this stew.

BEEF STEW WITH ANCHOVIES AND THYME

I love this with mashed or baked potatoes (with sour cream) and some cold-sour fat gerkins, sliced, or little cornichons just as they are. I sometimes make (and see Weekend Lunch page 294) a horseradish-fromage-frais raita sauce to go with it, too. It doesn't need anything to spruce it up in itself, but stews are useful in this way: what you do to them, with them, when you eat, entirely changes the mood of the meal. You could just as easily use lamb here, by the way.

3–5 tablespoons olive oil or good beef dripping
1½kg stewing beef, preferably shin, cut into about chunky strips approx. 6 x 3cm
1 large onion, halved then finely sliced
3 cloves garlic, minced or finely chopped
3 medium carrots, cut into batons the size of fat matchsticks
4 inner stalks celery, finely sliced
2 teaspoons dried thyme or 1½ tablespoons fresh thyme leaves
6 anchovy fillets (or half a tin), well drained and chopped up or minced fine
2 heaped tablespoons flour
3 tablespoons Marsala
500ml robust red wine
300ml beef stock
1 tablespoon tomato purée
½ teaspoon mace

Preheat the oven to gas mark 2/150°C. Put the casserole in which you will cook the stew on the hob with 3 tablespoons of the oil or beef dripping. Heat and then brown the meat briskly in batches; if you overcrowd the casserole the meat will steam rather than sear. Remove the meat to a plate and then, first adding more oil or dripping if necessary, toss in the vegetables, anchovies and thyme. Cook, turning frequently, on medium heat for about 10 minutes or until the mixture is beginning to soften. While this is going on, heat the Marsala, wine and stock in a saucepan and remove when it reaches boiling point.

Return the beef to the pan and then stir in the flour. After a couple of minutes or so, pour in the wine–stock mixture and stir well, then stir in the tomato purée and then the mace and some pepper. Taste to see if you want to add salt.

Put on a lid and then cook in the preheated oven for 3 hours. Remove, cool and then keep in the fridge until needed. I tend to reheat in the casserole on the hob.

Serves 6–8.

I love game birds roasted; I like them plain, with bread sauce, a port-fortified gravy perhaps, some salty bacon fried to a bronzy puce, with English mustard and nutty fried breadcrumbs. But a girl's got to have a casserole under her belt, too, if only because game birds tend quite often to be beyond roasting. This way of casseroling pheasant is a recipe – unfancy, reliable and just what you need – of the estimable Anne Willan's (from *Real Food: Fifty Years of Good Eating*) and is great with birds that have dwindled into toughness.

Ask the butcher to cut up the pheasants for you, and you can get the bacon or pancetta from him at the same time. I like using half veal and half chicken stock (I tend to buy in my veal stock), but if I've got some game stock in the freezer I'll use that. You will have lots of little bits of bird here, so each portion will be very small of course: you should get enough for about 8 people out of 3 birds. If you want, substitute guinea fowl for the pheasant and white wine for the red.

BRAISED PHEASANT WITH MUSHROOMS AND BACON

1 tablespoon vegetable oil
2 tablespoons butter
3 pheasants, weighing about 1kg each, cut into 6 pieces each
375g mushrooms, quartered
20–24 baby onions, peeled
250g piece unsmoked streaky bacon (or pancetta), cut into lardons
30g flour
600ml red wine
600ml veal or chicken stock, or more if needed
2 cloves garlic, crushed
bouquet garni

Heat the oil and butter in a casserole and brown the pheasant pieces, a few at a time. Take them out, add the mushrooms and cook until tender: about 5 minutes. Remove them with a slotted spoon, add the onions and cook until brown, shaking the casserole so that they colour evenly. Remove the onions, add the bacon and brown it too.

Discard all but 2 tablespoons fat, stir the flour into the bacon and cook gently, stirring until brown. Stir in the wine, bring to the boil and simmer for 5 minutes. Add the stock, garlic, bouquet garni, salt and pepper, and replace mushrooms, onion and the pheasant pieces. Cover the casserole and simmer on top of the stove, or cook in a gas mark 4/180°C oven until the meat is very tender when pierced with a two-pronged fork. Cooking time varies from 1 to 2 hours depending on the age of the pheasants. Stir from time to time, especially if cooking on top of the stove, and add more stock if the meat begins to stick. Wing and breast pieces may cook before the legs; if so, take them out first.

Discard the bouquet garni and taste the sauce for seasoning. Now, you can let the casserole cool, then put it in the fridge and take it out when you need it, up to 3 days later. Reheat it on top of the stove or in a gas mark 4/180°C oven for about 30 minutes.

BURGHAL

Instead of the usual mashed potato, this stew – and indeed any of them – is wonderful with burghal, or cracked wheat, bulgar wheat, however you like to call it. This has the advantage of being quicker and much less laborious to make, too; you can get on with it while you reheat the stew.

Try and think in terms of volume rather than weight (the same is true for rice and couscous): for 8 people, you need 4 American cupfuls (or up to the litre mark on a measuring jug) of burghal and 4 cups of water. Melt 3 tablespoons of butter in a heavy-based saucepan (which has a lid that fits) and stir in the burghal till all coated. Then add the water, bring to the boil, add a good pinch of salt, cover, and turn down the heat to absolute minimum. For preference use a heat-diffuser. Cook for about 30 minutes or until all the water is absorbed and the burghal is cooked but not soft; it should still be nutty in texture. You can leave the burghal, when it's cooked, with the lid on but the pan off the heat, for 10 minutes or so without harm.

VEGETABLES

One could go on for ever with stews, braises, casseroles: the permutations are enormous, and I can't think of one that couldn't be cooked in advance. Vegetables are a different matter. Few vegetables take long to cook, and now you can get most ready-trimmed, chopped, and utterly prepared for you at the main supermarkets. I make three exceptions: ratatouille, aubergine moussaka and petits pois à la française. Of course there are other vegetable braises which you could add to this list – broad beans with bacon, certainly, stewed artichokes – but most vegetable dishes that can be left sitting around to be reheated later are variations (technically, at any rate) on this theme.

I know some would argue that you *can't* cook and then reheat ratatouille, that it will go mushy and lose its vibrant, just-cooked freshness. But I like it softened slightly in the pan, the flavours still discrete but mingling into one another, everything sweet and soused. But perhaps that's because my mother always had a bowl of ratatouille on the go in the fridge: I remember it beginning to go soggy in its garlicky syrup.

RATATOUILLE

I couldn't remember exactly how my mother made ratatouille and didn't know if I used 2 courgettes or 3, or how many minutes I fried them. Pinpoint accuracy disappears with recipes you do often, but somehow I felt even more at a loss in transcribing this one from memory. And so, working on the principle that my mother would have consulted her, I turned to Elizabeth David. I'm not sure what follows is something Mrs David would be pleased with, if only because I have ignored something she is very firm about indeed: I never bother with salting and draining aubergines, and am not now going to start degorging courgettes, either. Missing out this stage hasn't resulted in a hopelessly soggy mess, otherwise I'm sure we, *mère et fille*, would have done as we were told in the first place. But if you feel it's important, then by all means cut the aubergines and courgettes into unpeeled quarter-inch thick rounds, sprinkle with salt and put in a colander with a plate on top of them, a weight on top of the plate, and leave all that in place for an hour or so, then rinse the vegetables and wipe them dry with kitchen paper.

I have also boosted the number of courgettes in Elizabeth David's recipe and decreased the amount of aubergine, simply because I like courgettes more than I like aubergines. She suggests 2 coffeecups of olive oil, which I reckon is about 10 tablespoons.

2 medium onions

2 cloves garlic

1 aubergine

5 smallish courgettes

3 large sweet red peppers

4 large, flavoursome tomatoes (or 1 400g tin drained tinned plum tomatoes)

6–10 tablespoons olive oil

1 generous teaspoon coriander seed, pounded, or ½–1 teaspoon ground coriander

fresh basil or fresh parsley

Slice the onions (I peel them, cut them in half and then cut each half into thin, half-moon slices), mince the garlic – and for this I use my mezzaluna to chop it very very finely – and cut the aubergines into thin half-moons and courgettes into ½cm rounds. Cut the peppers in half, remove the cores and seeds, wipe them, and then cut into thin, but not straggly, strips or chunks as you like. Skin the tomatoes: plunge them into boiled water for a few minutes and slip the skins off. Then halve them, scoop out the seeds and cut each hollowed ½ into 2 crossways. Or if you're using tinned, just drain, squeeze the seeds out of the tomatoes or scissor them over a sieve.

The vegetables in a ratatouille are cooked in this order – onions first, then aubergines, courgettes, garlic and peppers, and lastly tomatoes. You can either prepare all the vegetables before you start, or one at a time, chucking them into the pan in the right order.

Heat 6 tablespoons olive oil in a thick-bottomed wide pan: a round Le Creuset casserole is good here, or I use my deep Calphalon frying pan, as, even though it isn't heavy-bottomed, it doesn't stick on a low heat. Earthenware dishes look authentic – the perfect Sunday supplement picture – but they do tend to stick.

Put the onions into this pan, whichever one you're using, and cook until they're soft but not brown. Then add the aubergines, cook for a minute or so, then the courgettes, stirring them into the oil for a few minutes. Carry on like this with the peppers and garlic. If you feel you need more oil, pour it in.

Cover the pan and cook gently for 40 minutes. Make sure, though, that it *is* gently. You don't want the bottom burning and the top steaming. Now add the tomatoes, coriander and season. Cook for another 30–40 minutes until all the vegetables are soft but not mushy. Stir in the basil or parsley and eat hot or cold. I think that cold it is rather good with chopped fresh coriander, too. And it's excellent as a side dish, served tepid, with cold roast chicken or pork, or hot roast lamb. It keeps in the fridge for 5 days, but remember to take it out of the fridge well before you eat it.

AUBERGINE MOUSSAKA

Turning back to Elizabeth David reminded me of the smoky, satiny wonderfulness of aubergine stews.

This is a Lebanese recipe, very different from the traditional Greek one of the same name. Boldly, strongly flavoured, but mellow, the spices and seasoning dovetail into a perfect, aromatic whole. The recipe is adapted from a wonderful book of Lebanese home-cooking by Nada Saleh, called evocatively enough, *Fragrance of the Earth*. The pomegranate molasses (or syrup) stipulated here is found in Middle-Eastern stores, or look at the list of mail order suppliers on page 506. If you can go to a Middle-Eastern shop, though, you will be able to get the baby aubergines at the same time. Otherwise use large ones, cut into 1¼cm cubes.

500g baby aubergines
5 tablespoons olive oil
1–2 onions (about 250g), peeled and sliced thinly
10–12 small cloves garlic, peeled and left whole or slivered thickly
150g chick peas, soaked, rinsed, drained and precooked (see page 88)
1½ tablespoons pomegranate molasses (optional)
500g tomatoes, rinsed, peeled, seeded and quartered
1½ teaspoons salt or to taste
½ teaspoon cinnamon
½ teaspoon allspice
¼ teaspoon freshly milled black pepper
200ml water
parsley or coriander or mint

Trim the stems of the aubergines. Peel to look like Edwardian circus tents, leaving lengthways stripes about 1¼cm wide. In a pan heat 3 tablespoons oil over medium heat and sauté the aubergines for a few minutes or until golden brown. With a slotted spoon, remove to a side dish covered with kitchen paper and reserve. To the pan add the remaining oil, the onions and the garlic and sauté, stirring constantly, until pale in colour and soft, about 5 minutes, adding more oil if necessary. Add the chick peas and stir occasionally for 5 minutes, then add the pomegranate molasses, if used. Return the reserved aubergines to the pan and add the tomatoes, sprinkle with the salt, cinnamon, allspice and black pepper and add the water, bring to the boil and quickly reduce the heat to moderately low. Cover and simmer for about an hour. If you're using a large shallow pan, you may find they are ready after 45 minutes.

Serve warm or cold, but either way thickly sprinkled with chopped parsley or leafy fresh coriander, even if Nada Saleh issues no such command. Mint works well, too. Eat with lots of bread. It keeps in the fridge easily for 3–5 days.

Cooking this sort of thing in advance enables you to make more of it later. You could cook this moussaka at the weekend and stash it away for a quick mid-week supper by pairing it with some noisettes of lamb, cooked for a few minutes on each side. For vegetarians, sprinkle when reheating with feta cheese.

These dishes can be meals in themselves or served as a vegetable accompaniment alongside meat. But if you want to do an all-purpose vegetable accompaniment to meat or fish, plain or fancy, petits pois à la française are useful. Everyone loves peas cooked like this, fragrant with the lettuce and syrupy with the butter.

PETITS POIS À LA FRANÇAISE

For the lettuce, I use either a little gem or part of a cos if I'm shopping specially for it, but otherwise I'm happy to make do with whatever I've got to hand. I use fresh peas when I'm in the mood to pod them and when they're available; otherwise I use a packet of frozen petits pois. Don't bother to buy fresh peas ready podded: there's no advantage here over frozen. If you are using frozen peas, you won't have to cook them for so long. I tend to thaw them first and cook them for about 10 minutes. I like using chicken stock in place of the water, but this is not classical.

3 tablespoons butter
1½kg peas, weighed in the pod, or 500g petits pois frozen
1 small lettuce or 8–10 leaves of a larger lettuce, shredded roughly
6 spring onions, chopped
1 teaspoon sugar

Melt the butter in a pan and stir in the peas, lettuce and spring onions. Let everything become glossy and buttery and then add 50ml boiling water, salt, pepper and the sugar; remember that the liquid will boil down, so the seasoning will taste more acute in the finished dish. You can always add more salt or sugar later, anyway. And you may need to add more water if you're using fresh peas. Put a lid on the pan and stew gently for about 20 minutes. The peas should be tender and the juices scarce but thick. Taste for seasoning. Let cool, put in the fridge – for a couple of days at most – and reheat on the hob when you want to eat them. You may need to add a little butter and water when you reheat.

When serving, I like sometimes to strike an unorthodox anglo note by sprinkling them with some freshly chopped mint. Basil is wonderful, too: to me it always smells of summer. Chopped flat-leaf parsley is always good.

The next recipe isn't exactly a vegetable course, but it is such a perfect example of the cooking in advance principle, that I don't want to leave it out. Actually, you can eat it as a vegetable, but it has wider uses and applications, as you'll see.

ONION MUSH

This may not be a very attractive sounding name for anything, but what it aims to describe is wonderful, a kind of savoury honey. Indeed, this sort of thing often goes, in restaurants, by the name of onion jam. What it is, simply, is onion cooked slowly and at a very low heat till it turns golden and soft, a mellow, caramelised gloop to be stirred into anything when you want depth and flavour. It does take a long time to make (but if you've got a food processor requires hardly any effort to prepare) but you need to do pretty well nothing while it's cooking: the odd peek, the odd prod. I make up a lot of this, then freeze it in weight-labelled bags, to be brought out when needed. You need to bear in mind that one 100g onion cooks down to 50g of this mush, so you can just freeze it in 50g packets and use each in place of an onion whenever a recipe stipulates one. In practice, I like this so much I use much more than any recipe calls for;

500g minced meat, cooked with even 150g of this, is out-of-this-world wonderful: sweet, creamy, deep-toned and softly hearty. And I love it plain, too, on sandwiches, with steak, with anything. It's OK for 2 weeks in the fridge, or I find it so, but it does make life easier to make a lot and then freeze it in those small, recommended portions.

1kg onions
1 heaped tablespoon lard or butter and 3 tablespoons olive oil, or 4–5 tablespoons olive oil
100ml Marsala

Peel the onions and slice them very, very thin, preferably with the food processor. Put a very large, heavy-based frying pan on a low heat, using a heat-diffuser if you've got one. You may need a couple of pans. Put in the lard or butter and oil and when it starts melting and warming up, but before any heat emanates or any sizzles can be heard, add the onions, press down with a wooden spoon, then sprinkle some salt over. Pour the Marsala into a measuring jug, then make up to the 175g mark with boiling water from the kettle and pour over the onions. Cut out some tin foil and press it down over the onions, shiny side down, to form a tight, low, lid. Then put on the pan's real lid and cook, very low, for a good 2 hours. Check after an hour: it shouldn't be hot enough for any burning or sticking. If using a heat-diffuser and a sound thick-bottomed pan, you may want to give it a third hour. When the onion tastes completely cooked, very soft, take the lid and foil off and turn the heat up high to let all liquid bubble and burn off. When it's reduced and evaporated, you should have a soft, thick, caramel-coloured mush. That's it.

PUDDINGS

It is perfectly honourable to buy a tart from a pâtisserie. But I have discovered that I love making puddings provided I can do them in advance. What I hate is having to get up from the dinner table to start fiddling with a pudding just as the evening is getting underway and I'm beginning to relax. Anyway, most of the sweet things I like need to be made a good day or so before they're eaten.

Any trifle needs a day to sit in the fridge or a cool place, everything melding, setting, the component parts becoming this one glorious whole: here are three such.

RHUBARB, MUSCAT AND MASCARPONE TRIFLE

I first made this, like so many good things, by accident. I'd cooked some rhubarb and had some juice left over and turned it into jelly (and see page 345). I then thought that the jelly itself would be mysterious and wonderful as part of a toned-down, but at the same time expanded, trifle. I had some mascarpone in the fridge, so used that in place of the custard and cream of an English trifle. The result is more of a dinner party trifle, but not affectedly so.

If you've got a suitable glass bowl or dish, use that, as the colours are ravishing: the dusty-rose pink of the rhubarb, the soft green of the pistachios, the soft squish of cream between. I find that the proportions are best if you use a relatively wide and shallow dish, but if a bowl-shaped bowl is all you've got then just prepare for deeper layers. It's best when you use forced, pink rhubarb, but I make it just as often with the coarser greener stuff. And as for the pistachios, you can buy them ready-ground in Middle-Eastern stores and keep a stash in a jar with a lid in the fridge; 2 or 3 tablespoons sprinkled over the top should be fine.

The first time I put this together, I made my own cake for the base, but I've since moved on to bought trifle sponges. Feel free to do the same, although I'll give the recipe for the homemade version just in case.

for the sponge
butter and flour for greasing and lining pan
2 eggs, separated
60g caster sugar
50g plain flour, preferably Italian 00

Preheat the oven to gas mark 4/180°C. Butter a small (500g or with a liquid capacity of 500ml) loaf-tin well, then dust with flour, tapping to shake off excess.

Whisk the egg yolks with the sugar (preferably with an electric mixer) until pale and thick and creamy. It should have the texture of extraordinarily aerated mayonnaise. Add a pinch of salt to the flour and then sift it (sift it twice if you're using ordinary plain flour) holding the sieve high above a bowl, so you get maximum lightness later.

Whisk the egg whites with another pinch of salt until stiff, then add a dollop to the egg-yolk–sugar mixture and sprinkle over a couple of tablespoons of flour. Fold in with a metal spoon. Then carry on, gradually and with a gossamer-touch, using up all the egg whites and all the flour until you have a creamily combined mixture.

Pour the cake batter into the prepared tin and bake for half an hour or until the surface is springy and the sides have shrunk a little away from the tin. Gently unmould onto a rack and leave to cool. Slice and proceed as directed below. You can of course make this even further in advance and either freeze it, wrapped tightly, or keep it in the fridge for a day or so.

for the rest of the trifle
1kg rhubarb, trimmed and cut into 3cm slices
325g sugar
the juice of 2 blood oranges (or failing that, 1 large ordinary orange)
approx. 300ml muscat
6 leaves gelatine
325g mascarpone
2 egg yolks
1 egg white
90g caster sugar
50g peeled pistachios (about 100g in the shell), chopped very fine

Preheat the oven to gas mark 5/190°C. Put the rhubarb into an ovenproof dish, squeeze over the orange juice and spoon over the sugar and then either put the lid on or cover tightly with foil. Cook in the oven for an hour – opening oven and lifting up lid to give a good, sugar-dissolving stir after 30 minutes – until the rhubarb's soft and floating in a pool of pink liquid. Remove from oven and let cool a little before straining into a measuring jug. Reserve the rhubarb pulp for the time being. You should have around 700ml. Add 200ml muscat – or however much you need – to take it up to the 900ml mark. Meanwhile, soak the gelatine leaves (you need 1 leaf per 150ml of liquid) in cold water till soft. Heat 250ml of the rhubarby liquid in a saucepan until boiling point, then remove from heat. Squeeze out the gelatine leaves and whisk them into the hot liquid. Then pour that hot liquid into the rest of the juice, and taste to see if you want more sugar or, to sharpen, a squeeze of lemon. Leave to cool.

Now get your dish: I find this amount does enough for an oblong shallow container measuring 30 x 20 x 5cm which would feed 12–14 people, though I'd use the same quantities for 8 and up; for 6–8, I do half-measurements and use a bowl 20cm diameter and with a capacity of about 1¼ litres.

Cut the sponge cake very thin and line the bottom of the dish with the slices, or use bought trifle sponges split horizontally. Next spread over the rhubarb pulp; but if it is very green and stringy then leave this stage out. Now, pour over the jelly and put in the fridge to set for 6 hours or so: poke and see, but I am happy to do this over a few days; indeed I prefer it.

To make the cream to go on top, whisk the egg yolks with the sugar and when pale and moussy (though it doesn't have to be quite as moussy as for the sponge, above) mix it into the mascarpone. When all's combined, whisk the egg white till stiff and then fold it into the egg–sugar–mascarpone mixture. Spoon over the jellied sponge and put back in the fridge for 12–24 hours. An hour or so before you want to eat this take it out of the fridge and before serving sprinkle with the ground or chopped pistachios.

PROPER ENGLISH TRIFLE

When I say proper I mean proper: lots of sponge, lots of jam, lots of custard and lots of cream. This is not a timid construction, nor should it be. Of course, the ingredients must be good, but you don't want to end up with a trifle so upmarket it's inappropriately, posturingly elegant. A degree of vulgarity is requisite.

I soak the sponge in orange-flavoured alcohol (I loathe the acrid dustiness of standard-issue sherry), infuse the custard with orange, and make an orange caramel to sprinkle over the top; this seems to bring out the fruity, egginess of it all, even if you are reduced to using frozen fruit. I've specified raspberries but you could substitute blackberries (maybe sprinkling with a little sugar and using blackberry jam with the sponge), and I have used, too, those packets of frozen mixed berries. They're fine, but they definitely bring a sponge-sousing reminder of summer pudding with them. You can use trifle sponges here, and I do, but for those who cannot countenance such an unchic thing, I suggest some brioche or challah, sliced; indeed, loaf-shaped supermarket brioche or challah, which have a denser crumb than the boulangerie-edition or *echt* article, are both perfect here.

In a way it is meaningless, or certainly unhelpful, to give exact measurements; as ever it so depends on the bowl you're using. Think rather of layers: one of jam-sandwiched sponge, one of custard, one of cream, and then the nutty, toffee-ish topping. So use the quantities below – which will fill a bowl of about 1½ litre capacity – as a guide only.

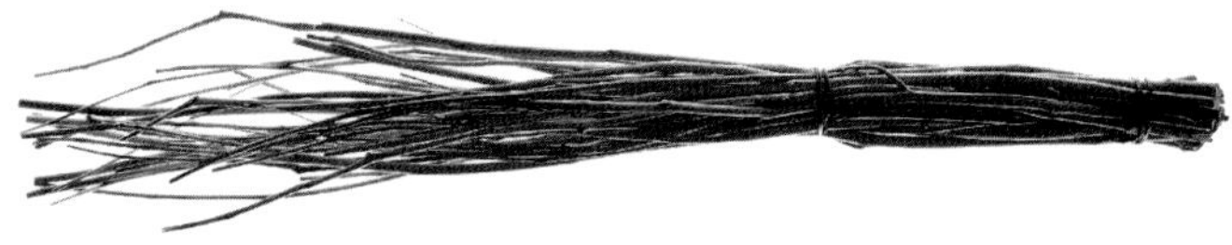

600ml single cream
zest and juice of 1 orange
100ml Grand Marnier
50ml Marsala
5 trifle sponges or 4–5 slices of brioche or challah
approx. 10 heaped teaspoons best quality raspberry or boysonberry jam
500g raspberries
8 egg yolks
75g caster sugar
450ml double cream
50g flaked almonds
1 orange
approx. 100g sugar

Pour the single cream into a wide, heavy-based saucepan, add the orange zest – reserving the juice, separately, for the moment – and bring to the boil without actually letting it boil. Take off the heat and set aside for the orange flavour to infuse while you get on with the bottom layer of the trifle.

Mix together the Grand Marnier, Marsala and the reserved orange juice and pour about half of it into a shallow soup bowl, keeping the rest for replenishing halfway through. If you're using the trifle sponges, split them horizontally, if the challah or brioche slices, take the crusts off and cut them each into two equal slices. Make little sandwiches with the jam, and dunk each sandwich, first one side, then the other, into the booze in the bowl and then arrange the alcohol-sodden sandwiches at the bottom of the trifle bowl. If you're using the challah or brioche, you might need to make up more of your alcoholic mixture, as the bread seems to soak it all in much more quickly and thirstily.

When the bottom of the bowl's covered, top with the fruit and put in the fridge to settle while you get on with the custard. Bring the orange-zested cream back to the boil, while you whisk together the egg yolks and sugar in a bowl large enough to take the cream, too, in a moment. When the yolks and sugar are thick and frothy, pour the about-to-bubble cream into them, whisking as you do so. Wash out the pan, dry it well and return the custard mixture, making sure you disentangle every whisk-attached string of orange zest; you will be sieving later, but for now you want to hold on to all of it.

Fill the sink with enough cold water to come about halfway up the custard pan. On medium to low heat cook the custard, stirring all the time with a wooden spoon or spatula. With so many egg yolks, the custard should take hardly any time to thicken (and remember it will continue to thicken further as it cools) so don't overcook it. If it looks as if it might be about to boil or split, quickly plunge the pan into the sink of cold water, beating furiously until danger is averted. But I find this yolk-rich custard uneventful to make: about 7 minutes, if that, does it; it's unlikely to need cooking for more than 10. When it's cooked and thickened, take the pan over to the sink of cold water and beat robustly but calmly for a minute or so. When the custard's smooth and cooled, strain it over the fruit-topped sponge and put the bowl back in the fridge for 24 hours.

Not long before you want to eat it, whip the double cream till thick and, preferably with one of those bendy rubber spatulas, smear it thickly over the top of the custard. Put it back in the fridge. Toast the flaked almonds by tossing them in a hot, dry frying pan for a couple of minutes and then remove to a plate till cool. Squeeze the orange, pour it into a measuring jug and then measure out an equal quantity – gram for millilitre – of sugar; I reckon on getting 100ml of juice out of the average orange. Pour the orange juice into a saucepan and stir in sugar to help it dissolve. Bring to the boil and let bubble away until you have a thick but still runny toffee: if you let it boil too much until you have, almost, toffee (and I often do) it's not the end of the world, but you're aiming for a densely syrupy, sticky caramel. Remove from heat, and when cooled slightly, dribble over the whipped cream; you may find this easier to do teaspoon by slow-drizzling teaspoon. You can do this an hour or so before you want to eat it. Scatter the toasted almonds over before serving.

This is certainly enough for 10, and maybe even more, though it certainly wouldn't swamp 8.

WHITE TIRAMISU

I wouldn't suggest a tiramisu, that Black Forest gâteau of the 1990s, in the normal run of things, but this coffee-less, chocolate-less, all-white confection is a rather chic take on it: it evokes, just by virtue of its name, the naff and overfamiliar, but elegantly, rather grandly, overturns that presumption, which I quite like. But even if it were to become the naffest, most overfamiliar and thus generally downgraded and despised *dolce* ever constructed, I would still stand by it: you'll see . . .

This pudding is always a success: it always works, and everyone always loves it. It is, once again, a recipe that bears the mark of Anna del Conte. I have made one slight alteration, which is to increase the liquid in which the biscuits are soaked. You must use the Italian savoiardi, not our lady's fingers. You need to go to a good Italian deli or see the Gazetteer. If you can't be bothered to make your own meringues, crumble some bought meringue nests.

small meringues, approx. 3cm in diameter, made with 2 egg whites and 120g caster sugar (see recipe on page 19)
2 eggs, separated
90g caster sugar
325g mascarpone
160ml white rum, such as Bacardi
200ml full-fat milk
18 savoiardi

Choose a dish about 10cm deep, suitable for holding 9 savoiardi.

Heat the oven to gas mark 1/140°C. Then make the meringues. Set aside 10 of them and crumble the others.

Beat the egg yolks with the sugar until pale and mousse-like. Fold in the mascarpone gradually and then beat until incorporated. Whisk 1 egg white (you don't need the second) until firm and fold into mascarpone mixture.

Mix the rum and milk in a soup plate and dip the biscuits in the mixture just long enough for them to soften. Lay about 9 moistened biscuits in the dish and spread over about a third of the mascarpone mixture. Sprinkle with the meringue crumbs. Dip another 9 biscuits into the rum and milk as before and then arrange them on top of the meringue crumbs. Spread over about half the remaining cream, cover with clingfilm and refrigerate. Put the remaining cream in a closed container and refrigerate also. Leave for a day. (I have left it for 2 days without any problem.)

Before serving, smooth the remaining cream all over the pudding and decorate with the whole meringue coins. I would offer a bowl of raspberries alongside.

Serves 6.

The white tiramisu is far less effort in the kitchen than it looks on the page. Another standby of mine is syllabub. You hardly have to do anything, although that isn't my prime motivation: it tastes fabulous, all that softly piled-up whiteness infused with nutmeg, the sort of pudding you imagine eating in heaven.

QUINCE SYLLABUB

This version is particularly fragrant, as the name suggests. The quince in question is not the actual fruit but the peachy-peppery breath of an eau de vie de coings (quince liqueur or quince brandy). Instead of the sherry you could use white wine, and instead of the quince liqueur, you could use ordinary brandy. The pudding might look rather lovely – to amplify the coral tones of the quince liqueur – if you chose one of those French dry rosés or *vins gris*. And if you want to play on the *Arabian Nights* feel of the creamy, quince-fragrant confection, then add a drop of rosewater (only a drop or it'll smell like bath lotion). I think I'd stop short of decorating with rose petals, though.

I normally hate things in individual portions, restaurant-style, but with a syllabub there's no getting round it. You have to eat it with a teaspoon. So, I pile it into separate glasses.

Since the alcohol, lemon juice and zest have to sit and steep overnight, you need to do this a little in advance, but I have happily done it rather a lot in advance and left the syllabub, made up and spooned into its glasses, on the floor in the larder for a couple of days before eating it. This amount makes enough to fit into 6 small glasses or 4 wine-glasses – the syllabub looks best piled right up to the top and swelling bulkily beyond.

8 tablespoons dry sherry
2 tablespoons eau de vie de coings
juice and grated zest of 1 lemon
4 tablespoons caster sugar
300ml double cream
drop rosewater (optional)
nutmeg

Put the sherry, eau de vie de coings, lemon zest and juice in a bowl, cover with cling-film and leave overnight. The next day strain the liquid into another bowl, stir in the sugar and keep stirring until it's dissolved. Keep on stirring as you gradually pour in the cream. Add a drop of rosewater and a grating of fresh nutmeg; I once tried cinnamon instead and, although I prefer the nutmeg, the cinnamon variant was well liked, so you may want to give it a whirl yourself.

Now whip the syllabub until it is about to form soft peaks. It should occupy some notional territory between solid and liquid, rather like the cool, buttery flesh of a newborn baby does when, touching it, you can't tell where the skin stops and the air begins. You don't want the cream to become too thick or, indeed, to go further and curdle. The answer is probably to use a wire whisk, but if you promise to keep the beaters going at the lowest possible speed and to be vigilant, then you can use an electric hand-held whisk. Jane Grigson, in her St Valentine's Syllabub (white wine and brandy, flavoured with honey and sprinkled with toasted nuts) talks of its 'bulky whiteness': that seems the perfect, poetic, description of the point at which you should stop whisking.

Spoon the syllabub into the glasses, and set by in a cold place or the fridge for 2–3 days. Sometimes I grate some more nutmeg over the syllabubs just before eating. And serve with biscuits, delicate, thin, light ones – tuiles, langue de chat (see page 20) or pistachio-studded Middle-Eastern pastry curls.

STEM-GINGER GINGERBREAD

Gingerbread is perhaps more of a cake than a pudding, but, with some sharp, damp but crumbly Caerphilly, Wensleydale or Lancashire cheese, makes a stylish ending to an informal meal. I include the recipe under cooking in advance because – to get the seductive, highly scented stickiness – the gingerbread must be wrapped in foil and kept for a day or so before being eaten. It is also good – if eccentric – in plain unbuttered slices with the aromatic spiced baked plums on page 130. And I love gingerbread with ice-cream: all you need is good vanilla ice-cream sprinkled with a little cinnamon, but if you really want to go for it you could serve, along with the ice-cream and gingerbread, some more stem ginger in its pungent syrup.

The recipe comes from *The Baking Book* by Linda Collister and Anthony Blake.

230g self-raising flour
1 teaspoon bicarbonate of soda
1 tablespoon ground ginger
1 teaspoon ground cinnamon
1 teaspoon ground mixed spice
110g unsalted butter, chilled and diced
110g black treacle or molasses
110g golden syrup
110g light or dark muscovado sugar
280ml full-fat milk
45g stem ginger. Drain off the syrup and grate
1 egg, beaten

Grease a 900g loaf tin (measuring 23cm x 11cm x 6cm) and line the bottom with greaseproof paper. Preheat the oven to gas mark 4/180°C.

Sift the flour, bicarbonate of soda and all the spices into a large mixing bowl. Add the diced butter and rub in with your fingers until the mixture resembles fine crumbs. (I use my free-standing mixer, with the flat beater in place.)

In a small saucepan, melt the treacle with the syrup, then leave to cool to blood heat. Meanwhile, in another pan, dissolve the sugar in the milk over low heat, stirring occasionally.

Add the grated stem ginger – it's easier to use a drum grater – to the flour mixture. Then whisk or beat the milk mixture into the flour mixture and next whisk in the treacle mixture, followed by the egg. When thoroughly blended, the mixture should be a thin batter.

Pour the batter into the prepared tin and bake for 1–1¼ hours or until a skewer inserted into the centre comes out clean. Start checking after 45 minutes. But be warned:

the mixture goes *very* runny before it is ready. Don't panic. The gingerbread will rise during baking and then fall and shrink slightly as it cools. Leave to cool completely in the tin, then turn out and wrap first in greaseproof paper and then in foil. Keep for a day before slicing thickly, then eat hungrily.

Serves 6–8.

ALMOND AND ORANGE BLOSSOM CAKE

For no real reason, I think of this as a summer version of the sticky gingerbread. It is wonderfully fragrant, not quite gooey, but dense with almonds and gently scented with oranges and orange-flower water. It is wonderful served with a compôte of cherries, or indeed with any fruit. I rely on cakes with berries for a dinner-party pudding and I'm particularly pleased with this one. Like the gingerbread, this almond cake has to be wrapped in foil (without the layer of greaseproof) for a day or so before being eaten.

225g soft unsalted butter
225g caster sugar
4 eggs
50g plain flour, preferably Italian 00
180g ground almonds
1 scant teaspoon almond essence
zest of 1 medium orange
juice of ½ medium orange
2 tablespoons orange-flower water

Grease a 21cm spring-release cake tin (if the only one you've got measures 23cm then that'll do, or anything between these figures, but no bigger) and cut out a circle of greaseproof paper to line the bottom. I lay the paper out on the table, put the tin on top, pressing down heavily on it with one hand and, using the other, tear the paper away from the base of the tin. What you end up with is a circle of the right size with maybe a few fuzzy edges, but what does it matter?

Preheat the oven to gas mark 4/180°C. Then cream together the butter and sugar until almost white. (Again, I use a free-standing mixer, with the flat paddle beater, for the entire operation.) Beat the eggs and add them gradually to the creamed butter and sugar, beating all the while. I put in a couple of tablespoons at a time, and with each addition, sprinkle on some flour. When all the eggs and flour have been incorporated, gently stir in the ground almonds, then the almond essence, grated orange zest, orange juice and orange-flower water.

Pour the mixture into the cake tin and bake for about 1 hour. After about 40 minutes you may well find you have to cover it, loosely, with foil; you don't want the top of the cake to burn. The cake is ready when the top is firm and a skewer, inserted in the centre, comes out clean. Take it out and let it stand for 5 minutes or so in the tin. Then turn it out on to a wire rack and leave till cool. Wrap it well in foil and leave for a day or two. Push some icing sugar through a fine sieve or tea strainer over the cake when serving.

Serves 8.

You can stew plums a few days in advance, and they freeze very well in their aromatic syrup. This is a favourite pudding in my house.

BAKED SPICED AROMATIC PLUMS

I am not normally the sort of person who bakes, bottles or otherwise prepares or preserves fruit: I like it ripe, fresh, as it is. I make a couple of exceptions: one for quinces, about which I can grow somewhat obsessive during November; the other for plums. We have a few trees in the garden and from them more fruit that we can eat. Even in a bad year, when the dusty blue, grape-black skins enclose disappointingly unyielding Pucci-green fruit, baking them like this transforms them.

1kg plums
300ml red wine
2 bay leaves
1/2 teaspoon ground cinnamon
2 cloves
1 star anise
seeds from 4 cardomom pods or scant 1/4 teaspoon ground cardomom
200g honey

Set oven to gas mark 3/160°C. Choose a baking dish that will fit the plums, halved, in one layer; if you haven't got one big enough you could use a couple, but make sure you fill whichever dishes you're using or there won't be enough syrup.

Cut the plums in half, remove the stones and put the fruit in the dish, cut side down. Then put all the other ingredients into a saucepan and bring to the boil. Pour over the plums, cover the dish tightly with foil (or a lid, of course, if you've got one that fits) and bake for about 1 hour or until the plums are tender.

Keep the cooled, covered fruit in the fridge for 3 or so days (and freeze them with impunity) until you need them. I find them easier to reheat, gently, on the hob.

Serves 6–8.

Opinions are divided in my household as to what goes best with these spicy, wine-dark plums. There is a custard contingent, but I veer more towards ice-cream or crème fraîche. But what I really love – and not just with this but with plain, uncooked blueberries (which you can now get all the year round, it seems) or most other berries – is something my grandmother used to make, called Barbados cream.

BARBADOS CREAM

It's difficult to be precise about measurements here: the idea is to stir together more or less equal quantities of yoghurt (and I always use Greek yoghurt) and double cream and then sprinkle over a good covering of brown sugar.

These are the quantities I use to fill a shallow bowl (and it must be a shallow bowl) measuring about 20cm in diameter. If you're having the Barbados cream as an accompaniment to fruit then this will provide enough for about 6, maybe more: it is delectably rich.

284ml double cream
300g Greek yoghurt
approx. 75g brown sugar (demerara, ordinary soft brown sugar or whatever you've got in the cupboard)

I know that the yoghurt and cream are not in exactly the same measurements, but since that's how they're sold in their cartons it seems silly not to use them as they are.

Mix them together and beat till fairly but not too stiffly thick. Pour into the bowl. Sprinkle over it a thick carpet of brown sugar, cover with clingfilm and leave somewhere cool for at least 12 hours or better still 24 hours.

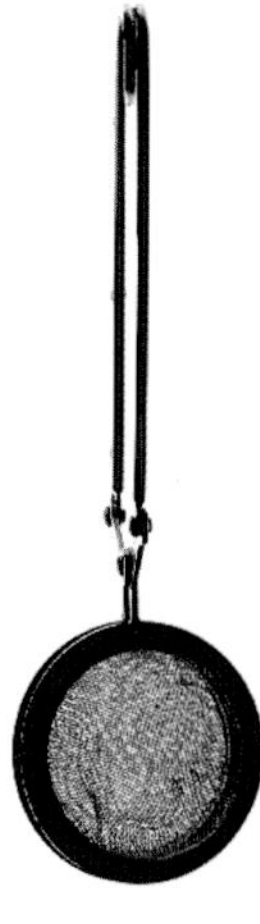

one & two

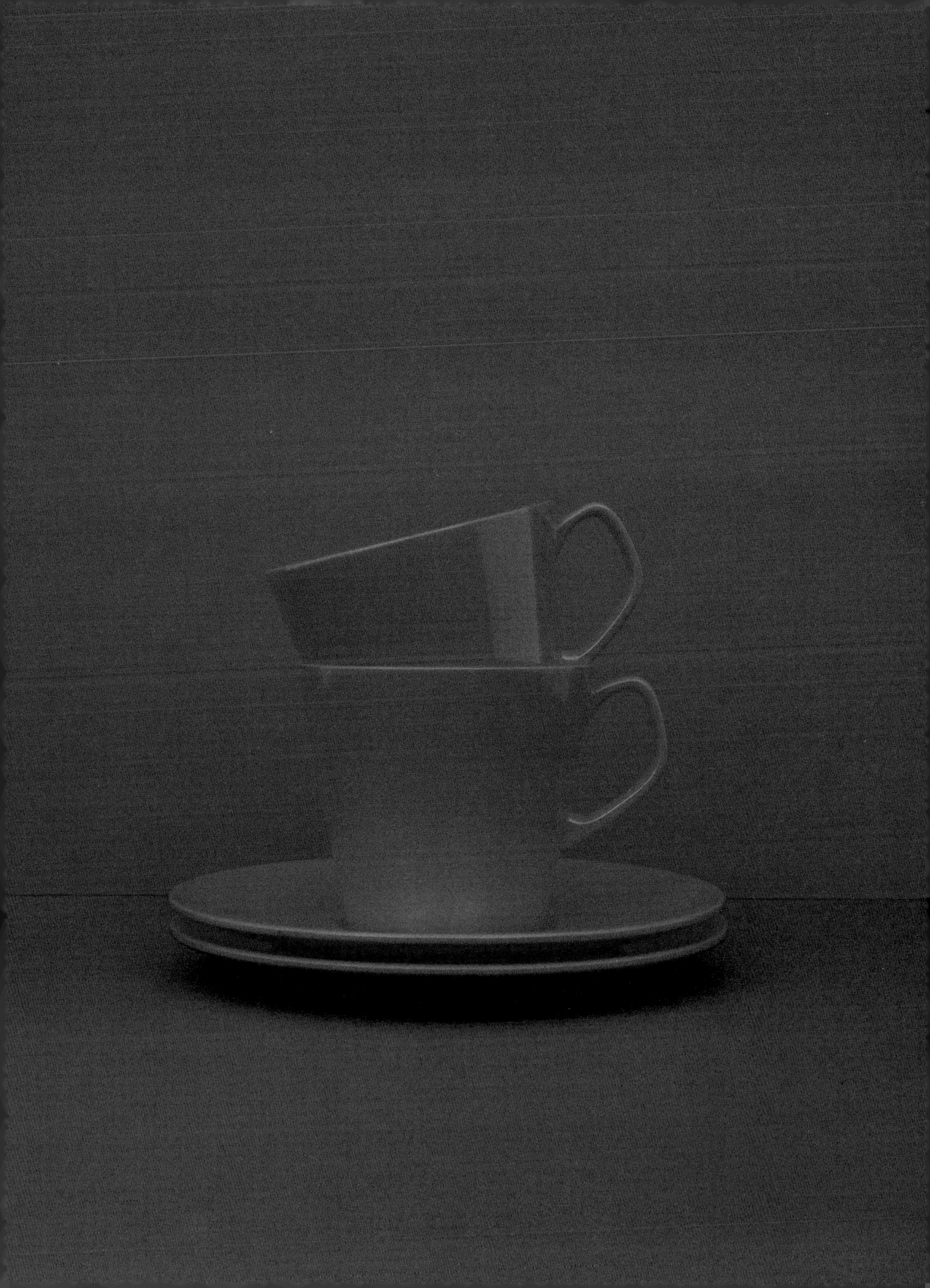

Don't knock masturbation,' Woody Allen once said: 'it's sex with someone I love.' Most people can't help finding something embarrassingly onanistic about taking pleasure in eating alone. Even those who claim to love food think that cooking just for yourself is either extravagantly self-indulgent or a plain waste of time and effort. But you don't have to belong to the drearily narcissistic learn-to-love-yourself school of thought to grasp that it might be a good thing to consider yourself worth cooking for. And the sort of food you cook for yourself will be different from the food you might lay on for tablefuls of people: it will be better.

I don't say that for effect. You'll feel less nervous about cooking it and that translates to the food itself. It'll be simpler, more straightforward, the sort of food *you* want to eat.

I don't deny that food, its preparation as much as its consumption, is about sharing, about connectedness. But that's not all that it's about. There seems to me to be something robustly affirmative about taking trouble to feed yourself; enjoying life on purpose, rather than by default.

Even in culinary terms alone there are grounds for satisfaction. Real cooking, if it is to have any authenticity, any integrity, has to be part of how you are, a function of your personality, your temperament. There's too much culinary ventriloquism about as it is: cooking for yourself is a way of countering that. It's how you're going to find your own voice. One of the greatest hindrances to enjoying cooking is that tense-necked desire to impress others. It's virtually impossible to be innocent of this. Even if this is not your motivation, it's hard, if you're being honest, to be insensible to the reactions of others. Since cooking for other people is about trying to please them, it would be strange to be indifferent to their pleasure, and I don't think you should be. But you can try too hard. When you're cooking for yourself, the stakes simply aren't as high. You don't mind as much. Consequently, it's much less likely to go wrong. And the process is more enjoyable in itself.

When I cook for myself I find it easier to trust my instinct – I am sufficiently relaxed to listen to it in the first place – and, contrariwise, I feel freer

one & two

to overturn a judgement, to take a risk. If I want to see what will happen if I add yoghurt, or stir in some chopped tarragon instead of parsley, I can do so without worrying that I am about to ruin everything. If the sauce splits or the tarragon infuses everything with an invasive farmyard grassiness, I can live with it. I might feel cross with myself, but I won't be panicked. It could be that the yoghurt makes the sauce, or that the tarragon revitalises it. I'm not saying that cooking for seven other people would make it impossible for me to respond spontaneously, but I do think it's cooking for myself that has made it possible.

Far too much cooking now is about the tyranny of the recipe on the one hand and the absence of slowly acquired experience on the other. Cooking for yourself is a way of finding out what *you* want to cook and eat, rather than simply joining up the dots. Crucially, it's a way of seeing which things work, which don't, and how ingredients, heat, implements, vessels, all have their part to play. When I feel like a bowl of thick, jellied white rice noodles, not soupy but barely bound in a sweet and salty sauce, I'm not going to look up a recipe for them. I know that if I soak the noodles in boiling water until they dislodge themselves from the solid wodge I've bought them in, fry 2 cloves of garlic with some knife-flattened spring onions and tiny square beads of chopped red chilli in a pan before wilting some greens and adding the noodles with a steam-provoking gush of soy and mirin, with maybe a teaspoon of black bean sauce grittily dissolved in it, it will taste wonderful, comforting, with or without chopped coriander or a slow-oozing drop or two of sesame oil. I can pay attention to texture and to taste. I know what sort of thing I'm going to end up with, but I'm not aiming to replicate any particular dish. Sometimes it goes wrong: I'm too heavy-handed with the soy and drench everything in brown brine, so that the sweet stickiness of the rice sticks is done for, and there's no contrast; I might feel, when eating, that the chilli interrupts too much when I'm in the mood to eat something altogether gentler. These aren't tragedies, however. And frankly most often I get satisfaction simply from the quiet putting together of a meal. It calms me, which in turn makes me enjoy eating it more.

NOODLES

GARLIC

SPRING ONIONS

CHILLI

SOY

SESAME OIL

But cooking for yourself isn't simply therapy and training. It also happens to be a pleasure in itself. Since most women don't have lives now whereby we're plunged into three family meals a day from the age of nineteen, we're not forced to learn how to cook from the ground up. I don't complain. Nor do I wish to make it sound as if cooking for yourself were some sort of checklisted culinary foundation course. The reason why you learn so much from the sort of food

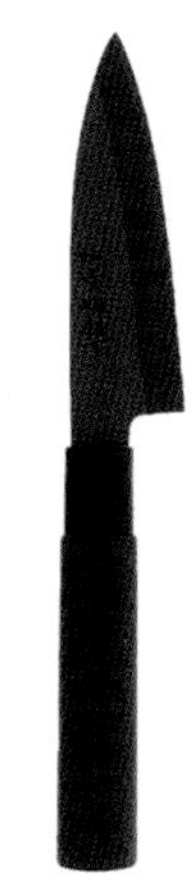

you casually throw together for yourself, is that you're learning by accident, by osmosis. This has nothing to do with the culinary supremacism of the great chefs, or those who'd ape them. Too many people cook only when they're giving a dinner party. And it's very hard to go from nought to a hundred miles an hour. How can you learn to feel at ease around food, relaxed about cooking, if every time you go into the kitchen it's to cook at competition level?

I love the open-ended freedom of just pottering about in the kitchen, of opening the fridge door and deciding what to cook. But I like, too, the smaller special project, the sort of indulgent eating that has something almost ceremonial about it when done alone. I'm not saying I don't often end up with the au pair special, a bowl of cereal, or its street-princess equivalent, the phone-in pizza. But I believe in the rule of 'Tonight Lucullus is dining with Lucullus.'

BREAD AND CHEESE

Eating alone, for me, is most often a prompt to shop. This is where self-absorption and consumerism meet: a rapt, satisfyingly convoluted pleasure. The food I want most to buy is the food I most often try not to eat: a swollen-bellied tranche of cheese, a loaf of bread. These constitute the perfect meal. A slither of gorgonzola or coulommiers sacrificed on the intrusive and unyielding surface of a Bath Oliver at the end of dinner is food out of kilter. Just bread and cheese is fine to give others if you've shown the consideration of providing variety. But I want for myself the obsessive focus of the one huge, heady *baveuse* soft cheese, or else a wedge of the palate-burning hard stuff: too much, too strong. If I'm eating a salty blue cheese, its texture somewhere between creamy and crumbly, I want baguette or a bitter, fudge-coloured *pain au levain*; with cheddar, real cheddar, I want doughier English white bread: whichever, it must be a whole loaf. I might eat tomatoes with the bread and cheese, but the tomatoes mustn't be in a salad, but left whole on the plate, to be sliced or chopped, *à la minute*. But, then, I love the delicatessen-garnered equivalent of the TV supper.

MUSHROOM-STEAK SANDWICH

I am pretty keen on the culinary ethos of the Greasy Spoon, too: bacon sandwiches, fried-egg sandwiches, egg *and* bacon sandwiches, sausage sandwiches; none requires much in the way of attention, and certainly nothing in the way of expertise. Even easier is a sandwich that on paper sounds fancier, a fab merging of caff and deli culture: get a large flat field mushroom, put it in a preheated gas mark 6/200°C oven covered with butter, chopped garlic and parsley for about 20 minutes; when ready, and garlicky, buttery juices are oozing with black, cut open a soft roll, small ciabatta or bap, or chunk of baguette even, and wipe the cut side all over the pan to soak up the pungent juices. Smear with Dijon mustard, top with the mushroom, squeeze with lemon juice, sprinkle some salt and add some chopped lettuce or parsley as you like; think of this as a fungoid – but strangely hardly less meaty – version of steak sandwich. Bite in, with the juices dripping down your arm as you eat.

There are other memorable more or less non-cooking solitary suppers: one is a bowl of Heinz tomato soup with some pale, undercooked but overbuttered toast (crusts off for full nostalgic effect); another, microwave-zapped, mustard-dunked frankfurters (proper frankfurters, from a delicatessen, not those flabby, mousse-textured things out of a tin). The difficulty is that if I have them in the house, I end up eating them while I wait for whatever I'm actually cooking for dinner to be ready. And my portions are not small to start off with. Two defences, other than pure greed: I hate meagreness, the scant, sensible serving; and if I long to eat a particular thing, I want lots of it. I don't want course upon course, and I don't want excess every day. But when it comes to a feast, I don't know the meaning of enough.

SOUP

FRANKFURTERS

Cooking for two is just an amplification of cooking for one (rather than the former being a diminution of the latter). To tell the truth, with my cooking and portion-size, there isn't often a lot to choose between them. Many of the impulses that inform or inspire this sort of cooking are the same: the desire to eat food that is relaxed but at times culinarily elevated without loss of spontaneity; the pleasures of fiddling about with what happens to be in the fridge; and, as with any form of eating, the need to make food part of the civilised context in which we live.

LINGUINE WITH CLAMS

My absolutely favourite dinner to cook for myself is linguine with clams. I have a purely personal reason for thinking of fish, of any sort, as the ideal solitary food because I live with someone who's allergic to it. But my principle has wider application: fish doesn't take long to cook and tastes best dealt with simply, but because it has to be bought fresh needs enough planning to have something of the ceremonial about it. I don't know why spaghetti alle vongole (I use linguine because I prefer, here, the more substantial, more resistant and at the same time more sauce-absorbent tangle they make in the mouth) is thought of as restaurant food, especially since most restaurants in this country ruin it by adding tomatoes. I have to have my sauce *bianco*.

The whole dish is easy to make. It is, for me, along with a steak béarnaise, unchallengeable contender for that great, fantasy Last Meal on Earth.

You can use venus clams, but palourdes or vongole are what you're after; at a good fishmonger's, you shouldn't have any trouble finding them. If you've got venus clams, add 1 tablespoon of bicarbonate of soda to the soaking water. If you've got the bigger palourdes, you may not need to soak them at all, a brisk wash may be enough: ask your fishmonger.

200g clams

150g linguine

1 clove garlic

2 tablespoons olive oil

½ dried red chilli pepper

80ml white wine or vermouth (Noilly Prat)

1–2 tablespoons fresh parsley, chopped

Put the clams to soak in a sinkful of cold water, if necessary, while you heat the water for the pasta. When the water comes to the boil, add salt and then the linguine. Cook the linguine until nearly but not quite ready: you're going to give them a fractional amount more cooking with the clams and their winey juices. Try and time this so that the pasta's ready at the time you want to plunge it into the clams. Otherwise drain and douse with a few drops of olive oil.

Mince or finely slice the garlic and, in a pan with a lid into which you can fit the pasta later, fry it gently (it mustn't burn) in the olive oil and then crumble in the red chilli pepper. Drain the clams, discarding those that remain open, and add them to the garlic pan. Pour over the wine or vermouth and cover. In 2 minutes, the clams should be open. Add the pasta, put the lid on again and swirl about. In another minute or so everything should have finished cooking and come together: the pasta will have cooked to the requisite tough tenderness and absorbed the salty, garlicky winey clam juices, and be bound in a wonderful almost-pungent sea-syrup. But if the pasta needs more cooking, clamp on the lid and give it more time. Chuck out any clams which have failed to open.

Add half the parsley, shake the pan to distribute evenly, and turn into a plate or bowl and sprinkle over the rest of the parsley. Cheese is not grated over any pasta with fish in it in Italy (nor indeed where garlic is the predominant ingredient, either) and the rule holds good. You need add nothing. It's perfect already.

COD WITH CLAMS

If you are afraid of tackling fish in general, and of cooking seafood in particular, just reading this recipe will show you how easy it is, but doing it is even better. Ease of execution is not the same as ease of attainment, of course: as with all fish, it is ruined by overcooking. This is one of those simple but essentially last-minute recipes that is easier to cook for one or two (or, at a pinch, four) than a huge tableful of waiting people. But if you want to turn this into dinner party food, choose a firmer (and more expensive) fish such as turbot; and strain the sauce to get rid of the stray bits of fishy detritus. I have nothing against cod, but it can disintegrate a little when it sits around.

250g palourdes clams (a good handful, about 12 in all)
1 piece cod fillet, cut from the top end of the fish, about 2–3cm thick (approx. 200g)
scant tablespoon cornflour
pinch cayenne pepper
1 fat clove or 2 smaller cloves garlic, chopped finely or sliced
about 1 tablespoon plus 1 teaspoon butter
drop of oil
4 tablespoons dry sherry
2 tablespoons water
approx. 1 tablespoon chives, chopped
approx. 1 tablespoon fresh parsley, chopped

Rinse the palourdes under the cold tap but don't bother to soak them. Throw out the ones that stay open. Dredge the cod lightly with the cayenne-spiked cornflour. You'll have some left over: just chuck it out.

In a wide, thick-bottomed pan which the cod will fit into flat, melt about 1 tablespoon butter and a drop of oil. Add the shards of garlic and cook for a bare minute, stirring all the time; above all, you don't want the garlic to burn or even burnish. Put the cod in, skin side down (I don't eat the skin; it's just that I find the cod is more likely to stay in one piece if I cook it like this) and cook for 2 minutes, then turn and cook on the other side. Flip back to its skin side, and throw in the clams, then add the sherry and water and put the lid on. Cook for about 3 minutes. Remove the cod and put the gaping-shelled clams around it on your plate. Don't eat any that stay shut. Then let the juices left in the pan reduce by bubbling away for 2–3 minutes. If you want – and I do – whisk in a small amount, about 1 teaspoon, of cold unsalted butter, divided into 2 or 3 tiny bits. Pour the juices over the fish on your plate. Throw over the chopped herbs. Eat with thickly cut bread that's good enough to be dunked without turning to pap. Serves 1.

If you've never cooked moules marinière, you might baulk at the thought: too fiddly, too unknown, too intimidating. But cook them once and you'll see that actually this is scarcely cooking at all. It is easy to buy mussels that have been pretty well cleaned, and there'll only be the odd barnacle to scrape off (itself oddly satisfying), then there's just an onion to chop, with some parsley and garlic, and the rest is about applying heat and liquid. Try this once and you won't need me to persuade you that it's easy. After that you will automatically start thinking of this as something you can cook quickly, with little effort and to great effect.

MOULES MARINIÈRE

I like a lot of winey mussel liquor here, so use more wine to start off with than you might find elsewhere. Traditionally, the onion or shallot, garlic and parsley are just simmered in the wine at first, then, after the mussels are in and steamed open, everything's removed to the bowls, the liquid strained and the butter whisked in. Do it that way, by all means, if you want to. More often I tend to do it as follows.

2kg mussels
50g butter
1 small onion or, better still, 2 shallots
2 cloves garlic
a good handful fresh parsley, chopped, to yield about 5 tablespoons
300ml white wine

Wash the mussels, scrape off any barnacles and pull off any beards. Throw away the cracked mussels or those that stay open after you've rapped rudely and insistently on their shells. (And when cooked, throw away any mussel that has stayed closed.)

On medium heat, in a pan which will take all the mussels later and which has a lid, put the butter in with the onion or shallot chopped very fine, the garlic chopped likewise or sliced thinly and about 1 tablespoon of the parsley. Stir about for a minute till the smell of the garlic rises and that particular, familiar fragrance wafts gloriously out of the pan. Add the wine, cook for another minute or so, with the lid on, but with the heat lowish.Then turn the heat up up up, throw in the cleaned mussels and clamp the lid back on. Give the pan a shake occasionally. Look after 3 minutes and remove all the opened mussels you see, then put the lid on again and give them another 2 minutes. Since you've got time while waiting for the rest of the mussels to open, I'd remove the empty shells of the already cooked mussels: it'll just make the plates a little less crowded, but it's hardly crucial. When the rest of the mussels are steamed open, remove them to your bowls (and you'll need huge ones). Take the pan off the heat, let the juices settle for a moment so any grit that might be in the mussels sits at the bottom. Then, pour the juices carefully over each bowl of waiting, gaping shells, leaving the gritty bits at the bottom. Sprinkle over the remaining parsley. On the table put another couple of bowls or plates for the empty shells and a baguette or other good white bread.

Serves 2.

As I say, I do think it's a good idea to get into the swing of cooking fish. When I've got a lot of people eating, I might cook a fish pie (see pages 267 and 397) but when there's just me, or two of us, I don't mind a bit of the necessary last-minute flash in the pan. Fish, I think, is best fried in bacon fat, which you can't easily buy (though my butcher sells, along with his organic, grass-fed beef dripping, some truly exceptional lard which comes in very useful here). If the bacon you get is good enough, you can provide the wherewithal easily enough. I always mean to keep the fat left in the pan after frying bacon (I've given up grilling it: apart from anything else, I can't wait that long for the grill to heat up), but the immediate pleasure of dunking a piece of bread in the pan to soak up the salty juices, the delectable grease, often prevents me.

EXCEPTIONAL SALMON

To cook exceptional but unfancy salmon for your supper, fry 2 rashers of streaky bacon, chopped fairly small (pancetta, cubed, would do as well) in a pan you've sprinkled with a little oil then heated. When they're beginning to go from crisp to hard brown, remove the bacon to a waiting strip of kitchen towel. Immediately put a piece of salmon in the pan with the bacon fat, sear on each side, then cook for a minute or so, depending on the thickness of the fillet, at a lower heat. Put together some green leaves – just lettuce, or varieties of, and some spring onions – and leave them be for a moment while you transfer the fish to a plate. Then squeeze some lemon juice into the frying pan and pour the juices over the waiting undressed salad. Toss the salad, add the bacon bits and toss again, and add to the plate with the salmon. Sometimes I leave the salad in a bowl, cut the salmon into pieces and add it, tossing, with the bacon. Apart from anything else, bacon lifts the relative flabbiness of farmed salmon.

If I'm feeling in the mood for excess, I boil 2 eggs for about 6 minutes (somewhere between soft and hard, yolk still oily but dense), peel and halve, and add them to the bowl of bacon and salmon salad. Or I take 2–3 tomatoes, briefly cover them in boiling water, then peel and deseed them and add them in fat strips to the salad. This is one of the few times I'd consider eating tomatoes with fish. The following suggestion is another.

SALADE NIÇOISE

The world doesn't need another recipe for seared tuna. But the only way I like salade niçoise is inauthentically: that's to say with fresh, not canned, tuna. This makes for good solitary eating: there's also enough cooking to make you feel that you're actually making something.

First, you have to see to your potatoes. If you can get Pink Fir Apples so much the better, but it's not an issue. What you want are boiled potatoes, or steamed, cut into thick coins while still warm, then dribbled over with olive oil and given a good grinding of pepper, preferably white, but again the colour is no big deal. Meanwhile you should have put your piece of tuna, cut into thick short strips, to marinade in a tablespoonful of olive oil, a good squeeze of lemon juice or red wine vinegar and a sprinkling of soy sauce. At the same time, put 1 tablespoon of capers, which have been packed in salt rather than brine, to soak. Cook some trimmed and halved green beans, drain, plunge into cold water and drain again. Put about 4 cherry tomatoes in a bowl, pour over some boiling water from a kettle and leave for a few minutes, then peel. Leave till cool, then quarter.

So: to the oil-drizzled potatoes in your bowl (I like a big shallow one, all to myself), add the tomatoes, green beans, some fresh marinaded anchovies (the sort that lie in bowls in the slope-windowed fridge counter at the delicatessen), the capers, drained well, and some torn-up bits of lettuce (or I like those bagged packs of baby spinach). Make a garlicky dressing, strong and astringent, pour over and toss the salad gently. If you want eggs, boil for 6 minutes. I like them still oily-yolked, a good dripping gold, not dusty yellow. And if you're in fancy mode, and are up to all that fiddly peeling, quails' eggs work well.

Meanwhile heat your pan to seething, add oil if you need it, then the tuna pieces and cook briefly but intensely on all sides. Throw in the marinade and let it bubble up, clinging stickily to the pieces of fish. Add the fish to the salad, toss and eat. And d'you know, if you *can* get those silver-skinned, ivory-fleshed, fresh, filleted anchovies, you don't even need to bother with the tuna.

SCALLOPS AND BACON

This is one of my favourites: it has just the right balance between nursery comfort and dining-room elegance and takes hardly any time to cook – and thus is just what you need after a hard day's work. Properly speaking, it is more of a starter or savoury, but when there's just two of you eating, it makes a perfect supper almost in its entirety; all I'd add is a dark and leafy salad, dressed with walnut oil and lemon juice.

You should aim to buy your scallops (unfrozen) from a fishmonger. And often I don't add the corals here, but stash them in the freezer and thaw at a later date to fry with some minced garlic and butter and eat, alone and greedily, mashed on pale and thickly sliced, real-bread toast.

1 teaspoon oil
4 rashers streaky bacon, cut in half lengthwise
10 scallops
1 tablespoon seasoned flour
15g butter
60ml dry sherry
fresh parsley

Put a teaspoon of oil in a thick-bottomed frying pan and when hot add the strips of bacon. Cook until crisp and remove. Separate the white flesh of the scallops from the corals and dredge the fat white discs all over in the flour. Add the butter to the pan and over a low to medium heat fry the floury scallops, turning after about 3 minutes and cooking on the other side for about another 2, or until they are cooked, but only just. Now add the corals to the pan and just turn them in the butter for a minute and remove. Put the scallops, their corals and the bacon on a plate. Over the heat add the sherry to the pan and pour it over the scallops and bacon. Sprinkle with freshly chopped parsley and there you have it. Serves 2.

When I'm in Italy, I love eating those small, fleshy prawns which are scarcely cooked, but just turned with garlic, chilli, wine and oil in a hot pan until they lose their grey transparency, becoming suddenly, shinily coral. You can't really reproduce that here, because we don't get the prawns: they're either cooked (in which case forget it) or raw and frozen, somehow acquiring an oversaltedness with their iced glaze. But my regular inspections reveal that in the better fishmongers the situation is improving, and frozen is a possible alternative. I am not talking about the near-ubiquitous tiger prawn for this recipe, but prawn prawns, the size that goes into the cocktail.

PRAWNS WITH GARLIC AND CHILLI

2 cloves garlic
½–1 fresh red chilli (according to size and taste)
2 tablespoons olive oil
200–250g raw unshelled prawns (400g when frozen)
100ml white wine
flat-leaf parsley

Peel and chop the garlic, and deseed and chop the red chilli pepper as finely as you can. Pour the olive oil into a wide, thick-bottomed pan. Then add the chilli and garlic and, on a moderate to low heat, to infuse rather than to colour, fry for 2 minutes, stirring all the time. Then turn the heat to high, add the prawns and stir-fry them for another 2 minutes or until they turn pink and are just, delicately, cooked: you want the flesh to stay tender. Pour in the white wine and let it bubble up. You don't want a liquid puddle around the prawns, just enough wine to let the juices ooze into a winey sauce. Another minute or so should do it. Taste for salt (as I say, the frozen raw prawns seem already saltier than normal) and then turn into your bowl and sprinkle generously with flat-leaf parsley. Eat with some good hunks of baguette. I eat these carapace, head and all: one of the reasons I designate them for solitary dinner.

If you want, and you keep some to hand anyway, you can add a tablespoonful or so of brandy before throwing in the wine.

Serves 1.

Along with every other greedy person in the country I have a growing collection of Australian cookery books. The following recipe – for prawns again – comes from Leonie Palmer's *Noosa Cook Book*, which is by way of being the food eaten at a small, paradisiacal-looking resort village on the Queensland coast. The chief drawback to anything deep-fried is that it has to be eaten straight away. If there's you at the stove cooking, sending plate by plate out to your friends waiting at the table, then life's not going to be much fun. If there are only two of you, you can both stand by the cooker and eat as the food comes hot and crunchy out of the pan. The quantities below make about 12 little patties.

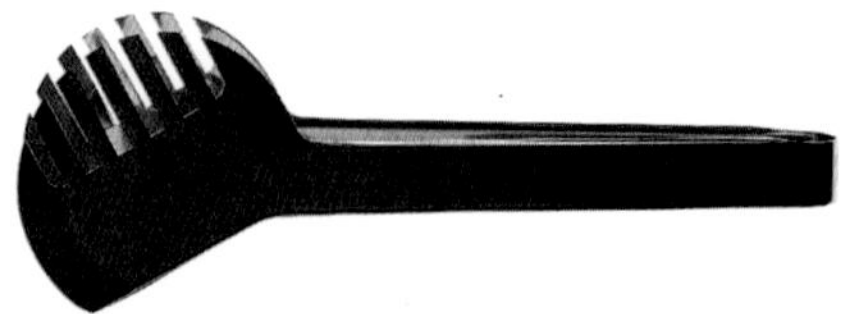

FRIED PRAWN CAKES

250g fresh raw prawns
1 clove garlic, chopped finely
2 spring onions, chopped finely
½ teaspoon salt
60g plain flour
4 teaspoons sherry
olive oil

Shell and mince the prawns. Mix or blend them with the garlic, spring onions, salt, flour, sherry and enough water to make a batter. Let stand, covered with clingfilm, for 1 hour. Then fry, in drops of 1 teaspoon, in olive oil (though not extra virgin) poured to a depth of 5cm in a pan, for about a minute each side.

These are delicious with a fierce mayonnaise (see page 13 for method) made by substituting lime juice for the lemon, and with a handful of fresh chopped coriander added at the end. But if the prawn cakes have exhausted your cooking capacity, then add some lime juice and chopped coriander to a bowlful of Hellman's. (Normally, I can't see why everyone is so keen on the stuff, but it lends itself well to this kind of adulteration; anyway, fried fish cakes of this sort seem to be able to handle the peculiar emulsification of factory-made mayo.) Or just squeeze the prawn patties with fresh lime as you eat them.

One of the great advantages of eating alone or with one other person is that you don't have to take into account the squeamishness of the average, unknown eater. By this I don't mean that you might otherwise be inviting strangers to dinner, but that there are always going to be some people (someone's boyfriend, a newish friend) whose tastes you can't test with strange bits of internal organs or the spookier meats. The fewer people you're cooking for, the more permissive and inclusive you can be.

Ever since a friend of mine told me about a wittily conceived warm rabbit salad with baby radishes and carrots she'd eaten at The French House in Soho, I've wanted to appropriate it. I've made up my own version here. If you know someone who likes rabbit and who will appreciate the joke, you're lucky.

You can buy boned portions of rabbit in most supermarkets (it comes from China as most rabbit sold over here does). Do: it makes the eating easier. Yes, this is very much an arranged salad, and normally I shun such restauranty displays of food. But when eating à deux, or indeed solo, you can generally get away with a greater level of cheffiness, if that's your secret desire, without losing your culinary integrity. Indeed, it's probably the best way to get it out of your system.

If you put the rabbit in the fridge to marinade when you get up in the morning, you won't have much to do when you get back from work in the evening.

PETER RABBIT IN MR McGREGOR'S SALAD

1 125g tub natural yoghurt
1 teaspoon best olive oil
2 tablespoons wine vinegar
1 tablespoon Dijon mustard
4 cloves garlic, crushed with flat of knife
½ teaspoon dried thyme
2 portions boned rabbit, approx. 150g each
2 tablespoons ordinary olive oil for frying

1 packet mixed lettuce leaves
1 handful radishes
1 handful smallest carrots possible

for the dressing
½ teaspoon Dijon mustard
scant tablespoon wine vinegar
salt and pepper
4 tablespoons olive oil

Make the marinade by mixing together the yoghurt, vinegar, mustard, garlic and thyme. Add the rabbit pieces, turn to make sure they're marinaded on all sides, cover and leave for 12 hours, or thereabouts, in the fridge.

At about the time you want to eat, preheat the oven to gas mark 6/200°C. Take the rabbit out of its marinade and wipe dry with kitchen towel. On the hob, in a pan (preferably one which will go in the oven) pour the oil for frying and, when hot, sear the rabbit a minute or so each side till golden, then transfer the pan to the oven and cook for 25 minutes or until tender. Remove and let cool a bit: you want this warm.

Divide the lettuce between the two plates, then chop up the radishes, in halves or quarters, or leave them whole, depending on their size. Or, if you prefer, you can slice them thinly into translucent white, crimson-rimmed discs. If you've managed to find those tiny spindly baby carrots, leave them as they are, even with their little bits of green attached, just wash and dry them. If you've managed to find only so-called baby carrots (and those ones no bigger than a girl's finger are not too hard to find now everyone's got a fixation with stunted veg), slice them down the middle lengthways, and into half again, if necessary. Arrange the radishes and carrots over the lettuces in any way which gives you pleasure. Make an emulsified dressing by putting the mustard, vinegar, salt and pepper in a bowl and whisking, and continue whisking while you add the oil. Dribble over the salad. Put the warm rabbit pieces in the middle of each plate.

Liver in general, and calves' liver in hands-up-in-horror particular, also belong to that genre of foodstuffs that cannot be served up confidently to a tableful of average eaters. But as I eat, so I write: and we often eat liver for lunch or dinner. To fry liver, melt a knob of butter in a frying pan with a drop of oil in it, and fry 2–3 pieces of thinly sliced calves' liver (I reckon just over 100g per person) in it, a minute or so a side, till still pink within, then remove to a plate, throw 2 tablespoons Marsala into the pan, let it bubble away until syrupy and pour over the liver. The mashed potato we eat with this needs more planning, but if I'm feeling lazy – and have the time – I just put 3 large baking potatoes in a gas mark 7/210°C oven a couple of hours before we count on eating and then, when they're thoroughly cooked inside, I scrape out the flesh and mash it with some butter and warmed milk to which I've added a good grating of fresh nutmeg, and some salt and pepper.

The last time we ate this, I see from my notebooks, we had some damson purée (made with 225g damsons, cooked with ½ cup sugar and ¼ cup water) and custard afterwards: just perfect.

LIVER WITH SWEET ONIONS

I can't remember what I'd been reading, some Italian recipe for duck, I think, with a sauce of pomegranate juice thickened with the mashed liver from the duck. But it made me want to try to use pomegranate in a low-key way in my cooking. You get pomegranate juice the same way you get orange or lemon juice: use a squeezer. I use one pomegranate here with an electric squeezer, but I suspect if I were using a normal hand juicer, I'd need a couple to provide the same amount of juice. In place of fresh pomegranates, you could get some of the divinely, darkly syrupy Middle-Eastern pomegranate molasses – which is sold in Lebanese and Greek shops and at some specialist food counters – in which case, I'd dilute a tablespoon in the same amount of wine or vermouth and a bit more of water (and taste), otherwise you'll have something much too sticky and strong. The extraordinary thing about the fresh pomegranate juice is how delicate and modestly fragrant it is.

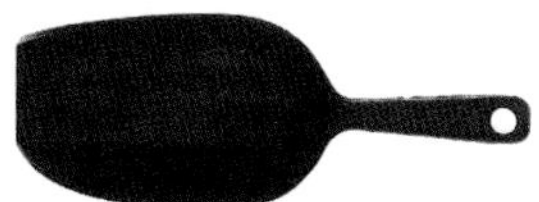

2 tablespoons butter
2 tablespoons olive oil
1 medium onion, sliced very finely
1 pomegranate
225g calves' liver
1 tablespoon flour

In a thick-bottomed frying pan on medium to low heat, heat 1 tablespoon each of butter and oil. Slice the onions finely (I use the processer) and cook in the butter and oil until they're soft – about 10 minutes. Pour over half the pomegranate juice and a little water, about 1–2 tablespoons, and cook for another 10 minutes or so until the liquid's absorbed and you have a soft, sweet and bronzy-puce tangle of onions in the pan. Remove to waiting, warmed plates and tent over with tinfoil to stop them cooling.

Add the remaining tablespoons of butter and oil to the frying pan, dredge the liver lightly in seasoned flour and fry in the butter–oil mixture for a minute or so on each side. Remove from the pan and put on the waiting plates with the onions. To the remaining pomegranate juice, add half its volume in water. Add the pomegranate juice and water to the hot pan and deglaze. Taste, and then pour over the liver and onions. I like this with plain boiled potatoes.

Serves 2.

DUCK WITH POMEGRANATE

You can roast a Gressingham or Barbary duck, if not actually a mallard, and baste it with reduced pomegranate juice. To make the sauce, sauté and purée the duck liver with some heat-softened rosemary and onion, some more pomegranate juice and the well-skimmed juices from the pan. And duck is perfect for two; there just isn't enough meat to feed four, as is often, shockingly, recommended. Magrets (duck breasts), fried, and with a bare sauce made from the pan juices deglazed with pomegranate juice and sprinkled with a few seeds, is a lower-effort take on the same theme.

The difficulty with giving quail to large numbers of people is that the scale's wrong: too many little bits. When there's just two of you, it suits somehow: less itsy-bitsy and failed nouvelle. I have a special fondness for the marinated quail below because I remember cooking it with my sister Thomasina. Not that the cooking is so involved that it needs two people; but chopping and cooking, the companionability of the kitchen, is always sustaining. She adored this, and I suppose it just became incorporated into our comfortingly repetitive, private culinary repertoire. Together, we ate bowls of chicken broth with leeks and boiled potatoes; roast chicken and leeks in white sauce with boiled potatoes;

spaghettini with tomato sauce and lots of fresh basil on top. On the evening of her arrival, at the beginning of any weekend she stayed with me, we always shared taramasalata eaten with warm pitta, with, alongside on the table, a plate of hot crisp grilled bacon and a bunch of spring onions.

MARINATED, FLATTENED QUAIL

4 quails
1 tablespoon olive oil
½ tablespoon fresh rosemary needles, chopped very finely
2 bay leaves, crumbled
1 fat garlic clove, finely chopped or minced
2 tablespoons red wine
150ml meat stock (see below)

You have to start this well before you want to eat. If you don't mind fiddling about with meat first thing in the morning (and I don't), do it before going to work; otherwise do it before you go to bed the previous night. With kitchen shears, or any good scissors, trim the wing tips from the quails. Then cut along both sides of the backbone and remove the backbone, so the quails lie flat, or flattish. I do love a bit of surgery. Give the quails a wipe all over with kitchen towel.

Mix together the oil, rosemary, bay leaves and garlic. Sprinkle the quails, both sides, with salt and pepper, then rub the herb mixture into the flesh. It looks as if there's not a lot of the herb mixture, I know, but what you have is enough. Remember, I said rub, not smear. Arrange in a single layer on a baking sheet or something flat that will fit in the fridge, cover with foil or clingfilm, and leave in the fridge for at least 6 hours, preferably twice as long.

When you want to eat, heat a large, heavy-bottomed frying pan (if you've got the wrists for it, a cast-iron affair is ideal here), or two if you don't think you can fit all four quail, flat-out as they are, in one. If you don't feel safe using the pans you've got without adding oil first, then do so, otherwise just wipe off the marinade and put the quails, skin side down, in the hot pan for about 5 minutes. Prod or move with a spatula every now and again to make sure they don't stick: you may want to turn the heat down after the first searing minute. When the skin's dark and meat juices start appearing on the upper side of the quails, turn them over for a moment, just to sear the bone side. Remove to a large warmed plate and cover with foil.

Turn the heat back to high and to the pan with its meat juices add the wine (and if you've got no wine open and won't be drinking with the quail, use Marsala), let half of it bubble away, and then pour in the stock. You can use stock cubes here: I use my Italian ones, gusto classico, and I make the broth up slightly weak; 150ml boiling water to ¼ cube. Let the stock bubble away in the pan until it is greatly reduced, becoming thick and syrupy. Pour these juices over the quail. To be frank, you can just use the wine with an equal amount of water and forget about the stock altogether. I like to eat this in my fingers, with bread, salad, tomatoes, spring onions, ham or bacon, maybe some beans, elsewhere on the table. This is picnic food. And obviously, you can alter the marinade: try chilli pepper, sesame oil, coriander, oriental basil, soy, the usual suspects, deglazing with sake and/or mirin.

Serves 2.

The fact that there might be only two of us eating would never prevent my roasting and eating a chicken (see page 8). Cold chicken sandwiches – bread, cut thick, chicken, mango chutney, just possibly mayonnaise, and lettuce – are the dinner I dream of, for myself, the next day, or any time. I might want a packet of crisps with it.

LEFTOVERS

Leftovers come into their own when you're eating alone: I love a really fruitful mopping-up exercise. The fabulousness of leftovers is their randomness. I'm the sort of person who can't throw away half a cold cooked potato or a tablespoon of yesterday's gravy. But, of course, it's impossible to know what might be lurking in anyone else's fridge. If you have leftover potatoes, slice and fry them up. Or mash them into a patty, with some softened onions, some chopped cooked greens, maybe an egg yolk, then fry and pour the heated, slightly diluted, leftover gravy over them. Or bind the potatoes with the gravy and top with the egg, poached. Or cut a slice of leftover meat into chips and make a salad with warm potato, gherkins, chives, lettuce and chopped hard-boiled egg. Whatever you have, eat it. Somehow, however lovingly I've done my shopping, it's the food I haven't planned on cooking that I want most to eat.

Other times, when there are two of you, you might want something not exactly fussier, but more elegantly composed, dinner rather than supper. Actually, I'd have no compunction about making this chicken with morels just for me: it's hardly difficult, and I don't know what there is about it, maybe the creamy old-fashionedness, that makes me sometimes, definitely and distinctly, yearn for it. I have a feeling, which memory doesn't actually ratify, that my mother or grandmother must have cooked something similar. Anyway, this is what I do.

CHICKEN WITH MORELS

15g dried morels
1 tablespoon butter
1 teaspoon garlic-infused olive oil, or ordinary olive oil
4 chicken thighs
1 small onion, chopped finely
1 clove garlic, minced (if not using garlic-infused oil)
2 tablespoons Marsala
1/3 Italian porcini stock cube, or 1/3 chicken stock cube, again preferably Italian
1–2 tablespoons mascarpone
freshly chopped parsley

Put the morels into a measuring jug and pour over hot (but not boiling) water to reach the 200ml mark. Leave for at least 1/2 hour.

Put the butter and oil into a pan which has a lid, and in which the 4 chicken thighs will fit snugly enough, and when hot put the chicken pieces in, skin side down. Cook for about 10 minutes, maybe slightly less, until the skin has lost its goose-pimply pallor and has become a warm golden brown. Remove to a plate, skin side up.

Into the pan now put the very finely chopped onion (and garlic, too, if you haven't used that incredibly useful standby, the garlic-infused oil) and cook at a low to medium heat until soft.

Drain the morels, reserving the soaking liquid (you'll have about 150ml). Strain this brown and aromatic water (I use a tea strainer) into another small saucepan and put on another hob: you want it hot. Inspect the morels (you can do this by feel, using fingers), remove any grit or gravel and add the morels to the pan with the onion. Put back the chicken pieces, this time skin side up, and add the Marsala. To the mushroom-soaking liquid in the nearby saucepan, add 1/3 stock cube, and dissolve. Pour this into the pan too and put the lid on. Let it bubble away, but not vociferously so, for about 20–25 minutes, by which time the chicken should be cooked through. Remove the chicken thighs to a plate while you reduce the sauce. You needn't remove the morels (though you can) but do push them to the edges of the pan so they don't get hit by the full blast of the fire. Using an ordinary dessertspoon, ladle out any fat you might see collecting about the edges of this still-fluid sauce; some chicken pieces can give off a lot of watery fat.

Turn the flame up high and let the mushroomy, chickeny, Marsala-deepened sauce thicken: depending on the dimensions of your pan, the material it is made of, the hob you're using, this could take 5 minutes or it could take 15. And it depends on how much sauce you want at the end. I stop when the sauces in the pan look as if they could be generously spooned over and around the chicken pieces without turning it into soup. When it's the right consistency to your mind (and this isn't a crucial decision: it will taste delicious whatever), add the mascarpone. One heaped tablespoon (and by tablespoon, of course, I mean the usual 15ml measure, which is not vast) should be enough, but add more if you want a paler, richer, more buttery sauce. Sometimes I add a glug more Marsala too. Taste.

Put the chicken pieces back in the pan, spooning the oaky-brown sauce over them. Sprinkle with freshly chopped parsley and serve – with plain boiled or steamed waxy potatoes or a floury and absorbent mash, or just plain boiled rice – and eat a pale, crisp and astringent green salad after.

Serves 2.

STEAK BÉARNAISE

The essence of eating for two exists in just one word: steak. I'm not saying I wouldn't cook it just for me, but there's something solid, old-fashioned and comforting about the two of you sitting down and eating steak. Too often when I'm at home alone I waft along, as you do, in a tangle of noodles, lemon grass and suchlike. Steak béarnaise is my dream. Fry a steak as a steak is fried, on a hot pan and for a short time. Turn to page 17 for a recipe for béarnaise. I don't do frites. Green salad made bloody with the steak's juices, and some real baguette, more than make up, in my book, for my chip deficiency; but then I live practically next door to a chip shop, so if I'm eating with someone who takes a less tolerant line, I'm safe. Just as I think that roast chicken is so good that I need a lot of persuading to cook it any other way, so I feel about steak that it is perfect simply grilled or fried. But steak au poivre, aux poivres, peppered steak, whichever handle you like to put on it, is, in shorn form, a forceful contender. For me it's better without the addition of cream; I like my steak butch, brown and meaty. This is hardly the orthodox approach, and I can see that you might feel a culinary classic ought to be respected. Sometimes I'd even agree. Just go cautiously. You don't want to feel you're having pudding at the same time.

I use either black peppercorns, half black, half white or, more often, a many-berried pepper mixture: some of the mixture isn't strictly speaking pepper at all, but I like its warm aromatic quality, rather mellower than the heat of pepper alone. I have been meaning for years now to buy a coffee grinder especially for spices, but still haven't managed to do so and use a pestle and mortar.

STEAK AU POIVRE

2 middle-cut rump steaks (or sirloin if you prefer), about 3cm thick
scant tablespoon olive oil
3 tablespoons peppercorns, ground coarsely (see above)
3 tablespoons butter, plus more if liked
3 tablespoons brandy

Using a pastry brush if you've got one, paint the steaks on both sides with oil; you should need not more than a teaspoon on each side. Then dredge the oily steaks in the mashed peppercorns: you want a good crusty coat. If the corns are too coarse, they'll just fall off; if they're too fine, you won't stop coughing when you eat them.

In a heavy-bottomed pan, put the remaining oil to heat up. Add the steaks, and sear on each side, then, over moderate heat, add the butter and another drop of olive oil and cook the steaks for about another 3 minutes a side or to requisite bloodiness. Remove to warmed plates. Turn the heat up to high again, then pour in the brandy, stirring well all the time to deglaze the pan. When you've got a thick syrupy glaze, taste it: you may want to add salt, and you may want to whisk in a little butter just to help it all taste and look smooth and amalgamated. This, too, is where you could add your dollop of cream if you wanted. I've also, instead of the brandy, used Marsala, without which I'm pathologically incapable of existing, and it was dee-licious.

Serves 2.

Real carpaccio, as invented by Harry's Bar, and served up in modish joints all over the northern and southern hemispheres, really is restaurant food – though for mechanical rather than culinary reasons. If you've got a slicer or can otherwise be sure of producing the correct, tissue-paper thin slices, by all means try it. Otherwise, do what any sensible, greedy person would do and work along the lines of the recipe in Richard Whittington and Alastair Little's seminal book, *Keep It Simple*. This is my adaptation: some quantities are changed, ingredients modified; I don't use the truffled oil the authors specify, because the first time I did this I didn't have any. Now I feel that it might interfere, so I use olive oil to dress the salad and replace their specified balsamic vinegar with lemon juice. And I use less cheese. But that's what you should do when cooking: you draw on your own tastes and adapt according to your personality. I wouldn't suggest substituting like for unlike, or not paying respect to the natural lie of a dish, but lemon, vinegar, oil, schmoil: don't get het up.

HOME CARPACCIO OF BEEF

250g beef fillet, cut from the tail end
4 tablespoons peppercorns
approx. 150ml olive oil
200g rocket (or other soft leafy salad)
½ lemon
85g piece parmesan

If the meat's been in the fridge, take it out a good ½ hour before cooking. Coarsely grind the peppercorns (see steak au poivre recipe, above); again I use my pestle and mortar. Put a griddle (smooth side) or cast-iron pan on to get really hot. Brush the fillet all over with a little oil, then dredge to coat with the coarsely ground peppercorns.

Fill a bowl with iced water, put the fillet to sear in the hot pan and give it 60 seconds on each side – and that's all six sides, the ends as well as the top and bottom, so that it's encased in searedness. Use tongs, ones that won't pierce the meat, to turn and hold the meat in place as you sear. Plunge the seared meat into the iced water, then take out, pat dry with kitchen paper and leave to cool. You can do this in advance, and put it in the fridge for a few days.

When you're ready to eat, take the meat out of the fridge and let it get to room temperature. Strew the salady bits on two plates. I never wash salad if I can get away with not, but if you suspect there might be even the slightest bit of grit, then do so. Dribble oil over the salad, sprinkle some salt and squeeze some lemon juice and, using your hands, turn to coat well but lightly.

Carve – cutting slightly on the diagonal – the fillet into thinnish but not wafer-like slices, but you can go chunkier if you want, and divide between the plates. Using a vegetable peeler, shave the cheese into thin curls and let them fall over the top of the steak and salad. I rather like this with some steamed waxy potatoes which, when cooked, are peeled and sliced into thick coins and laid, warm, on the plate with the salad, under the cold dull-ruby slices of fillet.

Serves 2.

Man cannot live on steak alone. Anyone who really likes eating likes stew. This one, which comes via Nigel Slater's *Real Cooking* is as wonderful as you'd expect anything of his to be. I love his writing, and his food: both of which inspire and comfort and at the same time, which is more than most of us deserve. This particular recipe has another virtue: it's the perfect amount for two slathering, stew-deprived people; or even one, as I can testify.

LAMB AND BEAN BRAISE

Apart from some initial rough chopping, this is an almost hands-free exercise – low effort, high yield. You do need to soak the beans and steep the lamb, but if you do them before you leave for work in the morning, you'll be ready for the off when you get back in the evening. I suppose you could always use tinned beans, but I can't honestly say that turning on the tap, and later the hob, are either of them fearsome strains.

300g dried cannellini beans
4 middle neck chops, about 6–7cm thick
1 medium-sized onion, cut into wedges
2 bay leaves
few springs thyme
2 sticks celery, sliced
2 carrots, sliced
3 cloves garlic, squashed
5 peppercorns
1 large dried chilli, or 2 small
1 orange
1 bottle red wine
3 tablespoons olive oil
2 large, flat, brown mushrooms, quartered
1 tablespoon balsamic vinegar

Soak the beans in cold water for a day, or overnight. Put the lamb, onion, herbs, celery, carrots, garlic, peppercorns and chilli in a large bowl. Shave off some orange peel – 6cm or so, it isn't crucial – with a vegetable peeler and add it to the dish of meat and vegetables, along with the rest of the orange, pith, peel and all, sliced. Pour over the wine to cover. I tend to use the whole bottle, since it's going to end up in the stew anyway. If you want to drink wine with the stew, get two bottles (or indeed more). Put the bowl of meat and vegetables somewhere cool or in the fridge.

When the beans have soaked and the meat steeped, drain the beans, put them in a saucepan, cover by about 10cm with cold water, bring to the boil and then let boil for about 20 minutes. Put the lid on and remove from the heat.

Strain the meat and vegetables over another bowl, in other words reserve the wine. Throw out the orange slices, but keep the strip of peel, and I get rid of the chilli at this stage, too.

Now get a thick-bottomed casserole which has a lid that goes with it and melt the oil in it. Pick out the bits of lamb from the sieve or colander and brown on all sides. Remove to a plate and put the rest of the stuff that you had marinading in the casserole to soften, adding the mushrooms. If the mushrooms are very big, cut them into eighths rather than quarters or, indeed, any old how: mathematical precision is not required. Cook for 10 minutes or so and then pour in the wine from the marinade (and the rest of the bottle if you didn't use it all earlier). Add the drained beans.

Bring to the boil over a medium heat, but turn it down just before it actually boils. Add the balsamic vinegar (though it's wonderful without, too) and put the lamb back in. Cover the pot with greaseproof paper. Stick on the lid tightly. This is to help stop the liquid evaporating.

Leave to simmer gently for about 1½ hours. The meat should be tender enough to come away from the bone and the beans soft enough to squish, at the push of a wooden spoon, against the side of the dish. Prod both meat and beans to check.

Turn up the heat and cook, uncovered, at a vigorous bubble until all of a sudden the juices thicken. This may take about 10 minutes, but be vigilant: it may not need to be much more concentrated than it is already. Taste for salt and pepper. I eat this in a shallow soup bowl, with a wodge or three of good bread, buttered or not as I feel.

Serves 2.

PEAS

Every day I thank God, or his supermarket stand-in, for frozen peas. For me, they are a leading ingredient, a green meat, almost. I don't eat them that much, straight, as a vegetable, but I'd hate to have to cook without them. The almost instant soup – a handful of peas, a jugful of stock, a rind of cheese, whatever's to hand – that I make for a sweetly restoring supper is itemised in Fast Food on page 180. The pea risotto that follows is another regular. Risotto is best suited to two. I like relative peace in which to cook it, and I prefer handling small quantities. It is also the world's best comfort food.

The quantities I use might be nearer those ordinarily specified for four; but when I cook risotto I don't want to eat anything else after. And I feel a pang if there's only enough for one middling-sized flat puddle of the stuff.

PEA RISOTTO

I specify frozen petits pois, simply because that's what I always use. I have used real peas, just podded, to make *risi e bisi*, the fabulously named Venetian slurpily soft risotto, or thick rice soup, however you like to think of it, complete with pea-pod stock. But to be frank, if you don't grow peas yourself, then there is not a huge advantage in using fresh ones. By the time they're in the shops, they're big and starchy and without that extraordinary, almost floral, scent; that heady but contained sweetness of peas just picked from the garden.

On the whole, I take the peas out and let them thaw before using them. But I don't see that it makes much difference.

As for stock: I haven't specified any in particular. When I can, I use ham stock which, because of my stock-making obsession, I usually have in the freezer; otherwise I make up some Marigold vegetable granules. I wouldn't use a dark beef stock here, but any chicken, veal or light broth would be fine.

60g butter
150g frozen petits pois
approx. 1 litre stock
2 tablespoons freshly grated parmesan, plus more for the table
grated nutmeg
1 small onion or, even better, banana shallot
drop of oil
200g arborio or Canaroli rice
80ml white wine or vermouth

Put about ⅓ of the butter in a pan and when it's melted add the peas, and cook, stirring every now and again, for 2 minutes. Remove half the peas and to the remaining half in the pan add a ladleful of the stock. Put a lid on the pan and let cook gently for about 5 minutes or so till soft. Purée this mixture – I use the mini electric chopper I used to use for baby food – with 1 tablespoon each of grated parmesan and butter and a grating each of pepper and fresh nutmeg.

Meanwhile, chop the onion or shallot very finely, and melt another tablespoon of butter, with a drop of oil in it, in a pan. Cook the onion, stirring with your wooden prodder, for about four minutes, then add the rice and stir till every grain glistens with the oniony fat. Pour in the wine or vermouth (last time I did this I used Chambéry and it was fabulous: it seemed to add to the grassy freshness of the peas) and let it bubble away and absorb. Then add a ladleful of the hot stock (I keep it on low on the neighbouring hob) and stir until this too is absorbed. Carry on in this vein, patiently, for another 10 minutes, then add the whole, just sautéed peas, and then start again, a ladleful of stock at a time. In about another 8 minutes or so the rice should be cooked and the risotto creamy. Taste to see if you need any more time or liquid. It's hard to be precise: sometimes you'll find you have stock left over; at others you'll need to add water from the kettle.

When you're happy with it, add the buttery pea and parmesan purée and beat it in well. Taste, season as needed, then beat in the remaining tablespoon of parmesan and any butter you may have left. You can sprinkle over some chopped flat-leaf parsley (and since I've got it growing in the garden I have no reason not to), but the lack of it won't give you any grief.

Serves 2.

The first time I made pea soufflé (in response to an urgent request) I had no cheese in the house other than some processed gruyère and emmenthal slices, and so had to chop those up small in place of the real grated stuff – and may I tell you they were absolutely delicious. I now keep them in the fridge and I always have egg whites in the freezer. Making a soufflé is no longer a kitchen requirement for the aspiring hostess; but it's always worth tackling recipes that scare you with their attendant mythologies, just so that you're no longer cramped by that lurking fear. Read carefully and you'll see that absolutely no culinary pyrotechnics are called for.

PEA SOUFFLÉ

85g gruyère, grated
120g frozen petits pois
30g butter plus more for greasing
15g flour, preferably Italian 00
125ml full-fat milk
pinch ground mace or freshly grated nutmeg
2 eggs plus 1 extra egg white

Preheat the oven to gas mark 6/200°C and put a baking tray in it to heat up. Butter a soufflé dish with about a 600ml capacity if you've got one. Otherwise any same-sized casserole or container, preferably round, should do. If you've got any parmesan to hand, then you could grate some over the buttered soufflé dish, tapping the dish so that it's lightly covered with it, much as you would when flouring a greased cake tin.

Put 15g butter in a pan and cook the peas till soft. Purée them with the grated cheese and set aside while you make the paste-thick white sauce. Melt the remaining 15g butter in a thick-bottomed pan and stir in the flour. Cook, still stirring, for 2–3 minutes, then, off the heat, very gradually whisk in the milk. When all is smoothly amalgamated, put back over a low heat and cook, stirring regularly, for about 5 minutes, or until the sauce is thick and all flouriness gone; if you're using ordinary plain flour you may find that you need another 5 minutes. Let the white sauce cool slightly.

Separate the eggs: put the yolks, unbeaten, aside for a while. If you've got a lemon in the house, slice it in half and wipe its cut side around the interior of a bowl – preferably copper or else other metal. Put in all the egg whites and a pinch of salt, and whisk until they stand in soft peaks. You want the whites firm, but not dry or stiff.

Leave them for a moment and then add 1 yolk to the white sauce, beating well, then add the other and beat that in. Then beat in the cheese and pea purée. Taste for salt and pepper and sprinkle on the mace or grate over the nutmeg. Remember the egg whites will damp down the intensity. Take a clean spoon and add a big dollop of the whisked whites to the now pea-green sauce. Beat this in as roughly as you like: you could use an electric whisk and it wouldn't matter; the idea is just to lighten the mixture to make it easier to fold the remaining egg whites in gently, which you should now do.

When the whites have been serenely and lightly folded in pour the mixture into the prepared dish – it should be about 3/4 full – and put it on the baking tray in the oven. Immediately turn the heat down to gas mark 4/180°C and cook for about 30 minutes or until the soufflé is risen to well above the rim of the dish. I'm presuming you've got an oven with a glass door and a light that works so that you can see the action inside.

Take out of the oven and eat immediately. This is intended to be supper in its entirety, it's not a delicate taster before something more substantial. Mind you, some prosciutto eaten alongside is not a bad idea.

Serves 2.

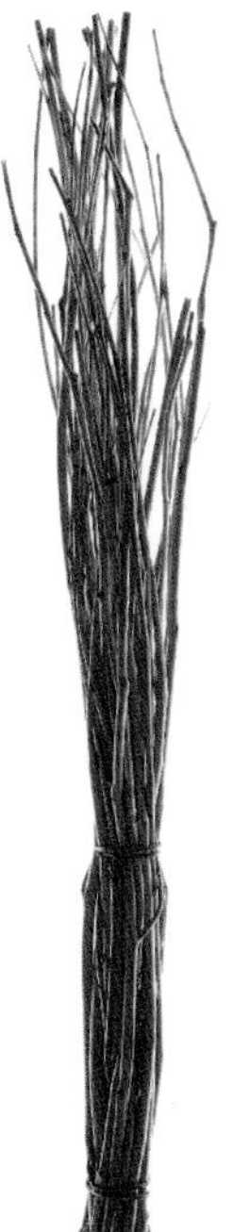

In theory, at least, I prefer meatier, chunkier soups (preferably with pasta in, too), but when I need soothing rather than bolstering, this nostalgic chicken soup is unparalleled.

CREAM OF CHICKEN SOUP

I use those spindly little dwarf – or baby – leeks (speciality of the sprauncier supermarkets), but ordinary, still slender, leeks, just *very* finely sliced, would do. In either case, discard most of the green part: you want this creamily white, not a pale, lurid lime green. I happily use my Italian chicken stock cubes here: half of one in 300ml water will be fine.

45g butter
200g dwarf leeks, sliced very finely
300ml chicken stock
300ml full-fat milk
2 bay leaves
1 clove garlic, peeled
1 free-range chicken breast fillet
1 tablespoon flour, preferably Italian 00
pinch ground mace
3–4 tablespoons double cream
1 egg yolk

Put 30g butter in a thick-bottomed saucepan, melt it and in it cook the leeks gently until soft. Meanwhile, put the stock and milk in a saucepan with the bay leaves, clove of garlic and chicken breast. Bring up to the boil, then turn down to a simmer and cook until the chicken breast is just tender. I know it sounds not very long, but about another 5 minutes should do it. A couple or so minutes before the chicken's ready, the leeks should be soft and cooked enough. Into the leek mixture stir 1 tablespoon of flour and cook on a low heat, stirring, for a couple or so minutes.

By this time the chicken should be ready to come out, so remove it and pour the milk and stock with the bay leaves and garlic into the floury leeks, stirring while you do so. Bring up to below the boil, stirring occasionally. While you're not stirring, shred or finely chop the chicken and add to the pan. Add a pinch of salt and keep cooking over a lowish heat, stirring occasionally, for 5 minutes. Add 15g butter and cook in the same way for another 5 minutes. If it looks as if it's getting too thick and white-saucey, just add a glug of full-fat milk or as much as you feel you need.

Pour into a blender in batches of about 10cm of liquid at a time and whizz and then push through a sieve back into the rinsed-out saucepan.

Put back on the heat, stirring until warm enough to eat. Mix the egg yolk and double cream together and, off the heat, stir into the soup.

Serves 1–2.

BUTTERNUT AND PASTA SOUP

This is robuster stuff altogether: I make it for lunch when it's cold and I want to cook something easy but with some distracting chopping involved. My usual, the Marigold vegetable bouillon powder, is pulled out here.

1/2 tablespoon olive oil
1/2 small onion, chopped very finely
250g butternut squash, peeled and cut in 1cm cubes
60ml white wine or vermouth
600ml stock
1 bay leaf
60g ditalini or other soup pasta

Put the oil in a biggish, heavy-bottomed pan on the hob and when hot add the onion. Cook for about 10 minutes, stirring regularly, until soft, then add the cubes of butternut and turn well in the pan for 2 minutes. Pour in the wine, let it bubble up, then add the stock and bay leaf. Bring to simmering point, then leave to simmer away for about 10 minutes. Take out a ladleful, purée it, then put it back in the pan. Turn up the heat and add the ditalini. Cook for about 10–12 minutes until the pasta is cooked, then ladle this thick, sweet stew of a soup into your bowl. Grate parmesan over as you eat.

Serves 2.

I see in my notes I've called this Sunday Night Chicken Noodle, and it's true I do often cook this, or a version of it, on Sunday nights. But if I do, I almost certainly have to have a rerun on Monday evening.

SUNDAY NIGHT CHICKEN NOODLE

4 tablespoons sake
3 tablespoons mirin
1 tablespoon soy sauce
1 fat clove garlic, crushed with flat of knife
1 dried red chilli pepper
1 free-range chicken breast
100g fresh noodles
handful choi sum or other Oriental greens
1 tablespoon oil plus few drops sesame oil
500ml chicken stock (a cube's fine)
fresh coriander

Mix the sake, mirin, soy, garlic and chilli. Cut the chicken into strips, put in a bowl and cover with this marinade. Leave for an hour.

Cook the noodles in boiling salted water and throw in the choi sum for the last 2 minutes' cooking. Drain. Heat up the stock.

Into a hot wok or frying pan pour the oils and, when they in turn are hot, throw in the pieces of chicken and toss about till cooked. Pour over the marinade and when it's bubbled nearly away and the chicken is glossy and dark, put the noodles in a bowl, pour the stock over them and top with the pieces of wok-bronzed chicken. Sprinkle over some freshly chopped coriander and eat. Serves 1.

SPAGHETTI AGLIO OLIO

Pasta is inevitably, these days, what one eats just in the normal run of things in the evening. You don't need a recipe for this any more than you do for bacon sandwiches, but this is not meant to be a manual to cook from so much as a prompt or companion guide to eating. These, then, are suggestions based on a presumption of interest rather than barked instructions to be carried out to the patronising letter. At home, alone, especially if I've been working late, I make a vast bowl of *spaghetti aglio olio* (sometimes, *peperoncino*): just spaghetti, or spaghettini, turned in some olive oil, in which some fat cloves of garlic have been turned till golden then discarded, with maybe a sprinkling of dried red chilli pepper. A glass of cold beer is wonderful with it. If you are so exhausted you want an even easier version, then I suggest you buy a bottle of garlic-infused olive oil.

LINGUINE WITH LARDONS

If you've got some lardons, make yourself a particularly good, particularly low-effort supper. Get in from work. Run your bath. Preheat the oven to gas mark 7/210°C. Put some fat lardons on a baking tray with a few cloves of garlic, peeled and roughly chopped. (Leave the garlic whole if you haven't the energy for even rough chopping.) Throw over 1 tablespoon olive oil. Put the water for the pasta on to boil and put the tray of garlic and lardons in the oven. When the water's boiling, add salt and throw in the pasta – linguine or spaghetti – and run up to your bath, taking with you the timer, set for 10 minutes (the pasta should take about 12 minutes). When the timer goes off, rush down in your towel, taste the pasta and, when it's ready, drain it, reserving a coffeecupful of water. Take the lardons out of the oven and toss the pasta in them, adding a drop or two of the cooking water if you think it needs lubrication. Decant into a bowl and, if you like, take it back up to the bath with you.

SPAGHETTI CARBONARA

This is my favourite – along with all my other favourites. I love the buttery, eggy creaminess of the sauce, saltily-spiked with hot-cubed pancetta: it's comforting, but not in a sofa-bound kind of way. It feels like proper dinner, only it takes hardly any time to cook. This is my most regular dinner for two: I keep, at all times, the wherewithal to make it in the house. You can add double cream to the egg-and-cheese mixture if you want – a couple of tablespoons, but then use 2 yolks only, rather than one yolk and one whole egg – but this takes it away from being something one can get together with ingredients to hand. On this ease-of-assembly principle, do by all means substitute 3 or 4 rashers of streaky bacon, cut into strips, for the pancetta. But it's not so hard to buy several 100g chunks of pancetta at one time and just bag them up and freeze them separately; this, really, is what I'd advise.

200g spaghetti
2 teaspoons olive oil
100g pancetta in one piece
4 tablespoons (60ml) Noilly Prat (or white wine)
1 egg yolk
1 whole egg
4 tablespoons (about 20g) freshly grated parmesan
black pepper and fresh nutmeg
1 mounded tablespoon butter (about 20g)

Put some water on and when it's boiling add a decent amount of salt and then, when it's boiling again, the pasta. Italians say the water pasta cooks in should be as salty as the Mediterranean. Cut the rind off the pancetta and put the rind in the pan with the oil on medium to high while you dice the rest of the pancetta, or cut into chunky strips. Then add it and fry for about 5 minutes, maybe more, until it is beginning to crisp. Throw in the vermouth and let it bubble away for about 3 minutes until you have about 2 teaspoons or so of syrupy wine-infested bacon fat. Remove from the heat, unless you have so brilliantly timed it that the egg mixture is prepared and the pasta cooked.

For the egg mixture, simply beat the yolk, the whole egg, the cheese, the pepper and the nutmeg (the pancetta or bacon and the cheese should provide enough salt) together with a fork. When the pasta's ready, quickly put the bacon pan back on the heat, adding the butter as you do so. Give the pasta a good shake in the colander (but mind it isn't too drained) and then turn it into the hot pan. Turn it with a spatula and a wooden spoon, or whatever works for you, and then when it's all covered and any excess liquid absorbed, turn off the heat (take the pan away from the hob if your stove's electric), pour the egg mixture over the bacony pasta and quickly and thoroughly turn the pasta so that it's all covered in the sauce. Be patient: whatever you do, don't turn the heat back on or you'll have scrambled eggs; in time, the hot pasta along with the residual heat of the pan will set the eggs to form a thickly creamy sauce that binds and clings lightly to each strand of pasta.

This makes two platefuls: it's up to you whether you conclude this is enough for one or two of you; I incline towards two for lunch and one for dinner.

PASTA WITH BUTTER AND STOCK-CUBE JUICES

The Italians do a wonderful pasta sauce which is really just the meat juices left in the roasting pan after their particularly flavoursome way of cooking rosbif. They make it with the rosemary-spiked juices left from a roast chicken, too, and you can adapt this to the last-minute, store-cupboard school of cookery by melting part of a crumbled stock cube in some rosemary-flecked butter. Again I like linguine here, but spaghetti's good, too.

While about 100g of pasta is cooking – I'm taking it you're eating this alone, but just double for two of you – melt 2 tablespoons butter in a saucepan, add 1 teaspoon olive oil and 2 peeled garlic cloves, crushed with the flat of a knife. When the butter starts fizzing, throw in the very finely chopped leaves from a finger-length sprig of rosemary. When the cloves of garlic turn brown, remove them and in their place crumble in about ½ a meat or chicken stock cube, preferably Italian. Turn in the pan, adding another dollop of butter, and then add 1 tablespoon white wine or vermouth and 1 tablespoon water and

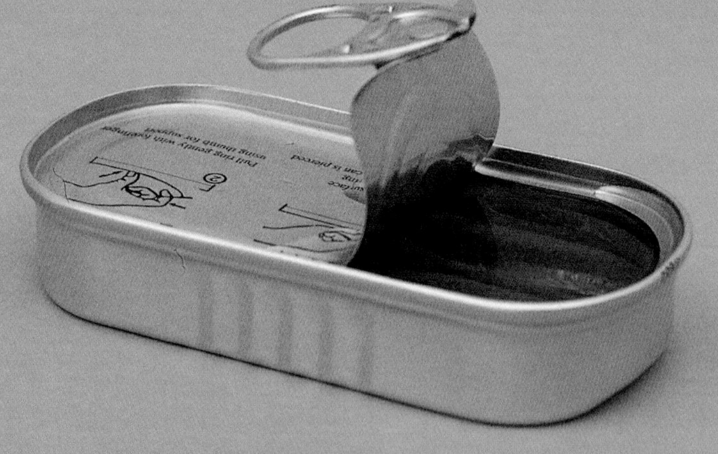
Pull ring gently with forefinger
using thumb for support
can is pierced

carry on cooking for a minute or so before spooning in another nut of butter.

When the pasta's ready, drain it, reserving a small cupful of water. Toss the pasta in the stock sauce, adding some of the water if the pasta absorbs too much of the liquid too fast. Grate over some parmesan and eat.

PASTA WITH UNPESTOED PESTO

In summer, when you might consider eating outside, make a large bowl, just for the two of you, of linguine with what I think of as pesto in its discrete parts: we're talking culinary deconstruction here. While the pasta's cooking, pour some, preferably Ligurian, olive oil into a large pan and throw in some peeled cloves of garlic. Cook over gentle heat until the garlic colours and its scent wafts upwards. Remove the cloves from the pan and the pan from the heat. Roughly tear up or shred a mound of basil leaves, set aside, and, in a dry frying pan, toast a handful or so of pine nuts. When the pasta's ready, drain it, toss it in the garlic-infused olive oil, then transfer to a warm bowl. Grate over some parmesan, then, using a vegetable peeler, shave in some pecorino (and, frankly, it doesn't matter if you use parmesan for both grating and shaving: who wouldn't, really?), and sprinkle with the toasted pine nuts. Toss well, throw over all but a small handful of the basil leaves, and turn again. Grate a little more cheese over and sprinkle with the remaining shredded basil leaves. Leave the bottle of oil within reach.

Mostly, when I'm cooking some pasta for myself I want it to take as little time as possible. But I don't mind that the recipe which follows is, well, not laborious, but time-consuming. I just love it. It's a version of the Venetian bigoli in salsa, the salsa in question being a pungent, long-cooked, almost emulsified sauce of onions and anchovies. Bigoli are the only pasta with an excuse for being wholewheat: that's how they are traditionally made. I made this the first time, though, to use up some spelt pasta I had. I'd been writing a piece for *Vogue* on farro and had been sent, as part of the requested consignment, some pasta made with this grain. I tried it once and loathed it. Then it occured to me that with a heartier sauce, something with real depth to it, it might work. I tried this, and was transported, converted. I've made it since many times with ordinary spaghetti – which works fine – and you can use any wholewheat version of pasta. And any long, hollow pasta, such as perciatelli or bucatini (in effect, non-wholewheat bigoli) is wonderful here. If you're intent on locating spaghetti di farro, turn to page 506 and the list of mail-order companies.

PASTA WITH ANCHOVY SAUCE

My mother always soaked anchovies in milk, just as she did kidneys and chicken livers, therefore so do I. The inclusion of Marsala is a non-Venetian innovation, but its dry, deep mellowness works well with the fierce saltiness of the anchovies.

What makes this ideal for me for eating alone is that I don't need to worry about any other person's tiresomeness about anchovies. An average-sized tin of anchovies should give you, when drained, 25–30g, or about 12 fillets.

15g anchovy fillets in olive oil (drained weight - about 6 fillets)
approx. 6 tablespoons full-fat milk
2 tablespoons olive oil
1 medium onion, sliced very finely (use a processor if possible)
2 tablespoons Marsala
100g pasta (see above)
2 heaped tablespoons freshly chopped flat-leaf parsley

Remove the anchovies from the tin, wipe with kitchen towel, put in a dish – a ramekin, say – and cover with milk; about 2 tablespoons should do it. In a heavy-bottomed pan, heat 1 tablespoon oil and then the onion. Cook uncovered over a low heat for about 5 minutes, then add the Marsala and cook for about 30 minutes, till you have a soft, golden, oniony mush. You may need to sprinkle in some water while it's cooking to keep it from drying up or sticking to the pan. If you make a lid out of foil and press down on the top of the onions (rather than the pan) this will help. Then turn up the heat and cook uncovered for a minute or 2, stirring to prevent sticking. While all this is going on, put on some water for the pasta.

Remove the anchovies from the milk and chop them finely. Add them to the onion mixture, stir well, pour in the milk in which they'd been soaking and keep stirring. When the anchovies have been incorporated into the purée, add 2 more tablespoons milk, the remaining tablespoon of oil and about half the parsley. Stir well and remove from the heat. Taste to see if you'd like some more milk; it will soften the taste and slacken the texture. When the pasta's cooked, drain it, and then quickly but thoroughly turn it in the warm anchovy and onion sauce. Transfer to your bowl or plate and sprinkle over the remaining parsley.

Serves 1.

When I'm cooking for myself, as you see, I want strong tastes. This kale with chorizo is one of my regular fast hot lunches.

KALE WITH CHORIZO AND POACHED EGG

Make sure you can get proper chorizo, and I mean here the fresh (or semi-dried, rather) sausages, not the larger cured salame. Sometimes these come in horseshoe-shaped linked sausage loops; in which case use half. If you don't like kale or it's not around, then a large packet of spinach and watercress salad, just wilted in the pan in which the chorizo's been cooking, will do – indeed more than do. It's a pleasurable variant rather than forced substitution.

175g kale
1 chorizo (approx. 100g)
1 egg
1 tablespoon ordinary oil

Put some water on to boil and when it boils, add salt. Remove the curly leaves of kale from the fibrous stems and tear the leaves into smallish pieces.

Cut the chorizo into slices about 5mm to 1cm thick and then cut these slices into quarters so that you have, finally, a chopping board heaped with oily orange confetti. Put the kale into the boiling salted water and cook till tenderish (kale is never going to be that tender and certainly shouldn't be floppy), which will take 5–7 minutes depending on its age.

Put 1 tablespoon oil in a heavy-bottomed, deepish frying pan and cook the chorizo pieces for a few minutes, stirring and pressing with a wooden spoon or spatula so that the paprika-red fat oozes out as the sausage cooks: 3 or so minutes should be fine. While all this is going on you should, as well as keeping an eye on the kale, be putting a pan of water on to poach the egg. I use that much despised thing, a shop-bought egg poaching pan with moulds. Drain the kale well and then stir into the chorizo. Put the egg in to poach and when it is ready, turn the orange-spliced kale on to a plate and turn out the poached egg on top.

Serves 1.

CHICK PEAS WITH SORREL

A comparable, desirable pungency is evoked by this bowl of chick peas and sorrel. If I've got some dried, cooked and soaked chick peas in a tub in the fridge (and I might have) I use them, but tinned, preferably organic (better textured) ones are fine. I first did this for the age-old reason that I needed to use something up, in this case some sorrel. There's a Middle-Eastern way with chick peas that I like, sour with lemon juice and thick with spinach. It occurred to me that using sorrel would provide the leafiness and the acidity: it does. For a drained 400g tin of chick peas, put 1 tablespoon olive oil in a pan and fry in it a small chopped onion – about 40g – with 2 finely sliced cloves of garlic and a good pinch of dried cumin. Crumble in ½ a dried red chilli pepper, sprinkle over a pinch of salt and cook, on a moderate heat, for about 5 minutes. Shred or chop a good handful, two-hands-cuppedful, of sorrel (about 50g) and throw into the onion pan. Throw in the drained chick peas after it and stir well till the sorrel's wilted and the chick peas are warm. I eat this from a large bowl with some more oil drizzled over it and warmed pitta. If this is supper, not lunch, I might make a cold plate of tomato salad to eat alongside, too.

INDULGENT DINNERS

I wouldn't want to suggest all cooking for one or two must necessarily be of the impromptu, quickly-thrown-together kind (and I say this as someone who is eating a Laughing Cow and plastic bread sandwich as she writes; very delicious it is, too). I don't mean it should be elaborate and minutely organised, but that cooking for two can be out of the ordinary in a way that a dinner party, unless you really are fabulously extravagant or very rich, just can't. The solitary diner can sometimes, if not often, eat lobster alone. I buy it cooked and cold and I fry some bacon to eat with it. I might make mayonnaise. I don't mind what I have to do to it or how I eat my lobster: salad, club sandwich (toast some brioche, just see), as it is in my fingers. The pleasure lies in the solitary indulgence.

My most intense solitary indulgence, without question, is grouse (see page 51); 12 August figures strongly in my diary. I'm not the type to go wading across moors, but I don't mind paying for my pleasures. Grouse are getting more expensive as they're becoming rarer, but my terrible worry is that soon they'll be extinct. This isn't an ecological concern, you understand, but a culinary one.

Plain roast grouse is wonderful enough; this is dreamlike. I'd never have thought of messing about with the perfect simplicity of the bird, but when we all went to the River Café on the eve of my sister Horatia and Inigo's wedding, we ate quail stuffed with mascarpone and thyme, and it was so deeply fabulous that I thought I'd try it with young grouse. The rest is culinary history – or it is in my house.

YOUNG GROUSE WITH MASCARPONE AND THYME

1 tablespoon butter
1 tablespoon olive oil
1 young grouse
approx. ½ a 250g tub mascarpone
3 tablespoons red wine (5 if cooking one grouse for two)
zest of ¼ of a lemon
small bunch fresh thyme (about 10 sprigs)

I am presuming the grouse is already draped in a couple of rashers of streaky bacon (that's how butchers seem to sell them now), but if it isn't then you can either get the bacon yourself or – as you don't necessarily want the taste and smell of bacon here – smear the breast thickly with butter to keep from drying out. Still, I kept the bacon on my grouse and it was delicious, so there's no crime in doing the same.

Heat the oven to gas mark 6/200°C. Put in a small roasting dish with the butter and oil in it. Remove the innards from the grouse and chop finely (I use my mezzaluna). Put the offally mess into a small bowl. Add 3 heaped tablespoons of mascarpone, a tablespoon of red wine, the zest of lemon and a vigorous amount of salt and pepper. Mix well: you should have a bowl of divinely pungent Biba-pink cream. Remove the thyme leaves from the sprigs – you want a good tablespoonful – and chop them finely. Again, I use my mezzaluna, but whatever you use make sure the thyme is well chopped, otherwise it will be woody and ruin the smooth aromatic creaminess of the sauce-stuffing.

Put the mascarpone mixture into the cavity of the grouse and put it in the roasting dish in the oven. Cook for 30–45 minutes. Some years the grouse are bigger than others, so it's hard to be specific about timing.

When it's ready, remove the grouse to a plate and put the roasting dish on the hob. Some of the mascarpone stuffing will have oozed out into the pan. This will form the basis for your sauce. Add to this gunge another tablespoon of mascarpone and a couple of tablespoons of red wine, stir well, scraping it all up. Let it bubble and then pour the sauce onto a warmed plate. Put the grouse on top and dive in. (If you're going to share the grouse with someone else you will need to double the final bit of wine and mascarpone to make enough sauce for the two of you.) I eat this with a big bowl of tender young kale with some butter stirred in and some nutmeg grated; mashed potatoes – for obvious reasons – are a pretty wonderful accompaniment, too.

Serves 1.

What, though, is in the back of my mind when I talk about the allowable and elegant excesses of eating for two is caviar. It would head my list of perfect dinners à deux. And this brings me to the subject of the seduction dinner. I am at the stage in my life when cooking for two is just about the shape of every day rather than the occasional lusty stab at culinary and extra-culinary conquest. But the seduction dinner is just a dinner party in miniature: the same constraints apply; and I advise those interested to turn to the Dinner chapter, with their calculator for ease of downsizing. For what it's worth, I still think (as I always do) that you can't go wrong with roast chicken. And I would be predisposed to respond warmly to anyone who had the cool grace to give me caviar to start. But, of course, I would prefer to buy my own caviar than be given it as part of the trade-off for a wearyingly unwelcome lunge.

And if a girl wants to eat caviar, a girl's got to know how to make blini. Sister, read on.

BLINI

SMOKED SALMON, CURED HERRING, SMETANA

First acquire your blini pan. In the context of caviar this is not a big expense (see Gazetteer for stockists). And I use my blini pan for much else besides: it happens to be the perfect size for a single, Cyclopean fried egg. Anyway, caviar is not obligatory with blini; I'm not sure they're not actually better with smoked salmon and salmon roe, pickled or cured herring, sour cream or smetana and a makeshift salsa of red onions chopped with capers. Really good caviar – and I like oscietra much better than beluga – needs nothing else but lightly toasted, heavily buttered Mother's Pride. But if you're going with the blini, provide some butter (unsalted of course, and either soft enough to be spread, or as the Russians do, poured in a little jug already melted) and either crème fraîche, sour cream or smetana; whichever you choose, use it in the blini batter.

The one difficulty with blini is not the yeast (though everyone seems phobically obsessed with that). Now that we have instant, or easyblend, yeast all you need to do is add it to the flour and proceed as normal – no frothing or any of that. And since all batters need to stand for a while, what does it matter that there's some yeast in it? I have tried, in the pursuit of science and reader-friendliness, to substitute baking powder, but without the yeast you lose that ethereal, moussy lightness. You just have buckwheat pancakes, which are fine enough, but they're not blini.

The real awkwardness is, I admit, to do with the yeast factor; you don't necessarily have a couple of hours to let the batter rise. So, I tried making up the batter in the morning and left it, not in a warm place for 2 hours, but in my fridge all day: it rose beautifully; they were the best blini ever. Which means that you can get back from work and take the batter out of the fridge, whisk up and add the egg white and you're ready to roll.

Before you start, preheat the oven to gas mark 2/150°C and put in a large plate. I like to make these when I've got a friend over. I make him or her sit on the stoop by my cooker, talking to me with a drink while I fry the blini and stash them, one by one, under a tin foil tent on the plate in the oven. I may throw one over while I'm making them, but the rest we eat at the table later: the perfect, companiable dinner.

This amount makes about 12 blini, which in my book (as this is) is just right for an entire meal, with additions admittedly, for two: you need to feel at the end that you *couldn't* eat another. Remember that as with all pancakes the first one is often a complete disaster. Once you've got the heat right and the feel of the pan, the rest will follow perfectly.

75g buckwheat flour
75g strong white flour
1 sachet easyblend yeast
½ teaspoon salt
½ teaspoon sugar
100ml milk
2 tablespoons crème fraîche (or sour cream or smetana and see above)
1 tablespoon butter, plus more for frying
1 egg, separated

Mix the flours, yeast, salt and sugar in a warm bowl (I let it sit, empty, in a sink of hot-tish water for a few minutes first). Pour 100ml of milk into a measuring jug and add the crème fraîche or the sour cream or whatever. Stir with a fork to combine well, and then add water so that the liquid comes up to the 250ml mark. Pour this liquid into a saucepan, add the butter and warm up till the butter melts. You don't want this actually hot, so leave it to cool slightly if, when you dip a finger in, it feels more than about blood heat.

Beat the egg yolk into the liquid and then pour this liquid into the flours and leave in a warmish place, covered with a damp tea-towel, for 2 hours (or all day in the fridge). Whisk the egg white till stiff but not dry, and fold into the batter.

Preheat the oven (and see above). Melt some butter and a little oil in a 10cm blini pan and, when hot, pour out the oil and start frying your blini. Each blini uses a couple of tablespoonfuls or so of batter; I dunk in my American quarter-cup measure and fill it about halfway. Fry the blini on the first side for a minute or two, until the batter starts bubbling on top, then flip it over with a spatula or palette knife and give about another minute. Don't whatever you do press down on the blini while it cooks. You want maximum fluffage here.

Of course, you can, without loss, make these in advance and keep them in fridge or freezer before reheating wrapped in foil in a gas mark 3/160°C oven, but nothing feels quite the same as making or eating blini hot from the pan.

If I had to choose a perfect, dream dinner, after the caviar and the roast chicken, it would have to be zabaione. It's not comfortable to make for any number larger than two.

Celestial though it is, it is not suitable for a seduction dinner. You don't want to have to stand up and start whirring away at a double boiler on the stove for a quarter of an hour at the end of dinner. Those of us who don't have such nervily romantic considerations to constrain us can plug ourselves into our electric mixers without embarrassment and for as long as it takes.

ZABAIONE

I use a stainless steel, round-bottomed bowl which I suspend over (but not touching) bubbling water in a pan. If you haven't got an electric beater, then just use a whisk: zabaione does, after all, predate the invention of the electric whisk; I dare say it predates the discovery of electricity.

2 egg yolks
25g caster sugar
60ml, or 4 tablespoons, Marsala

Put warm water in a pan on the heat, put the bowl you are using to construct your double boiler on top and in that bowl put the egg yolks and sugar. Start whisking them and continue whisking while the water heats up and starts to simmer: the egg mixture should become as thick as double cream and pale as butter; by the very end it should have tripled in volume. Continue whisking and slowly, slowly add the Marsala as you do so. When you have a soft, foaming, bulkily billowing mass, in short, when you have zabaione, you can stop whisking and spoon into a couple of glasses. This may be after a good ¼ hour's pneumatic whisking. Langue de chat are the biscuits to serve with it, or failing that, savoiardi.

Serves 2.

COMFORT FOOD

If you've got that lust for something soft and sweet, for babyfied comfort food, you might as well go flat out for it. Eating alone, I make what I remember my mother making for herself, bread and milk, in a large, cream china pudding basin. Put some torn up pieces of white bread in a bowl, sprinkle over some sugar and then pour in some hot milk. Eat, in an armchair, bowl on lap. If you keep vanilla sugar in the house, use that, but fiddle no further: this is not a dish which lends itself to great refinements.

BREAD AND MILK

BAKED SEMOLINA

More often than not I just make semolina as instructed on the back of the packet, the stirring kind: you just heat the semolina with vanilla and milk, adding sugar after it's thick and grainy and set, and dollop in jam once it's in the bowl. But baked semolina is just a snip above: comfort food with presence. You don't quite feel as if you're slobbing out on the sofa watching television and eating slops.

For some reason, I don't eat jam with this version of semolina, but drizzle from a gummy teaspoon a glowing, teak-coloured, dripping bead of honey.

vanilla pod or essence
500ml full-fat milk
3 tablespoons semolina
1 egg, separated
2–3 tablespoons sugar or vanilla sugar (to taste)
butter for greasing

Preheat the oven to gas mark 4/180°C and butter a dish with a 500ml capacity.

If you've got a vanilla pod, heat the milk in a pan and infuse it with the pod for 15 minutes. Otherwise just heat the milk, sprinkle in the semolina, stirring all the time to prevent lumps. After about 10 minutes the semolina should be cooked, swollen and thick. Leave to cool for about 10 minutes. Whisk the egg white till stiff: you may find this easier if you first wipe the bowl with the cut side of a lemon and sprinkle a little sugar into the whites.

Stir the yolk into the semolina and then the sugar and the vanilla extract, if you're using that. Add a good dollop of the whisked white, just to slacken the mixture, then fold the rest in gently. Pour into the waiting dish and bake in the oven for 35–45 minutes: the pudding will be risen, the top golden and blistered.

Serves 2.

I don't make puddings very often when there's just the two of us. I might do something with the plums or apples from the garden, maybe put together a crumble. The amount of actual crumble needed for a little pie dish is so small as not to be worth worrying about. You don't need to go dragging a machine into it.

APPLE AND WALNUT CRUMBLE

Crumble is a good way to start fiddling about with the idea of a crust: it's pastry really, only without the fear factor. Just plain, it's wonderful enough, especially on those grim days with saucepan-lid skies in late November and early February, but it's truly good as expanded here, with the nubbliness of the nuts and the almost honeyed crunchiness of the brown sugar. For two people who are wisely eating this with custard (see page 36 if you intend to make your own), ice-cream, crème fraîche or just old-fashioned cream in a jug (tick where applicable) but with nothing else before or after at all, use a pie dish of any sort with a capacity of about 500ml.

1 very large or 2 medium cooking apples
25g raisins or sultanas
3 tablespoons Marsala, warmed
100g plain flour
50g unsalted butter, cold and cut into little squares, plus more for greasing dish
60g walnuts (shelled weight), about 125g unshelled weight
45g light brown sugar, plus 1 heaped tablespoon

Heat oven to gas mark 5/190°C. Grease a pie dish with butter. Cover the raisins or sultanas with the warmed Marsala. Dark rum works well here, too: once it's cooked the rumminess ripens into something more aromatic than boozy.

Sieve the flour into a bowl and rub in the butter with your fingertips: the crumble should be like rubbly meal or porridge oats. Process the walnuts or chop very finely and stir them into the mixture. Then stir in 45g sugar. Set aside in a cool place – even stash in the deep-freeze – while you prepare the apples. This involves peeling, coring and slicing them and putting them in a heavy saucepan with the tablespoon of sugar and the Marsala and dried fruit. Put the lid on and cook for 5 minutes to soften, giving the pan a good shake once or twice in that time. Then put the fruit into the pie dish, cover with the crumble mixture, and cook for about 25 minutes.

There are times when real rice pudding is what's wanted, but it takes a good 3 hours to make one. It occured to me that you could proceed along the lines of a risotto: turn the rice in fat and then add hot liquid, ladleful by ladleful, until it's creamily absorbed. I did, and it worked – the perfect rice pudding for one. And all the stirring kept me occupied (without eating) until it was ready. This takes about half an hour. You need to give it about 10 minutes longer than the usual risotto as you want the rice rather less al dente.

RISOTTO-INSPIRED RICE PUDDING

700ml full-fat milk

1 heaped tablespoon butter

2–3 tablespoons caster sugar or vanilla sugar

60g (about 4 tablespoons) arborio rice

1/2 teaspoon good vanilla extract (if not using vanilla sugar)

2–3 tablespoons double cream, the thicker and fattier the better

Heat the milk in a pan that, preferably, has a lip. When it's about to boil (but don't let it) turn off the flame. (Or give the milk 4 minutes or so in a wide-necked plastic jug in the microwave.) If you're using the vanilla extract, add it to the milk now. Melt the butter and 1 tablespoon sugar in a heavy-based pan. When hissing away in a glorious pale caramelly pool, add the rice and stir to coat stickily. Slowly add the milk, stirring the rice all the time, letting each bit of milk – about 100ml at a time – get absorbed into the consequently swelling rice before adding the next bit. Start tasting at 20 minutes, but be prepared to go on for 35. You may want to add more milk, too. (And if the rice tastes cooked before all the milk's absorbed, don't carry on adding it.)

When the rice feels as it should, thick and sticky and creamy, take it off the heat, and beat in another tablespoon sugar (taste and see if you want yet more) and as much of the cream as you like. Think of this as the *mantecatura*: the final addition to a risotto, to thicken and add fat-globular volume, of butter and grated parmesan; indeed, just add butter if you haven't got any cream in the house.

Eat as is: no jam, no syrup, no honey, no nothing.

Serves 1.

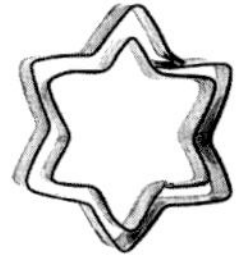

fast food

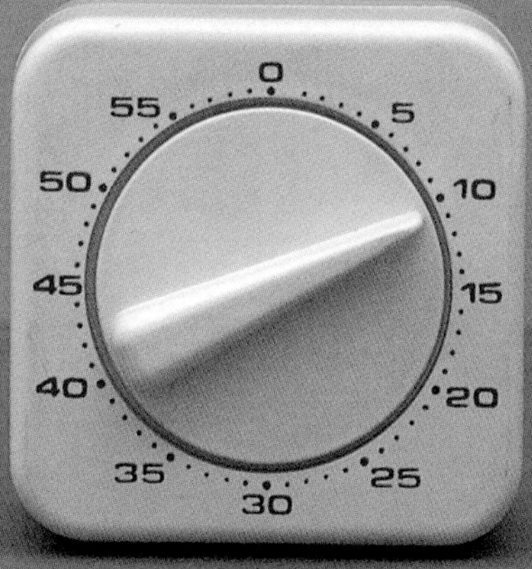
0
5
10
15
20
25
30
35
40
45
50
55

fast food

For the past few years I have written an annual round-up of cookery books and, putting aside fashions and fads, it is the subject of fast food which has recently begun to dominate. The reasons are understandable enough: we seem to have less time for cooking as we have more interest in food. Women have been traditionally the producers and providers of food in the home, but now that we go out to work there's no one to spend all afternoon making tonight's supper. But the disinclination to spend hour upon hour in the kitchen every night is not sex-specific. No one would want, after a long day in the office, to come back and start on some elaborate culinary masterpiece. Cooking can be relaxing (although it's interesting that it's men rather than women who tend more often to cite its therapeutic properties), but not if you are already exhausted. And since the working day seems to get ever longer, why would you want to be cooking a meal which isn't going to be ready for 2½ hours? What we all want is to eat something good and simple and soon.

POINTS TO REMEMBER

- Don't take short cuts with dishes that ought to be cooked slowly, to infuse and blend, to be cooled and added to. Choose instead food which is *meant* to be, *has* to be, cooked quickly, such as liver, fish or escalopes of meat.
- Remember to think not just in terms of actual cooking time in the oven, but of the amount of effort it will take you to put dinner together. I like shopping for food, and I don't work in an office: but on days when I'm really fraught, it's the shopping not the cooking that finishes me off. And when you're really exhausted, the easiest thing to cook is a roast chicken: it takes a while in the oven (see page xii), but demands a minimum of interference and energy from you.
- Quick, last-minute-assembly food can be the most stressful cooking of all. Its popularity is in part due to the influence of restaurants on our culinary imagination and repertoires. Restaurant cooking *has* to be quick; food has to be made fast, to order; chefs and their minions have to conjure up the finished dish within minutes. The constraints of cooking at home are entirely different: what makes life easier for a chef can make life hell for the domestic cook.

- I shy away from recipes which, however quick they may be to cook, require too much detailed attention in the preparation. Stir-fries are an example. In delicate moods, the idea of having to shred finely, dice, mince and slice into juliennes 7 different sorts of vegetable – even if the dish takes a mere 3 minutes to cook – could reduce me to tears.
- If you hate cooking, don't do it. You can certainly eat well enough just by learning how to shop. You can buy food that you don't need to cook – picnic food, cold food, things to heat up. Of course, trimmed vegetables and packaged salads are pandering to laziness and inviting extravagance on a ludicrous scale, but be grateful for them. If they taste good, don't worry about it. No one has to make themselves miserable over cooking.
- Make use of your store cupboard and fridge. You can rely on bought pasta sauces, on tins of white beans, anchovies and good tuna (in olive oil only) as well as small glass bottles of tapenade, green olive paste or goat's cheese in oil. Bacon is the easiest thing for the quick cook: grilling a piece of bacon is hardly cooking, and a few salty shards crumbled over or chopped into a pile of mashed potato, or mixed with beans and spinach, or chick peas and chilli-fried tomatoes and topped with a poached egg, make a better dinner than anything more elaborate and expensive from the chill cabinet.

REMINDERS OF AND IDEAS FOR HASTY IMPROVISATIONS

SALAD

You don't need to be reminded how to open a packet of designer leaves. But if you're in a hurry, salad can be useful, either as a starter to keep people quiet while you get other things ready, or as a main course if you are putting together a bought picnic supper (fruit, as well as cheese, good bread, pâtisserie). However, they can be just a little too flobby; you need texture, too. So just get a cos lettuce, tear it into large, crisp chunks and add it to any bought salad package (or mixture of packages). The quickest way of making a dressing is, at the last minute, to grind some salt over and then to drizzle some good olive oil and add the scarcest spritz of lemon (see also page 25).

To frisée or escarole, add hot, fried, diced pancetta or lardons. Make a dressing by adding Dijon mustard, more oil, and some red wine vinegar to the bacony juices in the pan. Then, onto the warm, tossed salad, shave some parmesan or other hard cheese and toss very lightly again. The chestnut and pancetta salad on page 362 is a slightly more solid variant. And you can substitute warm, just-cooked chicken livers, too.

To packets of spinach salad, add hot bacon and raw sliced mushrooms. Or make a spinach, gorgonzola and pine nut salad. Cut the gorgonzola (or whichever blue cheese you happen to like best) into crumbly cubes (don't worry about uniformity, size or even shape or you really will have a nervous breakdown) and toast the pine nuts in a hot oil-less pan until they begin to turn gold and fragrant.

To watercress and mâche, arranged on a plate not in a bowl, add some sliced, just-cooked-through scallops. Better still, fry some fat bacon first, then fry the scallops in the bacon fat. Chop the bacon finely and sprinkle over the scallop salad.

If you're in Germanic mood, then make a mustardy dressing for chicory – adding a stiff spoonful of crème fraîche – and buy thick slices of good ham from the delicatessen, cut them into batons and mix into the salad. You could do the same with warm potatoes, too: in which case you should really go the whole hog and add, instead of the ham, thickly sliced frankfurters, though please don't even think of using the flabby tinned sort with that moussy, lurid, loose-textured flesh.

A huge green salad, no funny turns, with a walnut oil dressing and a good cheeseboard, is one of the loveliest dinners I can think of: have a tumbling mass of grapes, too; good bread; thin and thick biscuits and, if you can ever find ripe pears, then make sure you have a dish of those, too.

SOUPS

PEA SOUP

The quickest and best soup you can make is to cook 450g packet frozen peas in 500ml stock made by adding 2 teaspoons Marigold bouillon granules to that quantity of boiling water. When the peas are tender, purée in the food processor or blender. Add some olive oil (preferably basil-infused, and see below) and season to taste. Serve parmesan to sprinkle over.

You can improve on this: if you've boiled a ham at any stage, then freeze the ham stock it's made and use here. Also, if you've bunged any hard, unyielding rinds of finished parmesan into the freezer as you go along, then salvage one now and throw that into the soup as it's cooking.

TOMATO AND RICE

Just as easy is a tomato and rice soup (see page 468, too) which you can make by adding water to a good, bought tomato sauce to make it liquid enough for rice to cook in. Bring to the boil. Throw in some basmati rice and 10 minutes later you've got soup.

Spinach, since you can buy it frozen and ready chopped, makes a good basis for a quick soup: chop and fry an onion first, then add spinach and, when it has more or less thawed, add 500ml or so of stock made from cubes or granules. After about 5 minutes, add a good squeeze of lemon and, if you want to make it richer when it's off the heat, whisk in some single cream beaten with an egg yolk.

SPINACH

PASTA

You need to wait for the water to boil, but you can lessen the overall time by buying fine egg pasta, which doesn't take very long to cook. Some butter, cream, parmesan and a few drops of white truffle oil make a wonderful sauce. Or don't even bother about the truffle oil. People shy away from cream and butter so much that, when they taste them, just as they are, warmed by a tangle of slippery-soft pasta, it comes as a surprise how transportingly good they are. And don't get anxious about the artery-thickening properties of such a sauce: you don't want to drench the pasta, just lightly cover it. I sometimes think that butter alone, with a grating of fresh nutmeg, is the best dressing for pasta.

BUTTER

CREAM

PARMESAN

TRUFFLE OIL

NUTMEG

And, finally, bear in mind Chinese egg noodles. They need a scant 5 minutes cooking, and a sprinkling of sesame oil.

FLAVOURED AND INFUSED OILS

I have come to the conclusion, having abominated them for ages, that infused oils are among the most important allies of the quick cook. I use basil oil mixed with lemon juice to make a quick, scented dressing for salads, or just as it is to anoint waxy boiled potatoes or peas or poached or fried meats. I have made a basil-rich version of the pea soup above by frying a chopped onion first in basil-infused oil, then adding some more of the basil oil at the end.

I habitually have an effort-free *spaghetti aglio olio* by just dousing the cooked pasta in 2 tablespoons of the garlic-infused oil. I use it for frying and marinading chicken pieces and coat diced potatoes with it before roasting them. I use it to warm through cans of cannellini beans, which I then let steep, so the garlicky oil penetrates the soft interior of the grainy beans, before sprinkling with chopped sage or parsley or both. In short, I have become a complete convert, with all the evangelical zeal which that implies.

CANNED PULSES

Canned pulses are obviously useful for fast-food preparation. If you want to heat them up you can, though they will need some help. Just put onion, garlic, a stick of celery, parsley (I don't even bother to remove the stalks), some bacon or pancetta in the food processor, blitz and throw the green-flecked, fragrant mound into a pan with 1–2 tablespoons olive oil.

When this mixture is really soft (remember you're not going to cook the pulses, just heat them up) stir in white beans, borlotti, lentils or chick peas. If I'm using lentils (which aren't quite as satisfactory as other tinned pulses) I add a carrot to the pulped mixture; chick peas can take the fierce rasp of a dried, or fresh, red chilli. And if you have lying around herbs other than parsley, then use them: rosemary and sage work particularly well with cannellini and borlotti, but you will need, especially with the rosemary, to make sure they are well minced.

When the pulses are warmed through, add more chopped fresh parsley and olive oil and, having tasted, probably quite a bit of salt. Pulses are best at room temperature, and taste all the better having sat around with the herbs and garlic and olive oil seeping stickily into them, so do them first thing when you come in from work, and leave them, reheating as necessary later.

ESCALOPES

Thin cuts of meat or fish need not much more than 1 minute each side in a frying pan or under the grill, and providing you don't leave them lying around to dry up and curl at the edges, are probably the best bet for the quick cook.

SALMON

Fresh fish is perhaps at its best grilled or fried quickly and served with lemon juice squeezed over it. Farmed salmon is much helped by lime.

You can buy the meat ready slivered: salmon is sold by supermarkets in similar escalopes, but unless you go to a fishmonger you are unlikely to get other fish cut as thinly. Whatever meat you buy, just fry it briefly in butter or oil, deglaze the pan with whatever you want, and pour the juices over.

PORK
VEAL

Pork or veal escalopes need just 2 minutes each side in a buttery pan (add a drop of oil first to stop the butter burning) and then a squeeze of lemon after. If you're cooking for more than two, then leave the escalopes as they are; otherwise snip each 1 into 3, so you have small slices about 6cm by 3cm. These will look better, more inviting, piled on a big plate. Lemon juice provides the simplest sauce, but by no means the only: use Marsala, white wine, vermouth or sherry glugged in at the end, with or without a dollop of cream. Calves' liver tastes wonderful in a buttery Marsala puddle. Dredge the slices first in some plain flour into which you've grated some nutmeg. This makes the sauce more velvety. Breaded escalopes are also worth remembering. If you're in a hurry, you might not want to bother with breadcrumbs. And I wouldn't get those bright orange ones in a box; buy instead some matzo meal. Dip the escalopes in egg, then in matzo meal, let them stand for a while to dry, and fry each one for 2 minutes or so in sizzling butter with a drop of oil in it.

CHICKEN

Chicken, especially the breast, needs to be paid quite lavish attention to keep it interesting, and I speak as someone whose favourite food is roast chicken. But when you're trying to get something together quickly, be careful. Everyone likes the idea of breast portions, but they can easily be bland or desiccated. If possible, let chicken breasts marinate for as long as you can, but at least 20 minutes, in olive oil and lemon juice and some peeled, knife-flattened garlic cloves. For each portion of chicken breast, work along the lines of 3 tablespoons olive oil, 2 tablespoons lemon juice and 1 clove garlic. But this is just the loosest of guides.

OLIVE OIL
LEMON
GARLIC

Lie the chicken in the lemony oil, cover with clingfilm and turn at half-time. To grill the chicken, preheat the grill while the chicken's steeping. The cooking itself is quick enough: about 6 minutes under the grill each side; frying is even quicker, about 4 minutes a side. Let stand at the end to allow the heat to seep through. Sprinkle with herbs, adding more lemon juice and some sea salt.

If you don't want to bother with marinating, then consider adding fat while the chicken's cooking. Make any mixture of herbs and butter and, having slashed the chicken breasts with a knife, smear this over. Or, very easy, mix some good bottled pesto with some softened butter (75g butter and 3 tablespoons pesto should do for about 4 chicken breasts) and dollop this over both sides, making sure you press well over the slashed skin, so the mixture permeates. Cook for 10 minutes a side, but you may find you need a bit longer: you don't want the pesto mixture to burn too quickly (it will blacken slightly: that is part of the plan, so don't panic) so cook with a less fierce heat.

PESTO

Leg and thigh portions take longer than breast, and for that reason are perhaps not ideal for the quickest of quick cooking. The answer is just to get the butcher to cut up the meat into smaller portions. Chicken cut up already and swathed in clingwrap from the supermarket is tasteless. It annoys me that so many people prefer the white meat. The brown meat is better, and particularly so when cooked in portions.

WITH VERMOUTH

PARSLEY

You can make bland chicken portions more memorable by serving with salsa verde. It doesn't take long to poach chicken portions. Take some skinned and boned chicken breasts, preferably free-range or corn-fed, and poach them in some stock (and I feel relaxed about some liberally diluted cubes here, though I'd use Italian ones, which are better) mixed with white wine or vermouth, into which you put some parsley stalks, a drop of soy sauce if the stock isn't already salty enough, some celery and 2 bay leaves. Poach gently till just done – 10 minutes or so should do it. Serve with the salsa verde on page 200, a spoonful or so drizzled over, the rest in a jug or bowl with a ladle, to the side.

DUCK

GINGER AND SOY

HONEY AND ORANGE

Duck breasts are always worth bearing in mind when you have to get something together quickly. Follow a proper recipe, as below, or just slash the skin side diagonally at about 1cm intervals, douse with strained ginger marmalade which you've made runnier with soy sauce, or honey mixed with orange juice (the sharper the better, and if you cook this in January or February, you should try and get hold of Seville oranges), or grainy mustard mixed with a drop or two of pineapple juice and a pinch of brown sugar. Roast, skin side up, in a hot oven (gas mark 8/220°C for about 20 minutes). I work on an allowance of 1 per person if I'm slicing them up. The meat is rich, and you somehow taste the duck better, get the sense of its flavour and feathery-velvety texture, when it is sliced. I'd just carve into diagonal, thin, but not wafer-thin, slices and spread them out on a large plate for people to take what they want themselves. I wouldn't give people their own little portion of fanned-out slices on an individual plate. Of course, you can just serve the duck breasts whole, as they are, in which case it might be safer to cook 2 extra per 4 people in case some want seconds: overcatering is always better than not accommodating people's greed.

Don't worry about having leftovers. What could be nicer the next day than cold duck, thinly sliced, and stirred into warm rice, doused with soy sauce and studded with just-hot sugar snaps? Or just eat it as it is, with a fat clump of Japanese pickled ginger and waxy, warm new potatoes.

PUDDINGS

The first thing the quick cook can dispense with is cooking the last course. No French person would consider apologising for buying something from a good pâtisserie and neither should you.

ICE-CREAM

Otherwise, think along the lines of good, bought ice-cream eaten with good, bought biscuits or splodged with easily thrown together sauces. Warm some honey, pour it over, then sprinkle with toasted flaked almonds, or substitute maple syrup and pecans or walnuts. Throw over a cup of espresso to make what the Italians call an *affoggato* (or use rum). Spoon over stem ginger in oozing, golden, throat-catchingly hot and sweet syrup. Or, as in one of the suggested menus below, just grind some good, dark chocolate to powdery grains in the food processor.

AFFOGGATO

STEM GINGER

CHOCOLATE

And, as mentioned in Basics Etc, in regards to the deep-freeze and how it may usefully be stocked, keep a ready supply of frozen berries – raspberries, blackberries or mixed – to hand. Use as they are – removing all strawberries from the mixed bag – only add sugar. You can also add some glugs of liqueur, some finely grated orange zest, a few mint leaves or some orange-flower water. Serve with crème fraîche or ice-cream, as you like. Just before serving, sprinkle with icing sugar or ground pistachios. You can make a creamy, red-splodged mess by whipping up some double cream, crumbling some shop-bought meringues and stirring in a packet of thawed, sweetened berries. I think this is much better than using the meringues whole and going in for nest-like effects.

BERRIES

CREAM

MERINGUE

It is worth always bearing in mind the icing-sugar-and-tea-strainer trick. Somehow, giving any bought or hastily-thrown-together pudding a smart dusting makes it automatically look like the loving product of hours'-long labour in the kitchen. I don't suggest you *ever* pretend something bought is home-made. Nor do I advise forays into cheffy fiddling in general – I am not a garnish girl – but this small degree of finish pleases me.

A BRIEF NOTE ON EQUIPMENT

The microwave is the usually-cited without-which tool for the time-pressed kitchen survivor. But consider, rather, the pressure cooker. New fangled models (and see Gazetteer) don't explode, don't hiss or honk or emit clouds of threatening steam and cut cooking time, on average, by a third. And – by way of even more dramatic example – you can cook dried, unsoaked chick peas in 35 minutes. Another very useful piece of gadgetry, if you're going to be having people round for supper often when you haven't really got the time to cook for them, is an electric rice-cooker (see Gazetteer also). You'd be surprised how much food can be eaten with rice; and the whole after-work kitchen flurry is much reduced when you're not dealing with potatoes, too.

QUICK AFTER-WORK SUPPERS FOR FOUR

Individual recipes that take under 30 minutes to cook are dotted throughout the book (and are listed as such in the Index in the back); after all, in the normal course of cooking we all mix food which can be rustled together quickly with that which takes longer or needs more care or attention. But there are times when anything that can't be done fast, and without faffing, is out of the culinary question. If you don't get back from work till 7, and have got people coming over at 8, you need to get moving. And bearing in mind that planning – the sheer effort of exhausted thought required – can sometimes feel just as burdensome as the preparation, I've drawn up a list of quick and easy two-course, after-work suppers.

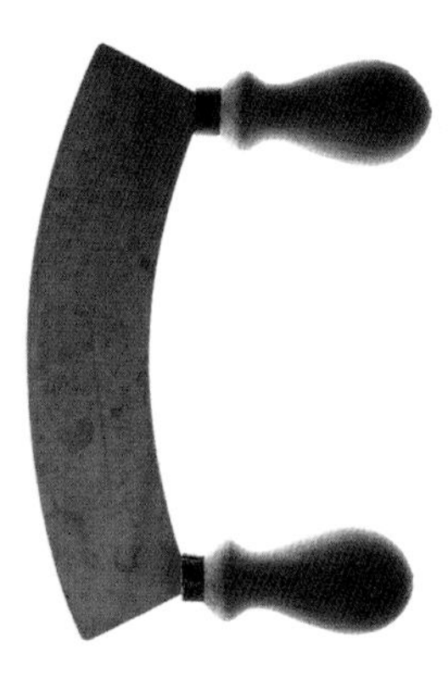

Nothing here takes more than half an hour to cook; most don't even take 10 minutes. And all recipes feed four.

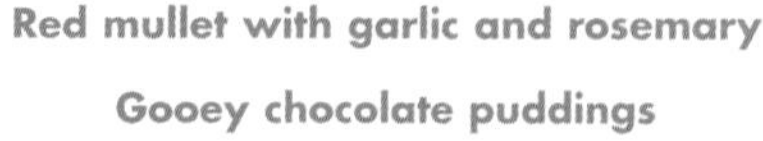

Red mullet with garlic and rosemary

Gooey chocolate puddings

This menu exemplifies my ideas for fast food: the fish itself takes a bare few minutes; the pudding you mix together when you get in and then just leave until the moment, more or less, you want to eat. You can thus appear the very model of serenity in the kitchen, however late or in whatever stressed state you actually got back.

The red mullet is fragrant, light, beautiful. The chocolate puddings, which are really Patricia Wells' recipe for chocolate gourmandise in *At Home in Provence*, provide a harmoniously voluptuous counterpoint: chewy and cracked like macaroons on top and on the base, with a thick, glossy goo of chocolate sauce in the middle.

RED MULLET WITH GARLIC AND ROSEMARY

Ask the fishmonger to leave the pearly-pink, crimson-beaded skin on the fish, but to remove the scales.

4 cloves garlic
needles from about 4 12cm sprigs rosemary
zest of 2 oranges
6 tablespoons olive oil
4–6 red mullet (depending on size), filleted
175ml vermouth or white wine

Finely chop the garlic, rosemary needles and orange zest: I pile everything onto the chopping board and use my mezzaluna. Put half of this mixture into a large frying pan with 3 tablespoons of the oil, heat, bring up to sizzling point, then add half the fish fillets, skin side down. Give them a couple of minutes a side, or until you can see that the flesh has lost its raw transparency. Remove the fish fillets to a warmed plate big enough to take everything later, and repeat the whole process with the rest of the ingredients. Add these fillets to the warmed plate. Deglaze the pan with vermouth, let it bubble up and when syrupy pour this, scraping up the chopped bits as you do so, over the fish. If you want to eat noodles with – and they do go well – then look at the noodle and mangetout stir-fry below (page 196) only missing out, I'd think, the mushrooms. The mullet is wonderful without noodles, too, just with some grilled tomatoes and good bread.

GOOEY CHOCOLATE PUDDINGS

125g best quality dark chocolate, finely chopped
125g unsalted butter
3 large eggs
150g sugar
35g plain flour, preferably Italian 00
butter and flour for preparing ramekins

Before you've even taken your coat off, put the chocolate and butter in a bowl and suspend over a pan of simmering water. Whisk every now and again until melted.

In another bowl, whisk together the eggs, sugar and flour until just blended. Gradually whisk in the melted chocolate and butter. Set aside to rest.

Grease four 250ml ramekins with butter and add flour to cover the butter, tapping the ramekins to get rid of excess. Preheat the oven to gas mark 6/200°C about half an hour before you want to eat pudding. And I'd leave cooking them until you've finished the main course. It doesn't matter if there's no food on the table for 10 minutes; and these do have to be done at the last minute.

So: pour the mixture into the ramekins and put them on a baking sheet in the oven for 10–12 minutes, until the tops are firm and cracking slightly and the edges set. Serve immediately and consider providing a jug of cold, cold cream for people to pour into their pudding's hotly deliquescing interior as they eat.

Beef stroganoff

Roast sugar-sprinkled peaches

Although beef stroganoff has to be cooked at the very last minute – which can often be the quickest route to a nervous breakdown in the kitchen – you can fry the onions and butter as soon as you get in. Then all you need to do once you're on the verge of sitting down is reheat them gently for a couple of minutes in a little butter, remove them again from the pan and then proceed with the meat. From that stage you're not more than about three minutes away from being able to eat, so this is worth bearing in mind for friends you just know are going to be late.

BEEF STROGANOFF

Most butchers can get you tail bits of fillet which will cost less and which you won't mind so much tearing into raggedy scraps. Cook a buttery mound of basmati rice to eat with.

90g butter and a few drops of oil
1 large onion, finely chopped
225g button mushrooms, sliced
fresh nutmeg
750 beef fillet, cut into thin strips
scant 1/2 teaspoon Dijon mustard
200ml crème fraîche
a few pinches ground paprika

Put 30g of butter in a frying pan with a drop of oil. Put on the heat, add the onion and fry gently, stirring frequently, until soft and beginning to colour. Add 30g more butter and when melted toss in the mushrooms and cook for another 4–5 minutes. Grate some fresh nutmeg and grind some pepper over the onions and mushrooms in the pan. Stir well and remove to a plate. Add the remaining 30g butter to the pan with a drop or two of oil and turn the heat to high. When the butter's hot, stir-fry the fillet for a couple of minutes, until it's just cooked but still very tender. Return the onions and mushrooms to the pan, stir well. Grate over some more nutmeg and stir in the Dijon mustard, then the crème fraîche. Sprinkle in a pinch of paprika, taste for seasoning and then pour onto a warmed plate. If you want, you can put the rice on the same plate, in a circle with the beef stroganoff in the middle (which is very much in keeping with the period in which this dish found most fashionable favour) or pile onto separate plates. Either way, dust a little more paprika over it once it's served up.

ROAST SUGAR-SPRINKLED PEACHES

This is scarcely a recipe: get 5–6 peaches (enough for 2 halves each and then a little more), split them in half, remove the stones and put them, cut-side up, in a buttered ovenproof dish in which they fit snugly. Into each cavity add a dot of butter and a tablespoon of sugar – vanilla, brown or ordinary white as you like – then another few dots of butter and roast in a preheated gas mark 6/200°C oven for about 20 minutes. Think about providing some good, bought ice-cream to go with. And you can substitute apricots or, of course, nectarines.

Squid with chilli and clams

Ricotta with honey and toasted pine nuts

This is the sort of dinner I cook when I've got girlfriends coming over, chapter meetings of the martyred sisterhood: even though quantities are enough for four, for some reason there are always only three of us, and I don't reduce amounts of ingredients correspondingly.

I'm not saying that this menu is necessarily unsuitable for mixed company, but my experience teaches me that this is more naturally girlfood. Your experience may be fortunate enough to make you feel otherwise.

SQUID WITH CHILLI AND CLAMS

I tend to get my fish from the fishmonger and get him to clean the squid; but you can buy it ready-cleaned at the supermarket. If you don't have any sake to hand (again, my supermarket stocks it) then use dry sherry.

40 palourdes or cherrystone clams (approx. 600g)
4 large squid (uncleaned weight approx. 225g each)
4–6 tablespoons olive oil
4 cloves garlic, squished with flat of knife
1 dried red chilli pepper
250ml sake
good bunch flat-leaf parsley or Thai basil

Rinse the clams under the cold tap, throwing out any that are cracked, damaged or which stay open. Slice the squid into rings. Put the oil in a wide saucepan (which has a lid, though you don't need it yet) on a high heat. When hot, add the garlic and crumble in the dried, whole, chilli pepper. Stir well, then add the squid and fry, stirring, for about a minute, until the glassy flesh turns a denser white. Add the clams, the sake and 250ml water (an easy way of measuring is to use an American cup measure for each in turn) and then clamp on the lid and turn the heat down a little. Cook for 4–5 minutes, shaking the pan a bit every now and again. Open lid to check the clams are all steamed open, then pour into a large bowl, and cover with freshly chopped parsley or Thai basil if you prefer.

It's idiosyncratic perhaps, but I find a bowl of plain basmati rice the perfect accompaniment. You might think of adding a couple of cardomum pods to infuse while cooking, but no butter or oil at the end, that's the point.

RICOTTA WITH HONEY AND TOASTED PINE NUTS

This doesn't really count as a recipe; it's more a suggestion.

Cut about 350g fresh ricotta into wedges or oblong chunks (fresh, unsalty goat's cheese, sliced, works just as well) and arrange them on a plate. Dribble a couple of tablespoons of good, clear honey over them and then sprinkle over about 50g pine nuts which you've first toasted till golden and waxily fragrant in a hot, oil-less pan.

Sole with chanterelles

Mascarpone, rum and lime cream

What I generally do here is make the first bit of the mascarpone cream when I get in (that's to say, everything up to the egg whites) and then whisk and fold in the egg whites just before I get started on the fish. It all depends how early you get in from work: if it's a bare half hour before you're expecting everyone else, just make up the pudding, egg whites and all, in its entirety.

SOLE WITH CHANTERELLES

I love the ecstatic saffron intensity of the chanterelles against the fine whiteness of the soles, but don't feel obliged to use them. I often substitute those surreally tinted pieds bleues (which for some reason my local supermarket stocks in profusion) and wild oyster mushrooms should be just as good.

600g chanterelles
125g butter, plus 1 tablespoon
1 tablespoon garlic-infused oil
4 soles, filleted
juice of 1/4–1/2 a lemon
125ml Noilly Prat (or white wine)
flat-leaf parsley

Cook the mushrooms, wiped with a kitchen towel first if they need it, in the 125g butter and garlic oil in a large, high-sided if possible, frying pan, adding salt and pepper to taste, then remove to a plate or bowl while you get on with the fish. You shouldn't have to add any more butter, but do, if you feel you need to; and you'll have to cook the sole in a couple or so batches. A couple of minutes on the first side, then another on the second should be all they need, but poke a knife in to check. Remove them as you go to a large, warmed plate (big enough to lie all 8 fillets on later), sprinkle with salt, then get on with the rest. When all the fish is on the plate, put the mushrooms back and heat up, adding a squirt of lemon juice and the Noilly Prat or wine; taste to see whether you want to add a little more lemon. Let the mushrooms bubble up and stir in the tablespoon of butter. Pour over the sole on the plate and sprinkle with freshly-chopped flat-leaf parsley.

I don't think you need to serve anything more than a bowl of green vegetables with this – given that the pudding is not a lean one – and I'd probably choose some purple sprouting broccoli when it's in the shops, or some frozen petits pois with a couple of handfuls of sugar-snaps thrown in for the last 60 seconds or so of cooking time.

MASCARPONE, RUM AND LIME CREAM

3 eggs, separated
6 tablespoons (90g) caster sugar
375g mascarpone
3 tablespoons dark rum
juice of 1–2 limes

Whisk the egg yolks and sugar together till light and moussily creamy. In another bowl, stir the mascarpone together with the rum and juice of 1 lime. Stir the egg mixture in gently but firmly, with a folding movement, and taste; you may want to add a little more lime juice. Don't worry about sharpness unduly: you need that to hold the egg-enriched mascarpone in check; what you want to end up with is the creamy tartness, the taste, of cheesecake, but with the whipped lightness of mousse.

Wipe the inside of the bowl you're going to whisk the egg whites in with the cut side of the lime. Then whisk them till stiff and fold them into the mascarpone mixture. Decant into glasses and keep somewhere cool till needed. I leave this blank and unadorned, but you could always pare a strip of lime zest, or even cut a twist of lime, holiday-cocktail style, for the top of each glass. But plain or prinked, you must get hold of some biscuits to eat with.

Lamb with garlicky tahina

Passion fruit fool

Again, you can more or less prepare the pudding when you get in – just leave the combining of the seed-studded pulp and sweetened cream till last minute – and you can put the lamb in its scant marinade and get on with the tahina garlic sauce at the same time. That leaves you with the lamb to cook: 15 minutes at most.

LAMB WITH GARLICKY TAHINA

with thanks to Steve Afif

I reckon on allowing each person a couple of noisettes, and further provide enough for half those present to have another one each. It's hard to say how big the noisettes will be as it depends on the time of year; you can always specify, though, the width you want the noisette cut. If you've bought them ready prepared and they're thinner than I've suggested, then remember to cut cooking time accordingly.

1 onion, peeled and roughly chopped
300ml best olive oil
zest of 1 lemon, and juice (separately) of 2
1/4 teaspoon ground cumin
10 noisettes of lamb, about 3cm thick
8 tablespoons tahina
4 cloves garlic

Put the onion into one large shallow dish in which all the noisettes will fit in one layer, or divide the onion into two medium-to-large freezer bags. Add the oil, lemon zest and cumin (dividing equally, obviously, if you're using bags). Give a good stir and then add the lamb. Cover dish or tie up bags and leave, turning or squishing respectively at half time. Leave the lamb like this as long as you've got, frankly, though it should be for at least 10 minutes and preferably not in the fridge. Preheat the oven to gas mark 7/210°C. Put a non-stick or cast-iron pan on the hob. Remove noisettes from marinade; you don't need to wipe dry, just brush off the bits of onion. Sear each side for a minute or two, then transfer to a roasting tray and thence to the preheated oven. Ten minutes should be right for pink, but not bloody, lamb; you may need a bit longer if the meat started off very cold. You will need to check for yourself, obviously, and when cooked as you want, remove to warmed plate.

For the sauce, put the tahina in a bowl and either mince or crush (this is one time I *do* use a crusher) the garlic and add, along with ½ a teaspoonful of preferably coarse salt. Stir with a wooden spoon, adding the lemon juice as you do; it will seize up here, but don't worry because it will loosen later. Slowly add some water (I find I can use about 150ml), pouring from a jug so that only a little goes in at a time, and keep stirring. When you have a smooth mixture the consistency of double cream, stop adding water. Put into a bowl with a spoon and sprinkle with ground cumin.

I like a plateful of lemony spinach with this – if you're buying it frozen, which I do, make sure it's leaf, not chopped, spinach – and a tomato salad. If you want carbohydrate, then burghal would be just right (and see page 114 for method).

PASSION FRUIT FOOL

The fragrant astringency of passion fruit is just right after the palate-thickening stickiness of the tahina. This recipe comes from Stephen Saunders' *Shorts Cuts* and is so good that I haven't even down-sized it from his specifications which are for 6: just use this to fill 4 glasses instead; your guests will thank you.

12 passion fruits
284ml tub double cream
100g icing sugar
juice of 1 lemon
2 teaspoons Cointreau

Cut the passion fruits in half and scoop out the pulp with a spoon and leave in a bowl. Semi-whisk the cream in a large bowl and leave it in the fridge. Put 4 glasses in the fridge too, though it won't hurt if they're not chilled. Sieve the icing sugar, and set aside.

Then, when you want to eat pudding, whisk the icing sugar into the double cream with the lemon juice and Cointreau. Fold in the passion fruits and pour the fool into the glasses. Serve whatever biscuits you like with.

Roast cod with upmarket mushy peas

Quickly-scaled Mont Blanc

The peas are actually a speeded up, simplified version of the garlic-breathy puréed pea crostini on page 334. If the quantities given seem to specify a lot, it's because people eat a lot of it. Though be grateful if you've got some left over: it makes lovely pea soup.

If you're getting the cod from the fishmonger, ask for it to be cut from the top end.

ROAST COD WITH UPMARKET MUSHY PEAS

for the peas

1 head of garlic

800g frozen petits pois

100g butter

4 tablespoons crème fraîche or double cream

for the cod

1–2 tablespoons ordinary olive oil

1 tablespoon flour

4 fillets of cod, about 200g each

Put separated but not peeled cloves of garlic in cold water, bring to boil, salt and then boil for 10 minutes. Fish out the cloves with a slotted spoon, push them out of their skins back into the water and bring back to the boil. Add the peas and cook for slightly longer than you would if you were eating them normally. Drain, then tip into the bowl of the food processor, add the butter and process. Add the cream and process again. If you've done all this when you get in, scrape back into the saucepan so you can reheat as and when you want it.

Now for the cod. Preheat the oven to gas mark 6/200°C. Get hold of a pan that will go in the oven later, if you can; otherwise use a frying pan and transfer the fish later to an oven tray. Whichever, pour the oil into the pan, put it on the hob and while it's heating up put the flour on a plate, add salt and pepper and dredge the cod fillets in it. Sear the cod fillets on each side then transfer to the oven and cook for 7–10 minutes depending on how thick they are and how cold they were before you started.

It's hard to cook potatoes in under half an hour, but if you get those teeny weeny miniature new potatoes you should keep within schedule. Or take more time but no more effort by putting 6 baking potatoes in the oven for 1½–2 hours (it all depends, of course, on your having that much time to play with), then scraping out the fleshy interior into a bowl. Warm up some milk and a huge amount of butter (I put both in a jug in the microwave) and fork into the potatoes with salt, pepper and freshly grated nutmeg.

You can do very easy sausages and mash, incidentally, by putting some sausages in an oiled pan for the last 50 minutes. Both worth remembering for those evenings you do get back a couple of hours before you want to eat, but without the energy to do anything in those two hours.

SAUSAGES AND MASH

The pea purée, while we're dealing with variations on a theme, goes just as rhapsodically well with noisettes of lamb (see above, only add some rosemary needles to the marinade in place of the onion).

QUICKLY-SCALED MONT BLANC

My mother often made this: at its most basic, it's just sweetened chestnut purée (from a tin) scraped into a bowl and some whipped double cream piled on top; you can add crumbled bought meringues, grated chocolate as you like, and whisk a tablespoon each of rum and icing sugar into the cream. If you can run to some actual marrons glacés, too, so much the better. This is so gloopy it's easier to do it in individual glasses, even if it's not my usual style.

Duck with orange salsa

Noodles with spring onions, shitake mushrooms and mangetouts

Ice-cream with stem ginger or figs

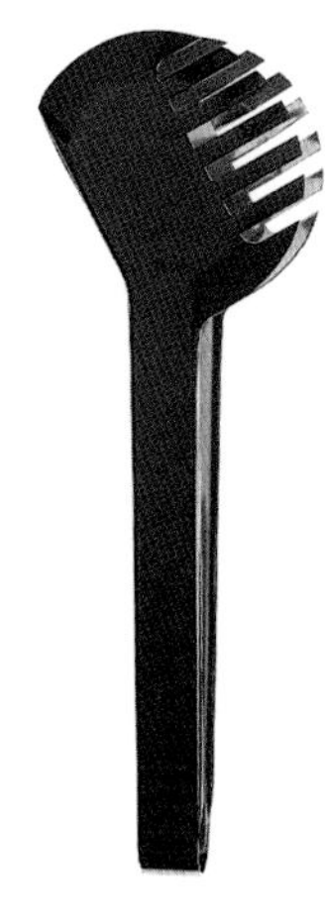

Prawn cocktail, Black Forest gâteau, coq au vin, duck à l'orange: there has been an insistent, cool-minded movement to bring these recently disparaged bistro specialities of the 1960s and 1970s back into culinary fashion. I have nothing against this in principle: if it tastes good, eat it. Fashionableness – ironic or otherwise – should not count against a food any more than its unfashionableness. The pairing of duck and orange can work (see page 184 also). And it can work quickly. The coriander-spiked citrussy salsa, an intensely-flavoured, swiftly-put-together relish, is a perfect foil for the sweet and rich flesh of the soy-sprinkled magrets. Blood oranges look spectacular, but tend to be hard to peel and chop. If you're in a hurry, choose a seedless, neatly-peeling Navel orange or substitute a pawpaw, though in which case don't bother about using the mint but do give a squeeze of orange along with the lime. Noodles are just right with this, and as usual you can boil them when you get in and finish them off later.

DUCK WITH ORANGE SALSA

4–5 duck breasts – magrets – approx. 200g each
soy sauce
2 oranges, preferably seedless
½ red onion
1 fresh red chilli
1 good clump coriander (to make about 3–4 tablespoons, to taste)
fresh mint (about half as much as coriander)
½ lime

Preheat the oven to gas mark 8/220°C.

Slash the skin of the magrets diagonally, about 4 times on each, then sprinkle with soy sauce and rub this over the skin with your hand. Arrange on a rack over a baking tray, skin side up. Cook for about 20 minutes, though do look after 15 minutes: the skin should be crisp, the flesh pinkly tender.

Meanwhile, peel the oranges, removing as much pith as possible. Slice the oranges crossways, and then chop each slice into small chunks. In an ideal world you might want to remove the membranes between each segment, but I don't. You may find it easier to use a grapefruit knife, if you own one: in which case, halve each unpeeled orange and use the knife to cut around the rim and through each segment, as you would if preparing a grapefruit. Cut each chiselled-out segment into 2 or 3 and then, after you've done all of them, squeeze the juice from the hollowed-out orange halves over the diced flesh. Chop the red onion finely. Cut along the chilli lengthways and deseed it (and see also the noodle recipe below). I think it is better to use your washing-up gloves for this, however unhygienic they may be, otherwise your hands will infuse everything with burning heat for the rest of the evening. Chop the chilli into tiny dice or shreds and stir into the oranges, along with the finely chopped coriander and mint. Sprinkle with salt and squeeze over the lime gradually and tasting as you do: you want the salsa to be sharp but not painfully so. Stir gently together and put aside until needed. Standing around for 15 minutes or so will do it no harm, indeed, on the contrary.

NOODLES WITH SPRING ONIONS, SHITAKE MUSHROOMS AND MANGETOUTS

Just as you can boil the noodles in good time – in other words, when you can still enjoy the privacy of your own kitchen – so you can chop all the bits to go in them. I know stir-frying can tax a girl's nerves, but this is serenely manageable.

250g egg noodles
2 tablespoons vegetable oil
1 teaspoon sesame oil
4 red chillies, deseeded and chopped
6 spring onions, chopped into 1cm lengths
240g shitake mushrooms, destalked and chopped
100g mangetouts, roughly chopped (in half or 3 pieces each)
2 tablespoons soy sauce
fresh chopped coriander

Boil the noodles in salted water according to the instructions on the packet, then drain, rinse in cold water and drain again. Heat the oils in a hot wok or large frying pan and stir-fry the chilli and spring onion for one minute, add the shitake mushrooms and stir-fry for another two minutes. Then add, stirring furiously, the mangetouts. Give them a minute, then add the noodles, lifting them up in the pan and stirring well so all is mixed in together, pouring in a couple of tablespoons soy as you do so. Toss well and quickly, then empty onto a big round plate. Sprinkle with coriander.

ICE-CREAM WITH STEM GINGER OR FIGS

All you need to do for pudding – following one of the suggestions in the hasty-improvisations section earlier – is put a tub of good vanilla ice-cream and a jar of stem ginger in syrup on the table. Tinned green figs – the stuff of sweet trolleys in provincial hotels, maybe – would also be just, delightfully, right after the zingily salsa'd duck.

Mackerel in cider
Buttered apples

Obviously, you can simply grill your mackerel: all you need then is a squeeze of lemon or orange juice over (a Seville orange if in season), and nothing could be better. Fish, especially oily fish, is always good when plain grilled. When I want to eat properly but in a hurry, I lunch on grilled trout, dry-fried herring, or mackerel fillets with pickled ginger and soy sauce. The reason I might want to cook fish in a way which might seem a little more elaborate is that cooking in the oven I find easy when I have people over.

Mackerel poached or steamed in cider, or sometimes cider vinegar, with a sauce which may or may not contain mustard, is a fairly common way of eating in Normandy and Brittany: this version happens to be reassuringly pared down. It helps, too, that mackerel (like trout) is easily bought at the fish counters of supermarkets. Obviously the cider intended is the French cider, made in the area, and it is relatively easy to buy over here now. But don't lose sleep over it: Bulmer's won't kill the dish. I'd stay if not in the region then within notional distance of it by having apples for pudding. The cider with the fish, and the apples after, do not cloy or bore; somehow the flavours seem to deepen rather than tire with the repetition.

MACKEREL IN CIDER

I know that the idea of cream, and quite so much of it, added to sauce that is to swathe such oily fish, might sound alarming. But when you're cooking quickly, something's got to give, and I find most often that something is the contemporary concern about cream and butter. Adding either or both of these is a way of adding instant depth, texture and accomplished finish to a dish. But if you want to add less, then I'm not stopping you.

3 mackerel, filleted (4 if small)
3 shallots, 1 banana shallot or 1 small onion, chopped finely
225ml dry cider
100ml crème fraîche or double cream
lemon juice (optional)
fresh flat-leaf parsley, chopped, to garnish

Preheat the oven to gas mark 6/200°C.

Put the mackerel fillets in a lightly buttered, shallow baking dish. Sprinkle with the shallots or onion and pour over the cider. Season with salt and pepper and cover tightly with foil. Bake for 20–25 minutes, until the fish is cooked through. Transfer the mackerel to a warm serving plate, remove skin and cover to keep warm.

Pour the cooking liquid into a small saucepan and boil, reducing to about half. Add the crème fraîche or cream and simmer with the heat low for a couple of minutes. Season to taste, adding lemon juice if you want.

Strain the sauce, pressing with the back of a spoon to extract all the liquid. Garnish the fish with parsley and serve with the cider sauce.

With this I can think of nothing better than plain boiled potatoes and spinach with a fragrant cocoa-brown dusting of freshly grated nutmeg. But frankly, you can put all your effort into the boiled potatoes (I think peeled large floury ones are more comforting here than the ready-washed and thin-skinned waxy ones, though I am prepared to accept them as an alternative) and then just make a quick salad with watercress (or one of those packets of watercress mixed with young spinach) and thinly sliced, medicinal, bulb fennel. This is the perfect foil to the pungent creaminess of the fish and sauce. A small amount of grain mustard in the salad's dressing will work well. I love my mother's cabbage with caraway here, too. Shred half a large white cabbage, either by hand or in the processor (using slicing disc). Melt 30g or so butter and a tablespoon of olive oil in a large, deep frying pan or wok. Scatter in a tablespoonful of caraway seeds, then toss the cabbage in. Keep stirring and tossing over high heat till the cabbage has wilted and shrunk a little (a couple of minutes or so) and then throw in about 200ml of hot stock (I use a pinch of vegetable bouillon powder in some boiling water) and toss, then clamp on a lid. In another couple of minutes or thereabouts, remove the lid, let bubble away for another minute and then serve: if you want to add more butter or more caraway seeds at this stage, do; anyway, sprinkle salt and grind pepper over generously.

CABBAGE WITH CARAWAY

Fry 3–4 coxes, peeled and cut into eighths, in about 60g butter until brown on each side. Sprinkle thickly with caster sugar until that too browns and then pile onto a plate and serve with ice-cream or cream (or add the cream to the juices in the pan and make a sauce that way). Ben & Jerry's Rainforest Crunch ice-cream is delicious with these buttery, caramelly apples.

BUTTERED APPLES

Chambéry trout

Salsa verde

With the herby, vermouth-poached trout serve a salsa verde, which is the perfect foil for the fish and an excellent idea for the quick cook anyway, since all you need to do is to put everything in a food processor and turn it on. The salsa verde is good with poached chicken breasts, too (see above, page 183).

With either the fish or the chicken, I'd go for some broad beans, which are perfect with the salsa verde, being, I suppose, an Italianate version of broad beans with parsley sauce which I ate often as a child. It's true that frozen ones tend to have rather a tough hide, but I can live with it. If you can't, take them out of the freezer before you go out in the morning. When you get back home in the evening they'll have thawed and you can then slip their skins off easily. Skinless, too, their cooking time will be reduced. Otherwise go for lentils, tinned if need be, with lardons, cubes of pancetta or strips of bacon, stirred into them. But remember that the bacon is salty and the salsa verde is salty and that tinned lentils tend to be salty, so go steady. That's why pancetta, if you can get it, is a better choice; otherwise remember that unsmoked bacon is generally (or at least I have found it to be so) less salty than smoked. For pudding: ice-cream slightly zhuzhed-up.

CHAMBÉRY TROUT

This is another easy way of cooking fish without touching it while you do so. I keep a bottle of Chambéry or Noilly Prat in the kitchen at all times, primarily because I am not much of a drinker and don't necessarily want to open a bottle of wine when I need just a little for something I'm cooking. Of course, if you've got friends coming for dinner you might want to drink white wine with the fish, so obviously use some of that rather than the Chambéry if you prefer. In which case, use 200ml wine, dispensing with the water.

butter or oil for greasing
4 trout, cleaned, with the heads left on
150ml Chambéry

Preheat the oven to gas mark 6/200°C.

Grease a baking dish – for 4 trout I use an old enamel one I have that measures about 30cm x 20cm – and then put the cleaned and seasoned trout in it. Pour over the Chambéry mixed with 50ml water, cover loosely with foil, making sure the foil doesn't touch the fish, and bake for about 20 minutes. When the fish is ready, the flesh should be beginning to be flaky and have lost its translucency. It's probably better to take the fish out before you think it is absolutely *à point*, as you can just let it stand, still covered, and to one side, for a few minutes, in which time it will continue to cook gently, which is the best way.

SALSA VERDE

I first had salsa verde when I was a chambermaid in Florence. I was there with a schoolfriend and we used to go, most evenings, to a trattoria called Benvenuto, and eat tortellini in *brodo*, their penne *al modo nostro*, which involved an intensely garlicky tomato sauce, then moussey-sweet *fegato* or, my favourite, tongue with salsa verde. Now I wonder how good the restaurant was, but then, when most of the time we were living on a bottle of wine, a loaf of bread and a kilo of tomatoes between us a day, it seemed like heaven. Anyway, after a while we came back mostly for the clientèle, made up in significant part by the local community of transsexuals and transvestites. The most beautiful of all of them, and the one generally held to be the glorious and burnished figurehead, the presiding force and icon, was a Bardot-esque blonde, only more muscular, known as La Principessa; those less appreciative of her aesthetic construction referred to her simply as La Romana. I felt I'd arrived when she huskily called out, 'Ciao bella' to me across the street one day.

Salsa verde has, since those days, become something of a menu commonplace over here, but the salsa verde that gets served up is often much fancier – with mint, basil, sometimes even coriander thrown in – than Benvenuto's version, which was just parsley, capers, cornichons, anchovy, oil and vinegar, making a semi-liquid, deep-flavoured and spiky sauce the colour of snooker baize. I, too, sometimes add to that basic mixture. I might throw in rocket, bought, not all limp in its expensively enveloped state at the supermarket, but in robust great bunches from the Greek greengrocer's; it gives a wonderful pepperiness (itself a good balance for the gratifyingly searing saltiness of the anchovies). At other times, tarragon, just a little, lends an aniseedy and hay-fresh muskiness.

After the salsa verde has emulsified, to make it creamier and more liquid I spoon or dribble in a good few tablespoons of the winey liquid in which the fish has been soaking. Normally, salsa verde has lemon added at the end if it's to accompany fish, vinegar if it's to go with boiled meats, but I tend to use vinegar more often, even with fish. And although it is not at all *come si deve*, I quite like borrowing a trick from *sauce gribiche* and adding some finely-chopped hard-boiled egg white, too, but for practical purposes, when the idea is to cook quickly, there's no call even to consider such innovations.

Now: I know most people put garlic in. But I thought I remembered that, when I had the salsa verde with tongue in Florence all that time ago, there wasn't any garlic in it. I couldn't be absolutely sure, so I asked Anna del Conte, the best Italian foodwriter in English, a great authority, utterly versed in her subject and a reassuring, illuminating recipe doctor. I felt doubtful suddenly only because every salsa verde I've eaten since has had garlic in. She reassured me, said that it most certainly wouldn't have had: salsa verde emanates from Lombardy (where the parsley is especially prized) and garlic was then anathema to the Lombardi. Breadcrumbs or some boiled or mashed potato (to thicken the mixture) are also traditional. Of course you can add garlic if you want, but I suggest not too much. I don't add breadcrumbs or potato simply because I use the food processor to blend it all, and the machine automatically thickens it. It is difficult to be specific about amounts, but what you should end up with is a green-flecked, almost solid liquid, which *looks* as if a spoon would stand up in it, even if, in fact, the spoon would, put to the test, soon sink gloopily into that thick, green, parsley-dense pond.

1 large bunch flat-leaf parsley
3 anchovy fillets
1 tablespoon capers
2 cornichons (miniature gherkins)
approx. 8 tablespoons extra virgin olive oil
approx. 5 tablespoons fish poaching liquid
approx. 1 tablespoon wine vinegar or lemon juice, to taste

Tear the parsley leaves from the stalks (don't worry about being too neat) and put them in the bowl of the food processor (don't even think about doing this sauce, or at least not if you want to get it ready quickly and with a minimum of effort, if you haven't got a food processor: just mix some oil and lemon together instead). Add the anchovy fillets (if they taste rebarbatively salty then soak them briefly in a saucer of milk), the capers (well rinsed in cold water and drained if they've been packed in salt) and the cornichons. Switch on and pulse, then scrape the bowl with a spatula and turn on again. Then, with the machine still running, gradually pour the olive oil through the funnel. Take the lid off to check how thick the sauce is becoming and dip in a finger to taste. Scrape down any mixture from the sides. Add more oil if needed, then when the fish is ready, spoon in some of the poaching liquid, all while processing. Taste after every small addition. Then pour the salsa verde into a bowl with a spoon and stir in the vinegar or lemon, a little at a time. And that's it. Keep whatever's left over in the fridge, covered with clingfilm. Eccentric though this might sound, I love it, sharp and cold and salty, with hot, fat, spicy, or even not spicy, sausages.

PUDDING

Again, this idea has been adumbrated earlier: to ice-cream you simply add some processor-pulverised chocolate. Break 100g of the best, most malevolently dark chocolate you can find into small squares and put them into the bowl of the food processor. Make sure they're cold before you start. Process and blitz them to dusty rubble. Empty onto a plate and put this plate in the fridge until you need it. At which time, pour the pulverised chocolate into a small bowl and put on the table alongside the tub of ice-cream.

Escalopes of salmon with warm balsamic vinaigrette

Bread, cheese and grapes

Any thin fillet of meat or fish will cook quickly, but salmon is particularly useful because its oiliness stops it from drying to rebarbative cardboardiness in the heat. But still, exercise caution: don't overcook; just dunk these fleshy, coral-coloured rags into the pan.

Balsamic vinegar is one of those ingredients whose fashionability leads people to disparage it. But the sweet pungency of the balsamic vinegar here is so right with the oily meatiness of the fish that its use is justified. After this, you can expand into a good plate of perfectly *à point* brie or camembert and another of aromatic, wine-toned grapes. Both *must* be at room temperature.

ESCALOPES OF SALMON WITH WARM BALSAMIC VINAIGRETTE

8 escalopes or thin fillets salmon, preferably wild, about 100g each
6 tablespoons balsamic vinegar
6 tablespoons olive oil
small bunch chives

Heat a thick-based or good non-stick pan or a griddle (using the smooth side) and cook the salmon for 1 minute on each side, then turn again for another 1 minute on each side. Put on a warmed plate and, when all are ready, sprinkle with chives you have snipped with scissors. Keep warm with tented foil.

In a small pan, heat the balsamic vinegar and oil until warm (but not hot) and dribble a little over the fish. Pour the remaining vinaigrette into a small jug (with a teaspoon near it, for stirring) and let people pour or spoon over as they wish. The measurements I've stipulated, strictly speaking, give you more than you need, but otherwise you will be producing such a mean-looking puddle.

Another way of doing this, and how I always do it if there's just me eating, is to pour a few drops of oil into the pan (you can't use a griddle here) and fry the salmon in it. Then, when the fish is cooked and on its plate, I pour a few drops of balsamic vinegar into the pan in which I've cooked the fish, swirl it about and pour it over the fish. Dot with scissored chives, and eat.

What works here is the gentle balance between the sweet acidity of the vinegar and the meaty oiliness of the fish. But you could elaborate on this theme with other vinegars, or the juices of lime, lemon or Seville orange.

If you're using lemon juice, fry the salmon in a small amount of olive oil and add (off the heat, at the end) parsley, feathery green wodges of the stuff, vigorously chopped but not minced by machine (unless you're using huge great quantities, the food processor is not the answer – you just end up with a damp green mess) in place of the chives.

If you want to deglaze the pan with lime, which makes for an intense and astringent dressing, cook the salmon first in a nut of butter. The sweetness of the butter counters the more invasively acid punch of the lime. Chop over musky, pungent, fresh coriander, but not much of it, just before serving. Or leave the salmon itself relatively unprinked and add the coriander, in relative abundance, to a couple of tins of drained, oil-dressed cannellini beans.

Before the cheese, you may want a green salad; or put all on the table together.

Cinnamon-hot rack of lamb with cherried and chick pea'd couscous

Baked figs

Lamb can be cooked very quickly indeed. Many people, however, stuff, prink and generally fuss about rack of lamb, but the truth is you need do nothing providing you buy good meat. Applying a little oil and spice will not take very long. It will make the fat crisp up better, which is a consideration, but frankly it won't matter if you don't bother. The figs afterwards offer sweet, plump, ripe fruitiness and appropriate exotic voluptuousness.

If you wanted, you could cook quail instead of lamb, in which case substitute 8 quail for the lamb and add some butter, also mixed with a little cinnamon, to put into the birds' cavities.

CINNAMON-HOT RACK OF LAMB

2 racks lamb
1 scant tablespoon chilli oil
½ tablespoon cinnamon

Preheat the oven to gas mark 8/220°C.

Mix the oil and cinnamon to a paste and rub over the meat. Place on a rack over a baking tin and cook for about 30 minutes. The skin should be conker-shiny and the meat within pink and tender. Let stand for 5 minutes or so before serving. Turn the oven down to gas mark 4/180°C for the figs.

CHERRIED AND CHICK PEA'D COUSCOUS

Couscous should, traditionally, be soaked and then steamed (see page 228), but you don't have to; if you're adding bits and pieces to it you can get away with this incorrect procedure, although expect aficionados to be shocked. It is difficult to give precise details for the couscous since different brands give slightly different instructions. I tend to use the Ferrero make of precooked couscous, which comes in a turquoise box with a picture of a comely Disneyish Middle-Eastern maid on it, and so the amount of liquid stipulated below is geared towards this brand. But even so, you may need to add a little more liquid if you think the grains are too stodgy.

Now, normally, I hate fruit in savoury concoctions, but the sour cherries here really do work. There is an authenticity to the mixture of sweet dried fruit and waxy nut and fragrant buttery grain. But if you don't like the idea of sour cherries, just leave them out.

The couscous will taste better if it has been steeped in stock rather than water, but by making stock I don't mean anything more arduous than stirring 2 teaspoons of Marigold bouillon powder or half a stock cube into boiling water.

2 teaspoons Marigold bouillon powder
350g couscous
40g dried sour cherries
½ teaspoon ground cumin
½ teaspoon cinnamon
60g pine nuts
400g tin chick peas
30g butter

Boil the kettle. Pour boiling water into a measuring jug to get 450ml, add the bouillon granules or crumbled ½ stock cube, then pour into a saucepan and bring to the boil again. Add salt. Put the couscous in a bowl, mix in the cherries, cumin and cinnamon and then turn into the pan of boiling water. Wait until it starts to boil again, put the lid on and take the pan off the heat. Meanwhile, put a thick frying pan on the hob and, when it's hot, toast the pine nuts. When they are beginning to turn golden, remove them.

Heat through the canned chick peas. When the couscous is tender and has absorbed the liquid, add the drained warm chick peas, stir in the butter, then half the pine nuts, and turn out on to a large heated plate and sprinkle with remaining pine nuts. You will probably have more couscous than you need here, but I feel that making less than this looks so miserable and unwelcoming. Anyway, it tastes good the next day. The best way of reheating it is either by steaming (a sieve suspended over a pan of boiling water will do it) or a quick burst in a microwave. Eat hot with some freshly snipped spring onions stirred into it and some harissa to the side.

BAKED FIGS

8 black figs
60g butter
4 heaped tablespoons honey
100ml red wine
4 cardomum pods, lightly crushed (or a couple of crumbled bay leaves)

Put the figs in an ovenproof dish in which they'll fit pretty snugly. Cut each one as if in quarters, only leaving the base intact. In a saucepan put the butter, honey, wine and cardomum and heat up. When the butter's melted, the honey's dissolved and you have a smooth, hot, sweet gravy, pour over the figs and put in the oven for about a quarter of an hour. Remove and let sit for 5 minutes or so before eating; and when you eat, make sure it's with a dollop of satiny, cold, Greek yoghurt to the side.

Chicken with spring onion, chilli and greek yoghurt
Seven-minute steamed chocolate pudding

During my time as a restaurant critic, I became obsessed with the insistent inanities of the fashionable menu. In the end, either someone can cook or they can't, either the food tastes good or it doesn't. I object, for example, to the term pan-fried. I mind because what are you going to fry something in, if not in a pan? But the thing about pan-fried is not so much that it is tautologous, as that it is a con-trick. Let me deconstruct: fried is greasy, heavy, fattening, old-style food which none of us eats any more; pan-fried is modern, light, clean-living, healthy. The distorted echoes of 'stir-fried' help formulate that image-by-association. But food, whether fried or pan-fried, is cooked in the same way. It's a brilliant wheeze. If you had read 'fried chicken', most of you would have immediately given a shudder. I could call it grilled (or even griddled) chicken and that would have been OK. But I have my doubts about the efficacy of the domestic grill, in the first place, and not everyone owns a griddle, in the second.

I cannot, just cannot, bring myself to call it pan-fried chicken. So, just chicken it is.

CHICKEN WITH SPRING ONION, CHILLI AND GREEK YOGHURT

The accompaniment borrows from the idea of tsatsiki and all those Middle-Eastern yoghurt salads; I have my friends Lucy Heller and Charles Elton to thank for it. I haven't put cucumber in this recipe, but sometimes I do. Coriander is, funnily enough, easier to come by than mint these days (although mint is certainly the traditional herb to use here) so you can use either of them. The point is to have a cool, pungent accompaniment to the tender, but not strongly flavoured, poultry. You can fashion it as you wish. If I use cucumber, I don't bother to salt and degorge it: it may, therefore, get watery if you leave it lying around, but, since this is a quick dinner, the trade-off is worth it. Use that unctuously creamy and solid Greek yoghurt: you want this sauce to be astringent but voluptuous; normal low-fat natural yoghurt is too thin, sour and depressing.

For this I would use the cut known as a supreme: a chicken breast which has usually been skinned, and is boned except for the small peg of shoulder bone. If it's easier, just buy breast portions, but in either case preferably from a corn-fed or free-range bird, and leave the skin on if you wish. It will look glorious if you happen to have a ridged griddle to put over the hob, but a thick-based frying pan is more than fine. Don't use a non-stick pan: you want a burnt-golden exterior and the non-stick pan pointedly can't give you that.

I think it's necessary to cook extra chicken, even if you have to fry it in two batches, just because I have never known people not to want more. And how could leftovers matter?

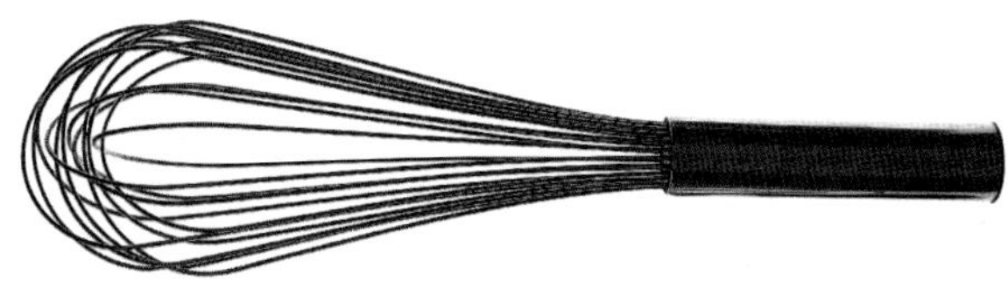

6 skinless chicken breasts
juice of 2 lemons
approx. 6 tablespoons olive oil
decent-sized bunch spring onions
1 green chilli
2 cloves garlic
1/2 cucumber (optional)
smallish bunch fresh coriander, to make about 2–4 tablespoons (to taste) when chopped
same amount of mint
400g tub Greek yoghurt

While you're making the sauce, marinate the chicken in the lemon juice and 3 tablespoons oil. Season with salt and pepper. If the breasts look fat and plump – you want them to cook fairly speedily – then put them between 2 sheets of greaseproof paper or clingfilm and bash them, using anything heavy you can lay your hands on – a can of baked beans, say – if you're not the sort to keep a meat mallet in the top drawer in your kitchen.

Slice the spring onions finely and deseed and chop the chilli finely, too. Peel the garlic cloves and cut each clove in very small pieces, preferably using a mezzaluna. If you are using cucumber, cut it up into small cubes. Peel it or don't peel it as you wish: I tend to use a potato peeler to shave off strips of peel so that there's a stripey dark-green, light-green effect; this was how my mother always did it. Chop the coriander and mint: again, the mezzaluna is the best way of doing this. Add everything to the Greek yoghurt. Stir, taste and add salt as needed.

Remove the chicken from the marinade. Add 2 tablespoons oil to a large frying pan and when it's hot, fry the chicken. Turn over after 5 minutes or so and cook the other side for about 5 minutes. It may be cooked, it may need more time. You may need to add a little more oil while cooking; you certainly will if you're frying in two batches. If you want, when the chicken is cooked, you can thrown the lemony marinade over it in the pan at the last minute. Arrange a large plate, and serve the yoghurt relish in a bowl with a spoon.

With this, I might give the couscous (see page 205 above) minus the cinnamon and minus the dried cherries. A tomato salad, with or without black olives, is all you need otherwise. If you can't find any tomatoes with flavour, then a crisp-leaved green salad will do.

SEVEN-MINUTE STEAMED CHOCOLATE PUDDING

I am not a particular fan of the microwave, except for defrosting baby meals and reheating cold roast potatoes (divine, though dangerous: I wish my Aunt Fel hadn't told me of this), but I had this chocolate pudding at the home of some friends one Saturday lunch-time and thought it was amazingly good: thick and rich and chocolatey. One thing, though: don't hide the fact that you're microwaving it: they do say the proof of the pudding is in the eating. This takes 2 minutes to prepare in the food processor, 5 minutes actually to cook in the microwave and 10 minutes' standing time after that. If you get everything ready in advance, just bung it in the microwave 15 minutes or so before you think you'll want to eat it.

This recipe comes from Barbara Kafka's *Microwave Gourmet* and I have kept to her quantities for 8 people because I am greedy. If you – unlike me – think 4 people won't eat enough for 8, then halve the quantities and cooking time and use a 750ml pudding basin.

150g unsalted butter
250g good quality dark chocolate
100g light brown sugar
1 teaspoon vanilla essence
125ml double cream
40g plain flour, sifted
½ teaspoon baking powder
3 eggs
double cream or crème fraîche for serving

Butter a 22½ x 10cm ceramic bowl or 1 litre pudding basin with 30g of the butter.

Grate chocolate in a food processor, then, with the normal, double-bladed knife fitting in place, add the remaining butter, cut into 8 pieces, and sugar. Process until thoroughly combined. Add remaining ingredients and process to a smooth mixture.

Pour into a prepared bowl. Cover tightly with microwave clingfilm. Cook at 100 per cent (Barbara Kafka refers to a 600–700 watt microwave as the norm. Mine is 750 watt but I leave cooking time as is) for 5 minutes, until set. Pierce film with the tip of a sharp knife, remove from the oven and cover the top of the bowl with a heavy plate; this will keep the pudding hot. Let stand for 10 minutes.

Put some double cream or crème fraîche – I prefer crème fraîche, as the sourness sets off the palate-coating sweetness better – in a bowl on the table.

Steak mirabeau

Raspberries and cream

The steak mirabeau is a recipe from one of my favourite cookery books, Ann and Franco Taruschio's *Leaves from the Walnut Tree* (the Walnut Tree was Elizabeth David's favourite restaurant), which is written with such love and quiet authority: you can trust this book; nothing is for effect and everything works. Innocent of illustration, *Leaves from the Walnut Tree* is far from being a chef-book. Often, when I'm wondering what to cook, and want to find something simple that won't take too long, I turn to it. This is just such a recipe. And it shows, too, the Taruschios' confident affection for the sort of food that glossier establishments with less secure foundations tend to eschew in a panic-stricken search for something ever new.

All you need after are raspberries and cream (and see below).

STEAK MIRABEAU

Buy good-quality anchovy fillets in olive oil and drain well. You could soak them for a few minutes in milk before draining well again, if you're worried that the fillets you've got are just too unbearably salty, but do remember that the particular fierce rasp of the anchovy is what's wanted here, so don't attempt to drown it out. I love anchovies with meat (see page 112 and 382) and, if you wanted, you could just as easily use some lamb steaks here. You could leave out the olives and the criss-crossing business, too. A tablespoon or so of cream at the end will make for a mellower concoction, but still a pleasurably bracing one.

1 tablespoon olive oil
2 tablespoons butter
4 sirloin steaks
freshly ground black pepper
20 anchovy fillets
18 pitted black olives, halved
1 glass red wine

Heat the oil and butter in a frying pan and when it's foaming add the steaks. Cook as preferred – I like mine bloody, so do them for 3 or so minutes a side – and season with freshly ground black pepper. When ready, remove to a large, warmed plate. Criss-cross the steaks with 4 anchovy fillets each and place the olive halves in the squares. (This doesn't look as dinky-do as it sounds.) Mash the remaining 4 anchovy fillets in the pan juices, add the red wine and reduce rapidly until a glaze appears on the sauce. Pour the sauce over the steaks and serve at once.

Perfect, sweet, waxy new potatoes are what you want with this; I love, too, the iron tang of some leaf spinach (frozen, to be sure) just buttered and nutmegged, soaking up the wine and olive brine of the steak.

RASPBERRIES AND CREAM

I suggest raspberries and cream for pudding: a mound of the fruit, a thick yellow bowl of the cream. If raspberries aren't absolutely as they should be at the moment, then stick to the same ingredients but treat them with less respect. Mash 300g raspberries (bar a couple of tablespoons which you've removed for later), tired fresh or just thawed frozen, sprinkled with a little icing sugar, in a bowl with a fork. Whisk 300ml, or thereabouts, double or whipping cream with 1–2 further tablespoons of icing sugar. Fold in the raspberries and spoon this rough fool into a bowl (or individual glasses if you prefer) and scatter the unmashed ones over the top. And you can always crumble in some shop-bought meringues, too.

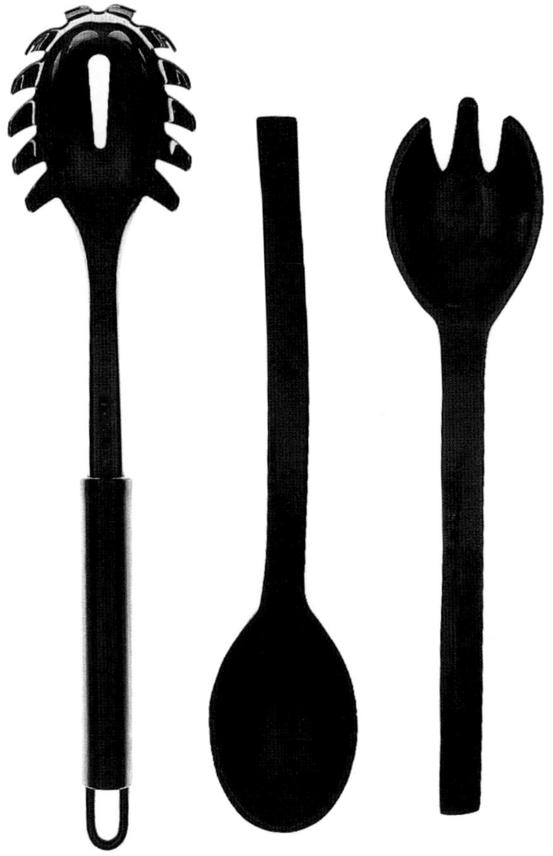

weekend lunch

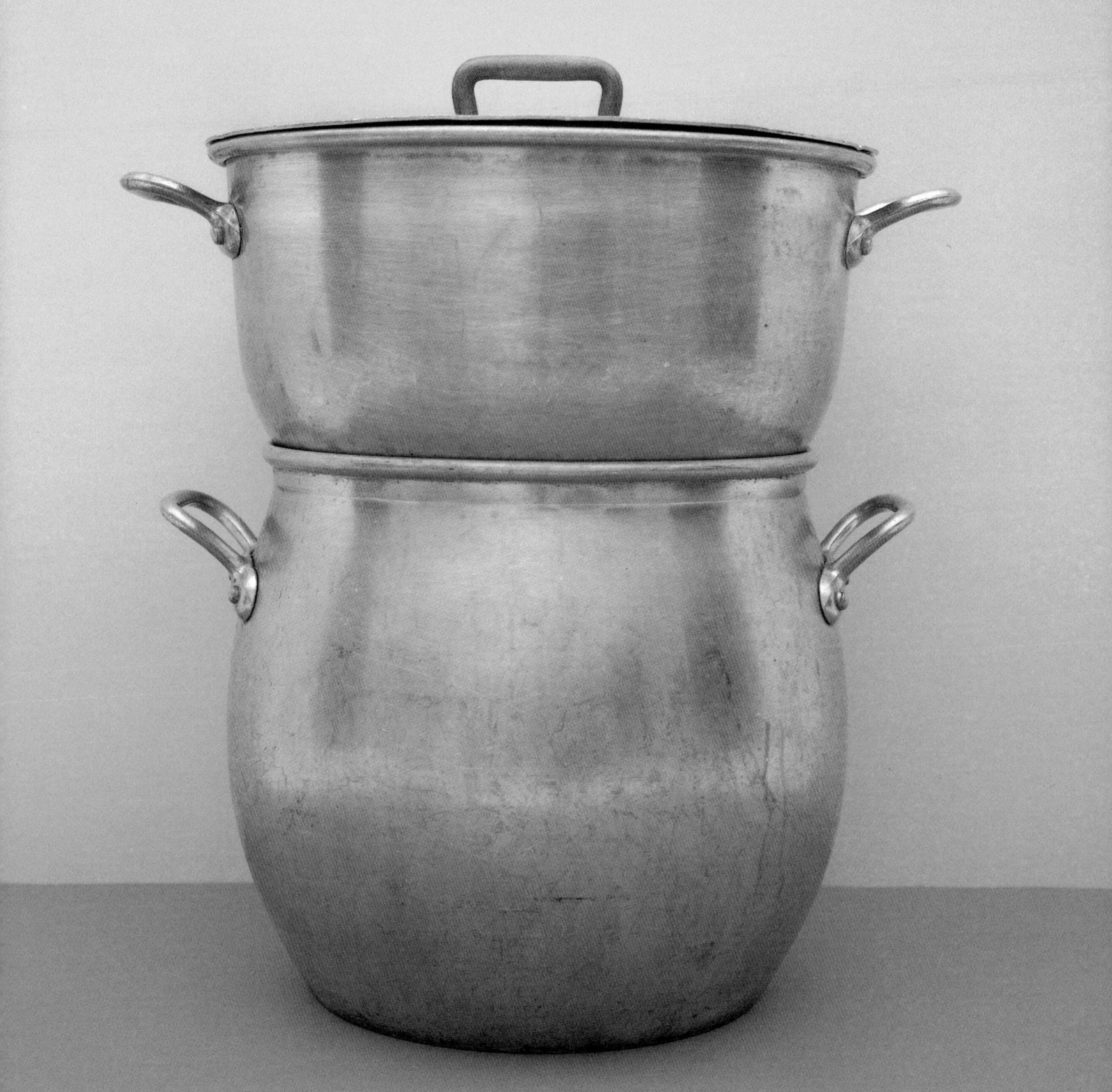

Although the dinner party remains the symbol of social eating, most eating in company among my friends actually takes place at weekend lunch. After a long day at work many of us are, frankly, too tired to go out and eat dinner, let alone cook it. And there is, as well, the baby factor. For many people of my generation, having to get food ready after the children have gone to bed explains the popularity of the Marks & Spencer menu. And even those who haven't got children are affected by the babysitting arrangements of their friends who have. When I was younger we stayed in bed at weekends until two in the afternoon: now that most of us are woken at six in the morning, there is a gap in the day where lunch can go. We have got into the habit of filling it.

AN INDOOR PICNIC

Lunch is more forgiving than dinner: there isn't the dread engendered by perceived but not-quite-formulated expectations: there's no agenda, no aspirational model to follow, no socio-culinary challenge to which to rise; in short, no pressure. Lunch is just lunch.

And if you don't want to cook it, you don't have to. Saturday lunch can be at its most relaxed and pleasurable when it is just an indoor picnic. What matters, then, is what you buy. These days shopping is nobly recast as 'sourcing' – and clever you for finding the best chilli-marinaded olives, French sourdough bread or air-dried beef: certainly no shame for not clattering about with your own pots and pans instead.

Shopping is not necessarily the easy option. It's certainly not the cheap one. But discerning extravagance (rather than mere feckless vulgarity) can be immensely pleasurable. Indeed, I can find it positively uplifting: not for nothing is shopping known as retail therapy. Shopping for food is better than any other form of shopping. There's no trying-on for a start. Choosing the right cheese, the best and ripest tomato, the pinkest, sweetest ham can be intensely gratifying. And in shopping for food which you are then going to prepare (even if that preparation involves no more than de-bagging and unwrapping) there is also the glorious self-indulgence of knowing that you are giving pleasure to others.

weekend lunch

Shopping is not a quick activity: you need to be prepared to proceed slowly, haltingly. Compromise can be ruinous. Of course, some of the time we all eat food that is less than perfect, less than enjoyable even, but you can't set out to buy inferior produce – what would be the point?

Good food doesn't have to be difficult to cook, and it certainly doesn't need to be difficult to buy. But you must know what you're after. The important thing is to be greedy enough to get what's good, but not so restlessly greedy that you get too much of it. Restrict your choices, so that you provide lots of a few things rather than small amounts of many. This is partly an aesthetic dictate, partly a practical one. If you buy 100g slices of six different cheeses, everyone is going to feel inhibited about cutting some off; however generous you have been, it is only the meagreness of each portion that will be apparent. Provide, instead, a semblance – indeed the reality – of voluptuous abundance. You don't need to buy more than three different cheeses, but get great big fat wodges of each. You want munificence, you want plenty, you want people to feel they can eat as much as they want and there'll still be some left over afterwards. Start by thinking along the lines of one hard cheese, one soft cheese and maybe a blue cheese or chèvre. You needn't stick to this rigidly: sometimes it's good just to be seduced by the particular cheeses spread out in front of you on a cheese counter. Keep your head, though: without ruling out whim entirely, don't be immoderately ensnared by fanciful names or the provocatively unfamiliar. One type of cheese no one has heard of might well be interesting, but not three. Anyway, the desire to be interesting is possibly the most damaging impulse in cooking. Never worry about what your guests will think of you. Just think of the food. What will taste good?

And you don't have to go through the ridiculous pantomime of pretending everything is homespun. If you're still getting your shopping out and unwrapping your packages when everyone arrives, who cares? Your kitchen doesn't have to look like a set from a 1950s American sitcom. It is curiously relaxing to be slowly creating the canvas – arranging the table, putting flowers in a vase, chopping up herbs and putting water on for potatoes – while talking and drinking unhurriedly with friends.

The shops nearest you will probably govern what sort of food you buy. I stick to the plainest basics: meat, cheese, bread; with tomatoes, a green salad, maybe some robustly salted, herb-speckled potatoes, the waxy fleshed, puce-skinned ones, cooked till sweet and soft then doused in oil, scarcely dribbled with vinegar or spritzed with lemon, and with a few feathery pieces of chopped zest on them, left to sit around to be eaten at room temperature.

ENGLISH HAM

PROSCIUTTO

If you're buying ham, get enough to cover a huge great plate with densely meaty pink slices. I sometimes buy both English ham, cut off the bone in the shop, and the cured Italian stuff. I like prosciutto di San Daniele better than prosciutto di Parma (the glorious, requisite, honeyed saltiness is more intense), but as long as it's well cut – and obviously freshly cut – so that each white-rimmed silky slice can be removed without sticking or tearing, that's fine: more than fine.

PORK PIE

SALAME

OLIVES

ANCHOVIES

There is internal pressure in my home to buy bresaola, too, but although I like eating it well enough, I never mind if I don't. I'd rather buy a big, unpacketed, butcher-made pork pie, one which has a short, short flaky crust lined with clear salty jelly and then, within, densely packed smooth and peppery pork. Salame, too, is good. I don't think you need both salame and pie, so choose which you prefer. If you buy a whole little salame, as with the large pork pie, you can introduce an all-important DIY element into the proceedings: put it on a wooden board with a sharp knife and let people carve off for themselves thick, fat-pearled slices of spicy sausage. This way, the individual act of cutting, slicing, serving yourself, becomes almost a conversational tool. It makes people feel at home when they're around your kitchen table. Allow yourself a few saucer-sized plates of extras – maybe some fresh, marinaded anchovies, olives steeped with shards of garlic and crumbled red chillies, astringent little cornichons, those ones that look like cartoon crocodiles in embryo, a soft, moussy slab of pâté – but, again, don't go overboard. I sometimes succumb to one of those Italian jars of olive-oil-soused blackened globes of chargrilled onions, sweet and smoky and wonderful with meat or cheese or a plain plate of bitter leaves.

SMOKED SALMON

TUNA AND BEANS

If you prefer fish to meat, go for the old-fashioned traditional option: a huge plate of London-cure smoked salmon – mild, satiny and softly fleshy – with cornichons, lemon and maybe a pile of blinis (see page 170 to make them, or buy the French ones in vacuum packs), potato pancakes (and see page 242), a loaf or two of sandy soda bread, or thinly sliced and already buttered brown. If you have a delicatessen or fishmonger near you that sells a good enough version of the stuff, then maybe you should get a tentacled mess of Italianish seafood salad. I quite like, too, that old-fashioned pairing of tuna and beans. My Great Aunt Myra, who was a wonderful cook, always used butter beans (just out of the tin, as was, of course, the olive-oil preserved tuna) and would gently mix the two, squeeze lemon over and cover with a fine net of wafer-thin onion rings. Yes, proper dried then soaked and cooked and drained real beans are always better, but there's something comforting and familiar for me in that quick and effort-free assembly. It tastes of my childhood.

BREAD

Smoked salmon calls for brown bread, but there's something reassuring about a thick wedge of white bread, heavy with cold unsalted butter and curved over a tranche of quickly grabbed ham to make a casual sandwich. But all that matters is that the bread is good: sweet, sunflower-seed-studded brown, English bloomer or French bread – which could be a just-bought baguette or, my favourite, the slender ficelle. I sometimes think if I see another ciabatta I'll scream.

TOMATOES

Frankly, if you can get good enough tomatoes, I'd just leave them as they are, whole, with a knife near by (a good, sharp, serrated one, suitable for the job) so that people can eat them in juicy red wedges with their bread and cheese, or cut them thinly and sprinkle with oil and salt to make their own private pools of tomato salad.

SALAD

A green salad needn't comprise anything other than lettuce. All you need for dressing is good oil, a quick squeeze of lemon and a confident hand with the salt, tossed with your own bare hands. You can, of course, supplement the torn leaves (and let's be frank, most of us will be opening one of those cellophane packets) with some thin tongues of courgette (the slivers stripped off with the vegetable peeler), chopped spring onions or a handful of not-even-blanched sugar-snap peas or whatever you want. There's one proviso: keep it green. There is something depressingly institutional about cheerfully mixed salads. I was brought up like this: my mother was fanatical, and her aesthetic has seeped into my bloodstream; my father takes the same line. Do not even think of adding your tomatoes: keep them separate. Cucumber tends to make the salad weepy. Give it its own plate, and dress with peppery, mint-thick or dill-soused yoghurt or an old-fashioned sweet-sour vinaigrette.

In the same way, I am fanatical about keeping fruit separate. There is, for me, something so boarding-housey about the capacious bowl filled with waxy, dusty bananas, a few oranges, some pears and the odd shrunken apple. I want a plate of oranges, another of bananas, of apples, of pears. I even put black and white grapes on separate plates.

An unfussy lunch sprawled out on a Saturday definitely doesn't demand culinary high jinks. Don't worry about pudding. You just need some tubs of good ice-cream – Rocombe Farm if you can get it (and the Waitrose organic vanilla is made by Rocombe Farm) or Ben and Jerry's or whichever make you like most. Or buy a tart from a good French pâtisserie.

I like just picking at food laid out in front of me, although I am alarmed at how much I can eat, and go on eating, that way. But somehow it can be good to have a full stop put on it. Sometimes, after a deli-to-table picnicky lunch, I feel I want to eat something, well, puddingy for pudding. A treacle tart or sponge (created in the food processor), a chocolate pudding or apple crumble, are a proper focus, reassuring after all that ambling about and fidgety grazing.

We all have our own fallback dishes: recipes we know so well that we don't even consider them recipes any more. I often cook the same thing for close friends at weekend lunch. In order of frequency these are roast chicken, just as it is, or cooked breast down in butter, with a lemon up its bottom and garlic littered around the pan; the effortless chicken with green chilli and herb yoghurt on page 207; linguine with lemon cream sauce (see page 253); and sausages and mash (see page 270).

The following ideas for weekend lunch are just that – ideas. I have suggested two courses. If you want to have bits of prosciutto or a bowlful of olives or designer crisps on the table while you're finishing off the cooking, do.

BASIC NO-EFFORT SATURDAY LUNCH

Roast chicken with green salad

Summer fruits and cream or ice-cream

A roast chicken is my basic Saturday lunch, Sunday lunch, any day, or even ceremonial dinner. This explains why I singled it out in Basics (page 8). You can use ginger to spruce it up instead of lemon. Rub the skin of a chicken with fresh ginger (make sure you've got a juicy tuber) and then cut some slices off the root and stuff the inside of the cavity with them. Gingered chicken makes for a wonderful chicken salad later: bring out that tin of water chestnuts from the bottom of the store cupboard if you dare, use lots of crunchy green leaves and some raw sugar-snap peas (or failing that, mangetouts) and sprinkle with some sesame seeds which have been briskly toasted in a fatless pan before generously dousing with an orientalish dressing. Use soy, use sesame oil, use rice vinegar –

GINGERED CHICKEN SALAD

one in a fairly normal vinaigrette or all three in conjunction as you wish – and eat in front of the TV.

Keep the green salad to go with either the ginger or the lemon chicken simple. Two small-to-medium chickens are fine for 8 and won't take long to cook. If you're on a particularly tight timetable, get the butcher to spatchcock the chickens for you (in which case ¾ hour at gas mark 6/200°C should do it). And all chicken is good eaten at getting-towards-room-temperature, especially spatchcocked chicken.

MIXED FRUITS

For pudding I often provide just a plate of mixed fruits: in winter out of a packet picked up from the freezer compartment; otherwise whatever's in season. Frozen berries are fine providing they're sufficiently thawed and you have removed every last strawberry. Sprinkle with some sugar, the finely chopped zest of ½–1 unwaxed orange (I use my zester to get the rind off, and then the mezzaluna to chop it finely, although I do sometimes leave the zest as is in thin little stringy ribbons) and a tablespoon or so of a liqueur of some sort. I throw all that stuff over while the berries are still frozen and then, just before eating them, I push over some icing sugar through my tea strainer so that they look beautiful. If I can't stop myself, I add a few tiny leaves of mint from the garden. Serve with good vanilla ice-cream or thick double cream. Normally for puddings I prefer crème fraîche, but here I wouldn't want any hint of sourness (the fruit, after all, has that), but might rather go for a bowl of cream whipped up with sugar and perhaps a drop of real vanilla extract. Work on the principle of one 500g packet of berries for 4 people.

ICE-CREAM

THE SLIGHTLY MORE THAN BASIC SATURDAY LUNCH FOR 6–8

Lemon chicken

Pecorino and pears, or sticky chocolate pudding

This lemon chicken is a not too anglo version of the Greek kotopoulo lemonato, that's to say chicken roasted in portions in the oven with wine and water to make an aromatic liquid to produce, along with eggs and lemon, a sharp but deeply flavoured avgolemono sauce. Obviously, you can serve it with just a green salad, especially in hot weather, but otherwise I'd do a bowlful of buttery basmati rice (quite the easiest rice to cook and the fastest, and see page 300) and some peas (which in my house means frozen petits pois, with some sugar added to the water along with salt and some basil with butter, a nut of which I add to the drained hot peas: chop the basil at the very last moment or else use some basil-infused olive oil). Or you could substitute for the rice and peas a large bowlful of broad beans. Fresh if you can, but if you are using frozen, thaw first and then slip off the skins. Then just steam the already soft beans or, better still, sauté them in some butter or olive oil with garlic and parsley, or mint, or indeed both.

PEAS

I cook the chicken in the oven just because I find it the most relaxing way to deal with it, but if you prefer to grill or sauté it, then do so.

If it's summer or an approximation of it, then, for pudding, provide a lemony, crumbly wedge of pecorino, and a bowlful of pears. Get the pears from a good greengrocer's or Marks & Spencer rather than the supermarket and buy them on the Wednesday before if possible (Thursday at the latest) to be sure they aren't tooth-breakingly hard.

PECORINO AND PEARS

The chocolate pudding wouldn't taste right in the heat, but in more customary English warmth it'll still work wonderfully.

LEMON CHICKEN

I prefer to go to my butcher for a proper, free-range bird, which he will then cut up into portions. I like the bird to be cut up small.

- 6 tablespoons olive oil (or more, see below)
- 1 large chicken in 8 or 10 portions or 2 small chickens cut into 6 portions each
- zest and juice of 1 large lemon or 2 small (preferably unwaxed)
- 1 tablespoon rigani or dried oregano
- 300ml white wine (or more if pan very large)
- 3 eggs

Preheat oven to gas mark 7/210°C.

Put a large baking dish on the hob (one big enough to hold the chicken, which should fit more or less over 2 burners) and pour in the olive oil. If you can't fit the chicken pieces in 1 pan and are therefore cooking them in 2 you may need more oil. Turn the chicken in the hot oil for a few minutes until the pieces are golden. Add the lemon zest and rigani. Pour over the wine, adding salt and pepper, let it bubble up a bit, then add 300ml water. Put in the oven and cook for about 30 minutes, more if the portions are large. (Check the individual pieces: you may want to remove the breast portions first.) Arrange the chicken pieces on a plate that can go back in the oven while you make the sauce. Turn off the oven.

AVGOLEMONO

To make the sauce, first pour the chickeny juices into a jug, and measure. You need about 300ml. You can make avgolemono straight in a saucepan, but you may feel safer using a bowl over (but not touching) gently boiling water in a pan.

In this bowl, put the eggs and lemon juice and start whisking. It's easiest to use a hand-held electric whisk, but any old thing will do. Keep whisking until the mixture's frothy. Pour in gradually, and still whisking, the chicken cooking juices. It shouldn't curdle, but if you're feeling nervous (or even if you're not, for it'll stop you needing to) put a bowl or pan of cold water next to you so that you can plunge the avgolemono bowl in if it begins to look as if it's thinking of overheating and splitting. It's ready when it's turned into a thin custardy substance.

Taste for salt and pepper. Pour some of the sauce over the chicken portions and put the rest in a jug or leave it in its bowl and just put a ladle into it. You'll have a nice big bowlful of it.

STICKY CHOCOLATE PUDDING

This is a variant on lemon surprise pudding, in which the mixture divides on cooking to produce a sponge above the thick lemony sauce which forms below. Indeed, it is known in my house as Lemon Surprise Pudding: the surprise being that it's chocolate.

Although I didn't actually eat this as a child, it is heady with reminders of childhood foods: the hazelnuts in the sponge bring back memories of Nutella, the thick, dark, fudgy sauce of chocolate spread. The proportions below are geared towards 6, but easily feed 8. It's heavenly with fridge-cold double cream poured over it.

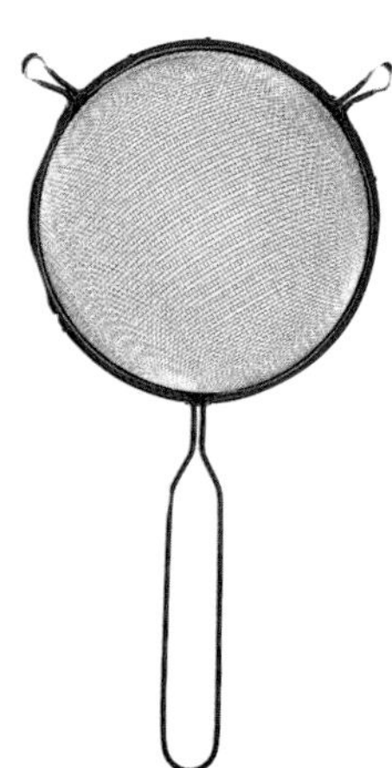

It is also child's play to make. Choose good cocoa and good dark chocolate and stick carefully to the exact measurements. (You can, though, use 200g flour in place of the 150g flour and 50g ground nuts, if you prefer.) I use one of those standard white soufflé dishes 20cm in diameter, or a shallow dish 30cm square. If you've got only a single oven, it makes sense to use the shallow tin: it will take less time to cook.

for the pudding
75g best dark chocolate or chocolate buttons
150g self-raising flour
25g good cocoa
50g ground hazelnuts
200g caster sugar
40g unsalted butter, melted
1 egg
180ml full-fat milk
1 teaspoon real vanilla extract

for the sauce
180g soft dark brown or muscovado sugar
120g cocoa, sifted

Preheat the oven to gas mark 4/180°C.

If you're not using the upmarket chocolate buttons, chop the chocolate roughly. I use my mezzaluna, but you could use a sharp knife. Don't use a processor since the pieces of chocolate will provide the chewy, melting lumps in the pudding: they need to be chunks and the machine will whizz them into dust.

Sift the flour and cocoa into a bowl, stir in the ground hazelnuts and the sugar, then add the chocolate. Whisk together the melted butter, egg, milk and vanilla and pour into the dry ingredients. Stir well, so it's all thoroughly mixed, then spoon into the buttered dish.

Now for the sauce, not that you make it yourself (the cooking does that for you) but you have to get the ingredients together. Put the kettle on. Mix the cocoa and brown sugar and sprinkle over the top of the pudding mixture in the dish. Pour the boiled water up to the 500ml mark of a measuring jug, then pour over the pudding. Put the water-soused pudding directly into the oven and leave it there for about 50 minutes. Don't open the door until a good 45 minutes have passed, and then press: if it feels fairly firm and springy to the touch, it's ready. If you're using the shallow dish, it'll be ready in 35–40 minutes.

Remove from the oven and serve immediately, spooning from the dish and making sure everyone gets both sauce and sponge.

AUTUMN LUNCH FOR 6

Ragoût of wild mushrooms with oven-cooked polenta
Cheeses with bitter salad
Stewed apples with cinnamon crème fraîche

You want mushrooms as fresh as you can get them. If you buy them in advance they'll probably be lying, ever more limp and bruised and unappetisingly damp, in their brown paper bag in the fridge and you'll get no pleasure at all out of the prospect of cooking them. So do your shopping on a Saturday morning.

This recipe for wild mushroom ragoût is adapted from a recipe in *From Anna's Kitchen* by Anna Thomas. I was sent it one year among many other books under review and was surprised to find myself utterly seduced by it. Any description undersells it: in America it would be described as a gourmet vegetarian cookbook. But it has none of the worthiness or pretentiousness which that might seem to suggest. It is fresh and alive and speaks directly and intimately to the reader. I could take so many recipes from it here, since I so often cook, if not exactly from it, then inspired by it (which is more telling).

This ragoût is a sort of woodsy stew, odoriferously autumnal. As for the cheese afterwards, I'd think about a really fulsome camembert or ammoniac gorgonzola; either paired with stringently dressed chicory. Deal with the apples by peeling, coring and segmenting about 4 bramleys. Put them in a pan, cover with 5–6 tablespoons sugar (or to taste), a tablespoon of butter, the juice (and perhaps the zest) of 1 orange and 2 cloves and/or a cinnamon stick. Cook, covered, on a low heat till the fruit is soft but not pulpy beyond recognition. Eat with crème fraîche sprinkled with cinnamon or bolstered with a whipped-in slug of Calvados. I love it with plain, sharp yoghurt and maybe some soft brown sugar.

STEWED APPLES

MUSHROOM RAGOÛT

800g fresh wild mushrooms, or a combination of wild and cultivated (obviously the more wild ones the better)
1 tablespoon olive oil
4–5 tablespoons butter
1 white onion, chopped finely
1 red onion, sliced finely
2 stalks celery, sliced thinly
3 cloves garlic, chopped
175ml dry red wine
75ml Marsala
1 bay leaf
½ teaspoon thyme leaves
pinch of cayenne
1 tablespoon flour, preferably Italian 00
500ml heated vegetable stock (I use Marigold bouillon powder or Italian porcini stock cubes, see page 506)
3 tablespoon flat-leaf parsley, chopped

Wipe the mushrooms thoroughly, trim off tough or woody stems, and slice the mushrooms or cut them into generous pieces.

Heat 1 teaspoon olive oil and 1 tablespoon butter in a non-stick frying pan or similar and sauté the onions and celery in it, stirring often, until they begin to soften.

I sometimes find I have to add more butter. Add the chopped garlic and some salt and pepper and continue cooking until the onions and garlic begin to brown. Add half the red wine and half the Marsala, the bay leaf and thyme. Turn down the heat and simmer gently until the wine cooks away.

Meanwhile, in another large non-stick pan heat 2 teaspoons olive oil with 2 tablespoons butter – again adding more butter if you like, though if you're patient it shouldn't be necessary. Sauté the mushrooms with a sprinkle of salt and a pinch of cayenne until their excess liquid cooks away and they begin to colour. Add the remaining wine and Marsala, lower the heat and allow the wine to simmer down. Then add the onions to the mushrooms.

Put the remaining butter in the pan in which you've sautéed the onions and let it melt. Stir in the flour and keep stirring over medium heat for a few minutes as it turns golden. Whisk in the hot stock and continue whisking as it thickens. Add this sauce to the mushrooms and onions, along with the parsley.

Simmer everything together very gently for about 10 more minutes. Serve with steamed or boiled rice – and I mostly just do a buttery pile of basmati – or polenta if you don't feel it's a bit too Notting-Hill-restaurant-circa-1995.

OVEN-COOKED POLENTA

This is the 'polenta senza bastone' (the bastone is the wooden baton traditionally used to stir the polenta while it cooks) from Anna del Conte's *Classic Food of Northern Italy*. It's much less work than traditionally-cooked polenta, and infinitely preferable to the quick-cook stuff.

Bring 1.8 litres water or stock to simmering point. Remove the pan from the heat and add 2 teaspoons salt. If you are using vegetable bouillon powder, here's where you add them to the water, in which case you probably won't need the salt.

Gradually add 350g polenta or, more properly speaking, maize flour, letting it fall in a fine rain through your fingers while you stir rapidly with a long wooden spoon. Return the pan to the heat and bring slowly to the boil, stirring constantly in the same direction. Boil for 5 minutes, still stirring. Now transfer the polenta to a buttered oven dish. I use an old and battered oval enamel casserole with a 2-litre capacity, but it doesn't much matter and you'll be able to see easily which of your various dishes will be the right size just by looking at the grainy porridge. Cover with buttered foil and cook in a preheated oven (gas mark 5/190°C) for 1 hour.

As for cheeses: keep in mind those that will crumble or meld into the salad on the plate. You are not looking for a cheese-and-biscuits kind of assortment. The salad should be mostly of chicory. Throw in one of those packets of mixed leaves (or maybe just half the packet) for ballast if you want and make a strong lemony, oily dressing thickened either with 2 pounded anchovy fillets or 1 teaspoon Dijon mustard mixed with a quick grating of orange zest.

And maybe put the apples and crème fraîche on the table at the same time as the cheese and salad.

I like this kind of aromatic, unstructured food: stews, braises, soupy mixtures of vegetables to be eaten with warm mounds of rice, couscous, pasta or just thick wedges of bread.

A thick, squashy root vegetable stew with couscous, an earthy, grainy, aromatic braise of carrots, turnips, parsnips and squash, is the ideal soothing Saturday lunch. Abroad (in Paris, mostly) I've eaten this with lamb, but I don't like the greasiness when I make it myself, unless I boil up the lamb (about 1–1½kg neck, generously covered with salted water) the day before and skim the fat off when cool (and see recipe for cawl on page 107). That way you get all the glorious sweetness of the meat, and the well-cooked stringiness (well, let's be frank here) that is so characteristic of this kind of stew. (See below, too, for a chicken couscous recipe.)

BOLSTERING SATURDAY LUNCH FOR 6

Golden root-vegetable couscous with chorizo, or chicken stew with couscous

Coconut crème caramel

I think of this as particularly good for Saturday lunch if you've been feeling rather fragile: the food is soothing and so, too, are the rhythms of its preparation.

You do need to do a couple of things in advance: put the chick peas in to soak (see page 88) and make the crème caramel. Neither of these activities should be too demanding even on a Friday (morning for the chick peas, evening for the crème caramel) after a long week at work. If you hate coconut (although the taste of it is subtle rather than pronounced here) then substitute the same quantity of full-fat milk. But after the warm spiciness of the stew, the lightly aromatic coconut custard is just right: it offers a gentle but resolute ending to the meal.

Each time I do this I use different vegetables in differing quantities, but if that sort of permissiveness makes you feel unsafe, then follow this recipe word for word the first time and then gradually, as you do it and redo it, you will find you loosen up. Don't think less of yourself for following orders to the letter. It takes time to learn when you can make free with a recipe and when it's best to rein in the improvisatory spirit. Most of my mistakes have been as a result of fiddling about with a recipe the first time I've cooked it, rather than doing it as written, and then next time seeing where I could improve or change or develop it.

I've specified already ground spices here: it is certainly better if you dry-fry and then grind your own, but actually I resort mostly to the dried ones when I make this, and I wanted to be honest rather than high-minded here. I do buy good spices, though, either French ones from the delicatessen or wonderful aromatic loosely packaged ones from the Middle-Eastern shop (see Gazetteer).

Use vegetable stock if you want this to be vegetarian: otherwise use any stock – chicken, beef, lamb – that you want. And the stock doesn't need to be strong: if you're using stock cubes or cartons of stock, then use extra water to dilute them.

I find it easier to chop all the vegetables before I need them. This recipe requires a lot of preparation, albeit of a basic and undemanding sort. I like a drink beside me and someone to talk to (or the radio to listen to). I peel, chop, assemble solidly and then that's it.

I use my couscoussier, but a big, deep pot will do. Obviously, you will need more or less liquid depending on the proportions of the cooking vessel, so be prepared to be flexible: do remember that you can use extra water; there's no need to have more stock on hand. Use a couple of pans if you don't have anything very capacious.

Chief among the virtues of couscous is the speed with which it is cooked. I love it for its sweet, soft graininess, which needs nothing more than a nut or two of butter by way of dressing. Try and resist the modern tendency to use oil instead. When I make couscous just for myself or for the children, I often cook it just by immersing it in an equal volume of hot stock but here I would soak then steam it.

Keep all the parts separate: the stew in one bowl, with plenty of juice; the grain in another; some harissa, that garlic-pounded paste of chillies, to the side. The culinary idea behind this is the contrast between spicy stew, spicier relish and the plain, comforting blanket of grain. You can moosh them all up on your plate, but if they were all mixed up on the serving dish, it would be both too sloppy in texture and too monotone in taste.

GOLDEN ROOT-VEGETABLE COUSCOUS

for the stew
3 carrots
2 parsnips
2 turnips
1 small kabocha squash (or failing that, butternut squash)
½ swede
3 courgettes
2 onions
2 cloves garlic
3 tablespoons olive oil
1 teaspoon each ground cinnamon, cumin and coriander
½ teaspoon paprika
generous pinch of saffron strands
1 litre stock
½ 400g can tinned plum tomatoes
grated zest ½ large unwaxed orange
100g sultanas
1½ 400g tins chick peas or 250g dried, soaked and partly-cooked chick peas (cooked as below in chicken stew but for 1 hour 50 minutes)
few drops chilli oil or 1 teaspoon harissa
fresh coriander or parsley to garnish

for the couscous
700g couscous
30–45g butter
100g pine nuts

Peel the carrots, parsnips, turnips, squash and swede and cut them into 3cm chunks. Peel strips of skin off the courgettes so that they are stripy dark and light green and then cut them into slices about 1½cm thick. Peel the onions, cut them into quarters and then thickly slice them. Peel the garlic and mince it.

Heat the olive oil in the pan and turn the onions in it for a few minutes, then add the garlic, the ground cinnamon, ground cumin, ground coriander, paprika and saffron. Stir over a low to medium heat for 5 minutes. Add the vegetables except for the chick peas (and tinned tomatoes) and turn briskly, but don't worry if you can't do this very efficiently: there are a lot of vegetables and not much space for them. After about 5 minutes add the stock, the tomatoes chopped roughly and drained of their juice (but keep it: you may need it later), the grated zest of orange, the sultanas (I love sultanas and hate raisins: if you feel differently, then do act differently) and the chick peas. Turn again so that, if possible, all get at least partially covered by the stock. Add the tomato juice from the tin and some more water if the liquid level is looking too low. Taste and, if you want to, add the juice of an orange. The stew benefits from an aromatic hint of orange, but don't be too heavy-handed.

Cook this fragrant, golden stew for about 20–30 minutes: the vegetables should be tender but not mushy (at least not all of them: some will be beginning to fray around the edges, and that's good) and the liquid a thin but not watery sauce. Taste and add a drop or two of chilli oil or a teaspoon or so of harissa if you want it to have a bit more punch. Pour the stew gently into a big round shallow bowl (and this should be warmed), with fresh, fragrant parsley or coriander snipped over the top. Put the pine nuts in a hot, dry frying pan and toast until they are golden and giving off a sweet resiny aroma. Set aside.

Read the instructions on the couscous packet. I tend to soak the couscous for 10 minutes, then steam it for 15 minutes, so get moving with it about 30 minutes before the stew is cooked. All you need to do is put the amount of couscous you need in a bowl and cover it with cold water by about 4cm. Then, when you want to steam it, drain it, put it in either a steamer basket or the top part of the couscoussier, add the butter on top of the grain, and put on top of the pan with the stew in it and cover. Leave for about 15 minutes; the butter should have started melting by the time it's ready. Transfer to a warmed dish or flat round plate, adding more butter if you like. Fluff up with a fork and scatter with pine nuts and you're done.

Though it's not strictly necessary, if you want some meat around, get hold of some chorizo. But make sure you buy the spicy, paprika-tinted sausages rather than salame. If you happen to live near a shop that sells merguez (which are actually more traditional here), then just grill them and serve them instead of the chorizo. Otherwise, use a cast-iron pan and cover the bottom with a film of olive oil. Prick the chorizo sausages, place them in the pan and turn them so that they are sealed on all sides. Throw in a glass of red wine, lower the heat and cook for about 10 minutes. Remove, and slice each sausage diagonally into 3 squat logs.

CHICKEN STEW WITH COUSCOUS

In the Middle East or North Africa chicken would be used primarily to flavour the broth, not to yield much meat to eat. But I reckon that, if people are expecting to eat the meat, you must have 2 small portions per person. Chicken is better if it is freshly jointed, so I get the butcher to cut one very large chicken into 12. You can, however, use thighs from the supermarket.

Don't worry if the stock isn't very strong: the broth should be light. The point of couscous is, I stress, to have the bland grains as a base for the vegetables and chicken, moistened by the gentle broth and given heat and intensity by the harissa.

You will need to start on this a good 24 hours in advance in order to soak the chick peas. If you prefer to use tinned chick peas, you can, but I think it's worth the effort (not in itself exactly arduous) of soaking and cooking the dried ones.

250g chick peas, soaked, or 1½ 400g tins
3 medium onions
1 bouquet garni
4 cloves garlic, unpeeled
2 tablespoons oil
1 teaspoon cinnamon
½ teaspoon cumin
¼ teaspoon cayenne pepper
12 chicken portions (see above)
500g carrots, cut in half lengthways then into chunks
4 celery sticks, 1 left whole, 3 sliced
1–2 teaspoons harissa

First cook, or part-cook the chick peas. Put them in a pan with 1 onion, halved, the bouquet garni and the garlic cloves, cover by about 10cm with cold water, add a drop or two of olive oil. Cover the pan, bring to the boil and then cook at a gentle boil for an hour. Leave in the pan.

Now for the chicken and vegetables. Pour 2 tablespoons oil into a big pot, add the cinnamon, cumin and cayenne pepper and 2 onions, finely sliced. Sprinkle with a pinch of salt and cook for a few minutes, until soft. Then add the chicken portions. (If you want them golden, fry them in a pan first, remembering to scoop up all chickeny juices by deglazing with some water.) Cover with cold water and bring to the boil. Skim off any scum that may rise to the surface. Drain the chick peas and add them with the carrots and celery, stir in a good teaspoon of harissa, and cook fairly gently for 1½ hours, maybe slightly less. If, then, you *really* feel the broth needs more flavour, don't panic: just add a stock cube or some stock granules.

As before, make sure you have read the instructions on the couscous packet to see when you should start cooking it; this is probably about ½ hour before the chicken and vegetables are cooked. Serve as for the vegetable couscous.

HARISSA

Since you can buy very good harissa, I make no apology for the fact that this home-made version is fairly labour-intensive. If, however, the idea of pounding the whole spices appals and yet you still want to make your own, then use ground spices (the caraway doesn't come ground, but can be dealt with in the processor later), reducing quantities slightly, and frying them first not in a dry pan, but one with a tablespoon or so of oil in it. The strength of chillies I tend to get for harissa register, on the heat scale, as 4/10.

60g dried unsmoked chillies
6 cloves garlic
2 tablespoons coarse sea salt
3 tablespoons coriander seeds
1 teaspoon caraway seeds
1 teaspoon cumin seeds
1 tablespoon sherry vinegar
3 tablespoons olive oil

Deseed the chillies, with rubber gloves on if I were you, especially if you wear contact lenses. Cut into thinnish slices – I use scissors for this – and put into a small bowl. Cover with boiling water from the kettle, and leave to soak for 1 hour.

Dry roast the coriander, caraway and cumin in a hot oil-less heavy-based frying pan, shaking and turning till lightly browned and beginning to give off heady fragrance – about 3 or 4 minutes – and then remove from the pan and bash to a powder with a pestle and mortar.

I finish off most of the operation in the processor, but if you want to be truly authentic I dare say you should continue pounding. Anyway, spoon the just-pounded spice powder into the bowl of the food processor. Pound the garlic and salt together with the pestle and mortar and then transfer that, too, to the processor. Add vinegar and the drained chillies, reserving the soaking water, and blitz till a fiery-red purée. Then, turn the machine on again and, with the motor running, pour the oil down the funnel. Stop, scrape up – or rather down – any mixture on the sides of the bowl, then switch on again, pouring in some of the chilli-soaking liquid; you want the texture thick but not stiff. Taste to see whether you want more salt or more vinegar, or indeed more chilli.

You can keep this, with a film of oil poured over the top, for ages in the fridge. And it's addictive stuff: once you start eating it, you'll want it with practically everything.

COCONUT CRÈME CARAMEL

Crème caramel is a soothing pudding to end with, and one that is not, contrary to appearances, very hard to make. It's easier to make the caramel alone in the kitchen, though. If there's anyone else there, they're almost bound to plead with you to take the darkly spluttering sugar off the heat before it's brown enough.

This version is not intensely coconutty, but after the third or fourth mouthful, a light, fluttery note of coconut begins to make itself heard. Think, too, of substituting ordinary milk, infused for 20 minutes with the zest of an orange, then strained. In which case, use orange juice not water to make the caramel.

I use an oval dish that has a capacity of 800ml. This makes a modest, though not too mean, amount for 6: boost quantities for exuberantly greedy people.

The canned coconut milk I use (because I had it in the larder the first time I made this) is called Thai coconut milk and it needs a good shake before opening and pouring over the eggs and sugar. Get the best eggs you can – not mass-produced.

4 eggs
4 egg yolks
45g caster sugar
1 1/2 400ml tins coconut milk

for the caramel
150g caster sugar

Preheat oven to gas mark 3/160°C, and put in the dish in which you are going to cook the crème caramel.

Put the sugar and 5 tablespoons of water in a thick-bottomed saucepan to make the caramel, stir to help dissolve, then put on a high heat. (Meanwhile fill the kettle up and switch it on.) Bring the sugar and water to the boil, without stirring – though I can never resist shaking a bit – and boil until it is dark golden and treacly. Get the warm dish from the oven, pour in the caramel and swirl it around so it coats the sides as well as the bottom. You need to use an oven glove or tongs (if you've got strong-gripping ones) to hold the pan because the caramel is extremely hot. You will have to work quickly but not hysterically so. Put the dish aside somewhere cool and let the caramel harden.

Then, in a bowl, whisk the eggs, egg yolks and sugar with a fork. Heat the coconut milk and, still beating with a fork, pour it over the egg and sugar mixture. Strain into the caramel-lined dish.

Get out a roasting pan and set the crème caramel container in it. Pour the recently boiled (but not boiling) water from the kettle into the roasting pan to come about halfway up the sides of the dish, then convey all of this to the oven.

Start testing (with your fingertips, press the top) after 45 minutes but reckon on about 1 hour before it is cooked enough. You want it set, but with a hint of wobble underneath. Remember, it will carry on cooking a little after you take it out.

Remove the dish when you judge the time to be right and let it cool. Then stick it in the fridge overnight. A bit before you want to eat it, take it out of the fridge, press with your fingers all around the edge to release the custard from the sides of the dish, then get a sharp, thin knife and trace along the sides, cutting down to the bottom of the dish. Keep calm: there is no reason why this shouldn't work. Place a flat plate (no bowl to it) over the top of the caramel dish and invert. Shake a bit, and remove the dish. In front of you should be a beautiful, gleamingly tanned mirror-topped custard, dripping with brown caramel down the sides and into a puddle around it. The crème caramel is always shallower on the plate than it looked as if it would be, but that's just what happens – or it does to me.

Put two spoons on the table and let people help themselves.

YOGHURT
HONEY
PASSION FRUIT
DOUBLE CREAM

If you want to make something that takes altogether less thinking about, then I suggest a glass-filling mixture of yoghurt, honey, passion fruit and thick, rich, yellow double cream. Passion fruit, like coconut, seems to go well after the sweet aromatic spices which waft from the stew.

It may seem to go against my usual ordinances to suggest making a pudding that is to be served already meted out in individual portions, but the mixture becomes quickly too gloopy to survive being served from a larger bowl. For each person, put into your chosen glass a big dollop of Greek yoghurt. On top of this pour in 1 tablespoon dark, clear, strong Greek honey, stir it in a bit, not so that it is completely mixed, but so that it isn't just sitting in a fat puddle on top. Now take a passion fruit, cut it in half and scoop the seeds and pulp out on top of the honey and yoghurt. Stir this in gently, but leaving most of it on top. Then on goes a generous tablespoon of double cream: not a runny one, nor a whipped up one, but one that is good and thick itself, as it comes. Now, drizzle a bit of honey over that, but only a tiny bit – the amount that comes off the sticky tablespoon you used last time. If your kitchen lunch is completely informal, and since this pudding is best done at the last minute, assemble it at the time. And if you wanted something even simpler you could use Jane Grigson's trick – which is to have a bowlful of passion fruits and another of good cream. Eaters lop off the top of the fruit, rather as if taking the top off a boiled egg, add a spoon of cream to the pulpy cavity – and then, pleasurably, eat.

EASY WINTER LUNCH FOR 6

Ham cooked in cider with leeks, carrots and potatoes

Baked wine-spiced plums with Barbados cream

The poet Paul Muldoon wrote wonderfully, in *Profumo*, of his mother going 'from ham to snobbish ham'. Plastic-wrapped, sliver-thin and pinkly shiny, it has its place. But the real thing is such a treat; such an ordinary treat, nothing fancy, but enormously uplifting. And it's just right for Saturday lunch: nothing to do except throw everything in a pan and then the whole house becomes imbued with savoury, clove-scented fog. Buy more than you want and then eat it cold for supper with poached eggs, or in a sandwich, or chopped in a pea soup cooked with the cidery stock the ham itself was cooking in. I love nothing more, on a Saturday night in, than a bowl of thick and grainy pea soup eaten with a spoon in my right hand while my left holds (for alternating mouthfuls), a ham sandwich, good and mustardy, made with unsalted butter and white bread, real or plastic (both have their merits). The leftover stock also makes the basis for excellent risotti (see pea risotto, page 156, and orzotto, page 353) and can be used to add depth and pungency to an ordinary chicken casserole.

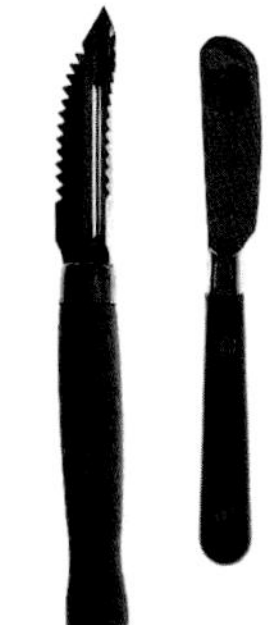

After the ham you want something not too filling, but a moussy little number would be striking the wrong note: the plums baked in spice-deepened wine are just right, warming and comforting but not bloating; and the Barbados cream is an optional accompaniment worth serious consideration. If you think it would make life easier, then just put some crème fraîche on the table instead. And, now I come to think of it, there's a very good case for custard. Still, I like the sugar-topped yoghurty cream: do it when you get up on Friday morning and then you don't even have to remember a thing when you get back from work. A good 24 hours will give everything time to meld fabulously. I'd do the plums in advance, too, although if you prefer you can cook them when you want to eat them. I know it might sound odd to specify a plum recipe for winter when these aren't winter fruits, but you can get plums (from South Africa among other places) in winter and they benefit especially from being cooked like this. Only the soft, juicy ones straight from the tree in August can be eaten as they are.

HAM COOKED IN CIDER

It is difficult to be specific about the size of the gammon you need: it depends how much you want left over. But I wouldn't consider getting a joint weighing under 2kg. What you're after is a joint of mild-cure gammon. I prefer to get my gammon from the butcher, but I have made more than respectable boiled ham from the vacuum-packed variety bought at the supermarket.

I don't soak my gammon: I just cover it with cold water, bring it to the boil, throw all the water out and put the gammon back in the pot and proceed. That gets rid of excessive saltiness, and probably doesn't add more than 40 minutes on to the cooking time. (But do ask the butcher: many gammons now need no soaking or precooking at all.) To calculate how much time the ham needs, work along the lines of 30 minutes per 500g plus 30 minutes. If it's come straight out of the fridge you could need to add a further 20–30 minutes.

I am basing this recipe on a 2kg joint, but armed with the information above, you can change the cooking time as you wish. Anyway, if the joint stays in the liquid for longer it'll be fine. And when you have finished lunch, put the ham back in the liquid until cool: this keeps it from going dry and stringy.

2kg joint mild-cure gammon (smoked or unsmoked as you wish)
2 carrots, quartered, plus 8 medium (or 6 large) carrots cut into half crossways then into half lengthways
2 onions, halved, each half studded with a clove
8 leeks
10 peppercorns
2 sticks celery or slice off, like a log, the bottom of the whole bunch
small bunch parsley, tied with a freezer bag wire
1 bouquet garni
1 litre dry cider
2 tablespoons light brown or demerara sugar

Get rid of any excess salt as needed (see above). Put the gammon in a large pot, add the 2 quartered carrots, the onions, the green end parts of the leeks (as long as they're not muddy), peppercorns, celery, parsley (if you keep the stalks together with a freezer bag wire it'll be easier to remove them later) and bouquet garni. Pour in the cider: I never mind which cider I use and I have profitably used apple juice, too. Then add cold water to cover and bring to boiling point.

Add the sugar, lower the heat and simmer briskly (or boil gently, depending on how you want to look at it) for about 1 hour 50 minutes. (And at about this stage you should start thinking about the potatoes, see below.) Remove the carrots, green parts of leek and parsley and put in the fresh carrots. After about another ½ hour, chop up the white bits of the leek. I would cut them into logs about 6cm long. Add to the pan and cook for about another 20 minutes. The ham should be bubbling softly in its liquid for around 2½ hours, all told. When it's all cooked, remove the ham to carve it, take the vegetables out with a slotted spoon and then put the ham on a huge plate surrounded by the leeks and carrots. Or carve it to order at the table and put the vegetables on a plate on the table by themselves.

Now: the potatoes. You can do either of two things: you can boil the potatoes in a pan of water while the ham is cooking, or you can cook them in the ham water itself. The advantage of cooking them separately is that they offer a distinct, appropriately plain, taste. And potatoes are really at their best when they are the bland but sweet bass note to sop up and support other, stronger, tastes. Added to which, you are left with a clear stock at the end; if you cook the potatoes in with the ham, all you can do with the stock, really, is make thick soup. And unless you have a very big pot, the ham, vegetables, and potatoes, all in together, will be a very tight squeeze.

Having said that, there is something wonderful about the sweet, grainy potatoes absorbing all that appley and salty stock. You decide. But whichever way you cook the potatoes, they should be the big floury sort, not the pebbly, waxy ones. I reckon on 1 potato (cut into 4) per person; I might even do 1½ per person, but then I like to have too much rather than not enough.

The recipes for both the plums and Barbados cream are in Cooking in Advance on pages 130 and 131.

GOOD, THICK WINTER PEA SOUP

As for the leftovers: there are pea soups, risotti and the like, mentioned throughout (check the Index too), but for a good, thick winter pea soup, all you need to do is throw into the cold stock a couple of handfuls of split green peas and boil away until you have a sludgy purée. A bright green fresh-pea soup is obviously not a winter meal, but if you cheat and use frozen peas (I always do) then it can be. But the grainy potage produced by the split peas is wonderfully satisfying – and you can just as well use the yellow split peas. In fact, you can use just about any pulse you want: it's just that split peas need no soaking. But if you don't feel like eating a ham-based pea soup immediately after lunch, then pour the stock (in labelled quantities) into containers or plastic bags and put them in the freezer. Don't stick it in the fridge with the intention of doing something or other with it over the next few days. You won't and you'll end up throwing it away, which would be too much of a waste for me to bear even on your behalf.

You could thaw some of the stock to make my next suggestion for a kitchen-bound Saturday lunch: minestrone. I haven't actually ever used ham-cooking liquid for it, but I've used chicken, beef and vegetable stocks and all have tasted wonderful. Strangely, the best minestrone I ever made was with a stock cube (a Knorr one made for the Italian market: *gusto classico*, which indicates a beef and chicken broth; and see Gazetteer for UK stockists). I think a soup like this makes one of the best sorts of weekend lunch. I love it not hot hot but a flavour-deepening lukewarm. Yes, you could serve cheese after it if you're worried that it isn't enough as it is for a main course but you'd be wrong. This is perfect for lunch: it's so nice, apart from anything else, to be able to have bowlfuls and bowlfuls of it rather than only a politely small amount in order to make room for a main course you're almost bound to like less. For dinner, fine: have something after the soup; but for lunch – and supper, indeed – you don't need to make a multi-coursed assault on people. To be frank, I'd be happy with just an orange afterwards, but I will suggest a more proper pudding, in the knowledge that you don't need a recipe for peeling an orange.

MOROCCAN ORANGE AND DATE SALAD

If you want to do something even simpler than the recipe that follows for baked Sauternes custard you could think of doing my Great-Aunt Myra's Moroccan orange and date salad. Oranges are peeled, depithed and then cut into thin discs; dates are halved, stoned and laid alongside. All you do is make an orangy syrup by boiling up some water, sugar, zest of the orange and some juice, plus orange-redolent alcohol if you like, though it wouldn't be very Moroccan. Still, I don't know if there is anything really Moroccan about this salad anyway. Sprinkle a small amount of syrup over the salad and then scatter with slithered almonds. And I rather like it without the syrup, but just with orange juice and a bit of orange liqueur sprinkled over, as well as the blanched (toasted or not) and slivered nuts and maybe some ground cinnamon. I have to say, though, that I find the custard (which involves just gentle whisking and stirring) rather easier to make than the orange salad with all that fiddly pithy business. No cooking should ever be undertaken with the single and vulgar aim of impressing anyone, but it's worth remembering as you make your choice that most people will presume that slicing a few oranges is as close to doing nothing as you can get whereas baking a fragrantly grapey and wine-resonant custard counts as making an effort.

I think of this menu as being particularly suitable for a weekend away: chopping and preparing vegetables are ideal work to do with either a lot of people doing bits of it each, or a lot of people sitting around to talk to while you do it. Don't be put off by the formality of the term Country House Lunch: I mean no more by it than to evoke a lazy, long weekend with friends.

COUNTRY HOUSE LUNCH FOR 6

Minestrone

Baked Sauternes custard

MINESTRONE

There has been something of a fashion recently for season-specific minestrone – a spring one majoring on peas, an autumn one containing porcini and so on – and while all these can be fabulous, the recipe here is for a plain, basic one (if such exists) that shouldn't be too hard to throw together all the year round. I doubt, however, if you'd really want to cook this in high summer; it tends to be on the menu as far as I'm concerned any time between September and May. As ever, the list of ingredients is not meant to be interpreted too strictly: any vegetable, more or less, can argue its case here. I am, however, unpersuaded by tomatoes. Yes, it is normal to include them, but I resolutely (along with the Milanesi) prefer not to. The only drawback is that the soup, after all that cooking, turns out an undeniable khaki. But it tastes so good, with an almost honeyed savouriness, that it really doesn't matter.

I have listed tinned beans below, but if you want to use dried ones then soak and cook them first. The added work is not burdensome in itself, but I do understand that activities-to-be-undertaken can take up psychological space, so to speak.

As for the work of chopping and preparing the vegetables: I like to chop the first one needed, then proceed to the next while the first is cooking, and so on. But if you want to be brisk and efficient, chop everything up in advance so that you've got an army of ingredients ready and facing you before you start.

I always freeze the rinds of old used-up chunks of parmesan, and throw one, or two if they're only little, into the minestrone while it's cooking; this brings a flavoursome unctuousness to the carroty-oniony liquor. (I sometimes bung a rind into pea soup, as well.) You should discard the cheese rind before serving the soup: I dredge it out and then chew on it as soon as it's bearable; I love its elastic stickiness. Last: the oil. I use Ligurian oil, which is sweeter and milder than the peppery Tuscan variety.

8 tablespoon olive oil, preferably Ligurian
40g butter
3 large onions, sliced thinly
5 carrots, diced
2 sticks celery, chopped fairly small
300g potatoes, peeled and diced
3 courgettes, diced
100g French beans, cut into 1cm lengths
225g Savoy cabbage, shredded
1 1/2 litres stock, beef, chicken or vegetable as you wish
rind of a finished piece of parmesan cheese, optional
120g dried white beans, soaked and cooked, or 400g tin cannellini beans
150g small tubular pasta, such as ditalini
40g parmesan, grated freshly

Get a big pot and put in the oil and butter and sliced onion and cook until the onion is softened but not browned. Add the chopped carrot and cook for about 3 minutes, stirring a couple of times. Do the same with the celery, potatoes, courgettes and French beans, cooking each one for a few minutes, stirring a few times. Then add the shredded cabbage and cook for about 6–8 minutes, stirring now and then.

Add the stock. Put in the end-bit of cheese if you've got one, give a good stir and taste to see if any salt is needed. (The cheese rind will give a small saline kick of its own, and remember if you're using stock cubes that they can be very salty.) Cover the pan, and cook at a gentle boil for 2–2 1/2 hours. The soup should be thick, so you have to cook it for long enough to lose any wateriness, but it has to have enough liquid in it at this stage for the pasta to absorb while it's cooking. If the soup is too thick when you've finished cooking it but before you put in the pasta then add some water.

Now remove the lid, add the white beans and cook for 5 minutes, then turn up the heat slightly and put the pasta in. It should cook in about 15 minutes. When it's ready, take out the parmesan rind, grate in the fresh parmesan and give the pan a good stir. Serve with more cheese.

First time around I love to eat this with a slug of soft, light Ligurian oil poured into it, but afterwards, when it's been left to get thicker and sludgier in the fridge, I like it heated up so that it's warm (just) but not hot and with some tube-clearing chilli oil – known to the Italians as *olio santo* – to punctuate its satiny depths.

I don't want to sound too fussy, but when you serve it, if you can, give people proper soup bowls (in other words, wide and shallow rather than deep and cupped): I don't know why it should make a difference, but it does.

BAKED SAUTERNES CUSTARD

I first ate this custard at Quaglino's: it's one of the best things I've ever eaten in a restaurant, and I say that after about twelve years as a restaurant critic. There, it's cooked in caramel-bottomed individual dariole moulds and turned out, a golden-topped shivering tower of the stuff on the plate, and served with Armagnac-soaked prunes. My version, based on the then chef Martin Webb's recipe, is somewhat simpler. I don't know why I still call it Sauternes custard, except that it sounds so luxuriously evocative, since it is only if you're feeling extravagant or generous (depending on how you look at it) that you will actually use Sauternes. Restaurants don't have to worry about opening a bottle just for the odd 200ml of it. You can get a cheapish ordinary Sauternes, but then you will find it lacks distinction in general and in particular that musky, scented note of botrytis, which was the point of using Sauternes in the first place. If you've got guests who you can count on appreciating a bottle to go with the pudding, then it is worth it. You need a little for the custard, but the rest will get pleasurably and more or less immediately used.

I like this warm, spooned straight from the dish it's cooked in (eaten about 45 minutes to 1 hour after it comes out of the oven), but it is also wonderful cold, as long as you remember to take it out of the fridge a good hour before eating it. The cold option has two things going for it: first, it makes more of a contrast with the warm soup; and second, you can do it all the day before. Of course, it would look better unmoulded, but that's something I can't manage and wouldn't advise trying. Yes, I know that the gleaming construct of an unblemished, unmoulded mound of smooth custard is a wonderful thing, and a gloopy scoop of it from a large oval dish is at best homely. But this is partly because we have all been too much influenced by restaurant preparation. If a dish looks homely, well then, that's how it should be when eaten at home. The taste is so wonderful, so subtle but resonant with it, that any amount of visual inelegance is irrelevant.

POACHED APRICOTS

Cold, especially, it would be wonderful with poached apricots. The apricots that are sold in this country are generally in no fit condition to be eaten, but poaching will help. Otherwise, just soak and cook some good dried apricots. Hunza ones, those little, brown, wrinkled, round fruits, are the ambrosial best. Soak them in water, enough for the fruits to swell and become juicy again, and leave for a few hours. Then transfer fruits and soaking liquid to a pan, add water to cover (if necessary), bring to the boil and then simmer until soft. Remove the apricots to a bowl and then boil down the liquid in the pan to a syrup. Hunza apricots need no extra sugar. Pour over the syrup and leave till room temperature or cold (but not fridge cold). Or you can prepare ordinary dried apricots along the lines of the eastern Mediterranean recipe for them on page 355, or indeed the poached peaches I suggest as an accompaniment to the Sauternes custard ice-cream on page 377. If all this is sounding a little complicated, then fresh raspberries or strawberries doused in some of the wine you're using for the custard would do as well. But don't start thinking that you absolutely have to be doing anything; this custard is good enough alone. No, more than good enough: sublime. In some moods any accompaniment is a distraction.

2 whole eggs
4 egg yolks
75g caster sugar
350ml whipping cream
180ml Sauternes or dessert wine
1 vanilla pod, or substitute vanilla sugar (see page 82) for the caster sugar

Preheat the oven to gas mark 2/150°C. Fill up the kettle and put it on. Whisk the eggs, egg yolks and sugar in a large bowl, and put the cream and vanilla pod, if using, and Sauternes or dessert wine, into 2 separate pans. Bring the cream with the vanilla pod to just below boiling point and then remove from heat, cover and let infuse for 20 minutes or so. Then, at around that time, bring the Sauternes or dessert wine to just below boiling point. If you are using a vanilla pod, remove it after it has sat in the cream for 20 minutes.

Start beating the egg and sugar mixture again. Pour the wine over it and continue beating while you then pour in the cream. Don't go mad with the whisking. If you beat too much air in, it'll go frothy and you will have a layer of bubbles on top, which you don't want. Strain the mixture (this will help remove some froth) and pour into the dish; I use an oval one with a capacity of just under a litre. Put the dish into a baking pan and pour the recently boiled (but not boiling) water into the baking pan to come about halfway up the sides of the dish. Cover loosely with baking parchment or waxed paper.

This will take about 1 hour to cook. The custard should be firm but not immobile: when you press with your fingers it should feel set but with a little wobble still within. When you eat it it should be just warm, soft and voluptuous, like an eighteenth-century courtesan's inner thigh; you don't want something bouncy and jellied. A bit of dribble doesn't matter: it might not look defined on the plate, but it will taste resolutely good on the palate.

On my last birthday, I went to the pub for lunch. I should amplify: the pub in question is the Anglesea Arms, whose kitchen is presided over by Dan Evans, a one-time protegé of Alastair Little. His food is fresh, strong, modern, but not caricaturedly so, and eclectic but not vertiginously so. I suppose because it's a pub rather than a restaurant – although there is a properly designated restaurant space – the food is bound to be more informal, nearer to the food you would like to eat at home.

I had six oysters, then potato pancakes with blitz-marinated smoked haddock, which lay on top of each pancake with a splodge of crème fraîche beneath and a flurry of snipped chives on top. This was heavenly. And, I have since found out, not hard to make. You can replace the haddock with smoked salmon, but somehow it seems to signify 'no effort'. Although the smoked haddock is easily prepared once you get home, you do need to go to a fishmonger to get the fish cut into the requisite thin slices. If this is too much trouble you can wander off towards other things: these pancakes are good topped with chicken livers sautéed in butter, and the pan deglazed with Marsala, sherry or muscat. Or you might consider a tranche of just seared salmon (or a silky layer of the smoked stuff) with a poached egg on top.

These pancakes – crêpes Parmentier – are named in honour of the man who forced the potato into the affections of the French, and who persuaded, to that end, Marie Antoinette to weave potato flowers into her hair. They aren't difficult, but you need a blini pan which is about 12cm in diameter.

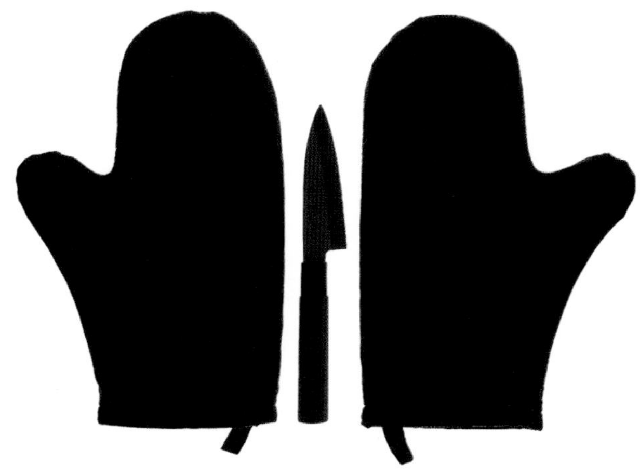

THE SMALL BUT PERFECTLY FORMED LUNCH FOR 4

Crêpes Parmentier with marinated smoked haddock

Poires belle Hélène

CRÊPES PARMENTIER WITH MARINATED SMOKED HADDOCK

for the potato pancakes
500g floury potatoes
4 teaspoons plain flour
3 eggs
4 egg whites
50ml crème fraîche (taken from tub, below, for the haddock) or double cream
50ml milk
vegetable oil for frying

for the haddock
500g smoked haddock (weight before slicing, etc.)
3 tablespoons good olive oil
juice of 3 lemons
sea salt and freshly ground pepper
1 250g tub crème fraîche
small bunch chives, snipped
very small bunch coriander, chopped

When you buy the haddock, ask the fishmonger to cut it into very thin slices rather like smoked salmon. It won't be quite so thin, but you want him to be thinking in that direction. Since the marinating is so brief, I will leave it for now and come back to it once the pancake mix has been made.

Peel and dice the potatoes and put them on a steamer basket or perforated container (a metal colander would do) over gently boiling salted water until tender. Try them after 20–30 minutes, and then keep trying. It depends, obviously, on the size of the dice. I usually cut the potatoes into 3cm x 2cm chunks. At about the time they're ready, preheat the oven to gas mark 4/180°C and put in a plate big enough to hold all the pancakes.

Now, put the cooked potato dice into a bowl and add the flour, mixing well. I tend to use a hand-held electric mixer for the entire operation. Then add the eggs, egg whites (not beaten, just as they are), crème fraîche and milk; mix well so that you've got a smooth, thick batter and add salt and pepper.

Pour a film of oil into the blini pan and put it on to the heat. When it's very hot add some batter, about a half ladleful or so. The pan should be slightly more than half filled. Keep it on the heat and watch: when the pancake is ready to turn, you'll notice the top beginning to bubble and the bottom will be brown; you can judge this by slipping a

spatula underneath the pancake and upturning it slightly. Having flipped it over, cook it for slightly less time than the first side. These pancakes are easy to turn anyway, so don't worry about it. And if you make a mess of the first one, just jettison it and proceed. I get 9 pancakes out of the quantities stated, so you've got room to lose one and still give people 2 each. If you think 2 each isn't going to be enough, then just boost quantities. As each pancake is cooked, put it on the plate in the oven to keep warm.

While you're cooking the pancakes, prepare the smoked haddock. In a shallow dish big enough to take all the fish, pour in the oil and lemon juice and sprinkle on some sea salt (I know you think the fish is salty enough anyway, but it will need salt, I promise) and pepper and place the thinly sliced fish in this basic marinade: 4–5 minutes is as long as it should be immersed. This means you can really wait until you've more or less finished dealing with the pancakes. By this time you'll be taking them in your stride so won't worry about having to fiddle with something else at the same time.

I like serving the component parts separately, for people to assemble themselves. On one plate place the lemony fish, on another the pancakes, in a bowl the crème fraîche and in a couple of others the snipped chives and chopped coriander.

ST JOHN'S SALAD

As for salads or something to eat with or after, I would roll out a salad from St John's restaurant of fresh, fresh flat-leaf parsley with red onion rings and soaked, drained and dried salt-preserved capers. A drizzle of oil with the quickest squeeze of lemon is all you need; it is important after the intense flavours of the haddock that the salad dressing should be light.

POIRES BELLE HÉLÈNE

Now for the pears. Old-fashioned they certainly are, and my grandmother used to make them for me when I was a child. But they're not nursery food and it isn't just nostalgia that makes me dredge them up. Pears are so rarely edible when raw. When they're good, they're wonderful, but I am beginning to think Ralph Waldo Emerson was being optimistic when he wrote, 'There are only ten minutes in the life of a pear when it is perfect to eat': most pears go from hard to woolly without ever passing through the luscious ripe stage. Poaching pears is one way of dealing with all those hard unyielding fruits in the shops: somehow, however wooden they felt raw, poached they become infused with a juice-bursting plumpness. In fact, it is a positive advantage to use what would in other circumstances seem rebarbatively firm fruit. (Actually, I have rather a soft spot for tinned pears; the dense graininess of the liquid-soused fruit is remarkably seductive.)

for the pears

4–6 firm pears, Williams or dessert variety which looks suitably pear-like

juice of 1 lemon

100g caster sugar (or vanilla sugar if you've got it)

1 vanilla pod or 1 teaspoon pure vanilla extract if not using vanilla sugar

for the chocolate sauce

200g bitter dark chocolate

120ml strong black coffee, or 1 teaspoon instant coffee made up with 120ml water

90g caster sugar

120ml double cream

crystallised violets, optional

Peel, halve and core the pears and sprinkle over them the lemon juice to stop them from discolouring. In a wide shallow pan (in which the pears will fit in one layer – otherwise cook them in batches) put 300ml water, the sugar and vanilla pod if using. Bring to the boil, stirring every now and again to make sure the sugar dissolves, then lower the heat slightly and simmer for 5 minutes. Put the pears into the liquid, cut side down, and raise the heat again so that the syrup boils up and the pears are covered by it. You may need to spoon the syrup over. After half a minute or so, lower the heat, then cover the pan and simmer for 10 minutes, turn the pears, cover the pan again and simmer for another 10 minutes. Carry on until pears are cooked and translucent: they should feel tender (but not soggy) when pierced. They may need more or less cooking time: it all depends on the pears themselves. Take off the heat, keep covered and leave to cool. To serve, arrange pears cut side down on a big flat plate and pour some syrup over. (Any remaining syrup will keep in the fridge or freezer and can be used to pour over apples or other fruit when making pies or crumbles. You can wash the vanilla pod, wipe it and put it in a canister of sugar.)

Now the chocolate sauce: place the chocolate, broken up into small pieces, in a thick-bottomed pan with the coffee and sugar and melt over a low heat, stirring occasionally. Then pour in the cream, still stirring, and when it is very hot pour into a warmed sauceboat or a bowl with a ladle.

Traditionally, on top of the ice-cream should go the pear, then the chocolate sauce and finally the violets. I'd rather put on the table a tub of ice-cream, a plate of poached pears, a jug of chocolate sauce and, if possible, a saucerful of crystallised violets.

People are wrong to be daunted by pastry, but there's no point in pretending they aren't. There is something unhelpful about suggesting you get to grips with it at the end of a long day's work, but at the weekend you can work calmly. And the weekend is just the time to eat simple, comforting food such as steak and kidney or rhubarb meringue pies or a soft and swollen, creamy crab tart. The following four menus all include a pastry factor.

SCHOOL-DINNER LUNCH FOR 4–6

Steak and kidney pie

Banana custard

If you can't stomach the idea of banana custard, substitute the trifle on page 123, or provide good ripe bananas and good thick cream and put them on the table with a bowl of soft brown sugar and let everyone mash their own.

STEAK AND KIDNEY PIE

Cook the meat in its liquorice-dark gravy first and then assemble the pie later with the made, cooled filing. The advantage of the two-pronged attack is that the meat is at its best when cooked, on low heat, for a good long time and the pastry needs a shorter time at a higher heat to keep it crisp but yieldingly rich. Another advantage is that you can cook the meat in advance. I make a suet crust here (as one would, indeed, for a steak and kidney pudding), rather than shortcrust, for two reasons. The first is the most compelling: it goes so well, it fits, tastes as it should; it somehow manages to give me a nostalgic glow of satisfaction about food I was never actually given to eat as a child. The second is simply that this is the easiest of all pastries to make and roll out: just stir all the ingredients together in the bowl, roll out and stretch any old how over the pie. Suet crust (unlike ordinary pastry, which benefits from hanging around) has to be used the minute it's made; and it makes for a bumpy, ramshackle-looking pie.

If you don't like kidney (and unless you've got a good butcher it can be bitter and somehow sawdusty and rubbery at the same time) then just boost the quantities of steak and add more mushrooms. These should be field mushrooms: you want all that leaky black pungency; button mushrooms can be just pretty polystyrene. I use stout rather than wine because I love it, and also because I make the pie filling in advance and don't drink enough to have an open bottle of red wine on the go. Use the best beef stock you can, but if you can't do better than a good cube, then don't lose sleep over it.

This is, you don't need me to elaborate here, a standard British dish, but I start it off as the Italians do their stews: with a soffritto of carrot, onion, celery and, less orthodox, sage. If the lovage is out in the garden, then I use that instead of celery, but to be frank, it isn't for long that the desire to eat steak and kidney pie and the seasonal availability of lovage overlap. You could, I suppose, add garlic too, as the Italians would, but I don't. Not because I think it would be disastrous, but because I just instinctively don't.

2 medium onions
1 medium carrot
½ stick celery or small handful lovage leaves
3 sage leaves
4 tablespoons oil or dripping
200g field mushrooms
small handful fresh parsley (to make about 1 heaped tablespoon when chopped)
2 tablespoons butter, approx. 30g
4 tablespoons flour
fresh nutmeg
500g stewing steak, cut into approx. 3cm chunks
250g kidneys, cut into chunks of approx. 3cm
200ml beef stock
200ml stout or red wine

for the crust
200g self-raising flour
2 teaspoons baking powder
fresh nutmeg
100g suet

Preheat the oven to gas mark 2/150°C. Finely chop the onions, carrot, celery (or lovage) and sage. I use the food processor for this. Put 2 tablespoons oil or dripping (and I get grass-fed beef dripping from my butcher, which is just wonderful here) in a thick pan and heat, adding the finely minced vegetables. Stir around on a medium heat for about 5 minutes or until softish. Remove to a thick casserole with a lid.

Slice the mushrooms and chop the parsley. Add 2 tablespoons butter to the pan and sauté the mushrooms for a few minutes, add the parsley, turn well and then add to the vegetables in the casserole. Sprinkle the flour onto a large plate and add an exuberant grating of fresh nutmeg and some pepper. Turn the steak and kidney in the flour and when all the pieces are done, heat another 2 tablespoons oil or dripping in the pan and brown the meat. Don't cram the pan or the meat'll be steamed rather than seared: just do 4–5 chunks at a time, removing them to the casserole as you go. If there's any flour left on the dredging plate add it to the frying pan, stirring as you do so. I use a flat wooden spoon-cum-spatula for this. Add the stock and stout (or wine) and stir well, scraping any bits from the base of the pan and pour over the meat and vegetables in the casserole. Season, cover and cook for about 2 hours. You want the meat to be tender but not falling apart. But you shouldn't have a problem at this low heat anyway.

When it's ready, leave to cool. If you can't cook the pie filling in advance, then you need to decant it to make it cool more quickly. I would just pour it into a roasting dish (or anything that will take it in as thin a layer as possible) and put somewhere cold. Later, transfer to a 20cm pie dish. Put a pie funnel (or up-ended eggcup) in the middle.

The pastry will need about 30–40 minutes to cook, so bear that in mind when you decide when to get started on the pastry. And how easy is that? Preheat the oven to gas mark 7/210°C. Put the flour, ½ teaspoon salt, the baking powder and another extravagant grating of nutmeg in a bowl. Stir in the suet and then, still stirring, add water, 100ml of it at first. You need a soft paste: add more water (or flour if you've been too heavy-handed with the water) as you think necessary. This is a forgiving kind of pastry, so don't worry about exact calibrations.

Sprinkle some flour onto a surface, some onto the rolling pin and some more onto the surface of the dough and start rolling. You need a fat disc, about ½cm or so thick (¼ inch in old money), slightly bigger than the diameter of the pie dish. You'll have rather more than this, so from the overmatter cut some strips and cover the rims of the dish with them. It helps to dampen the rims with a little cold water first. Now, lift up your circle of nubbly soft pastry and drape over the pie dish. Cobble together somehow if holes appear, and press down over the pastry rims. Put in the oven and cook for about 10 minutes, then turn down to gas mark 5/190°C and cook for another 25 minutes. Peep after 15: if the pastry looks as if it might stop browning and start burning then cover loosely with foil. Whip the foil off, though, for the last couple of minutes.

I think you have to serve peas with this: and since it obviously isn't summer food, I mean by this frozen petits pois. Potatoes aren't strictly necessary, I suppose, given the pastry, but even so potatoes mashed with an equal volume of parsnips (or swede) and more butter than anyone would like to own up to, would be just right.

BANANA CUSTARD

The first time I made a banana custard, it looked so pallid. The point is, of course, that everyone is used to eating it made with Bird's custard, so that one can't help but expect to see that bouncy canary-yellow. The next time I added saffron to the custard (as long as you don't add too much the note it strikes is intriguing rather than intrusive), which turns it from palest primrose to a yellow that would do honour to the most dazzling tartrazine. It is more than just a culinary joke, though, enjoyable as that is in itself. And for once powdered saffron may be a better choice than strands. Saffron strands leave little red strings, which are beautiful enough, to be sure, but what we are after is an uninterrupted blanket of unarguable yellow.

If you hate the idea of the saffron, then leave the custard pale and uninteresting: there's no mileage in adding food colouring and no point in using Bird's.

You could also bake this custard (see page 377).

600ml full-fat milk
good pinch ground saffron
8 egg yolks
60g caster sugar
4–6 bananas, firm but ripe

Fill the sink with cold water: you may need to plunge the custard pot into this later to stop it cooking quickly.

Put the milk in a pan, sprinkle in the saffron, and bring to boiling point. Meanwhile whisk together the egg yolks and sugar with a fork, and just as the milk is about to come to the boil pour it over the eggs and keep on whisking. Pour into a wide, heavy-based saucepan (I use the largest one I've got) and cook on a low heat, stirring constantly with a wooden spoon. In about 10 minutes the custard should be cooked. Remove from the heat and plunge the pan into the cold water in the sink and stir until cooled. If, indeed, at any stage you think the custard is about to boil or curdle, then immerse the custard pan in the cold water and beat vigorously.

Slice the bananas into a dish. I do them in coins of lengthening diagonals, rather like at school. When the bananas are arranged as you like them, strain the custard over and leave to cool and form a skin. This is imperative. I don't even like skin on custard, but I recognise that. You can make the custard in advance, sprinkling icing sugar on top to prevent it forming a skin, but the bananas cannot be cut and the whole assembled till the last minute.

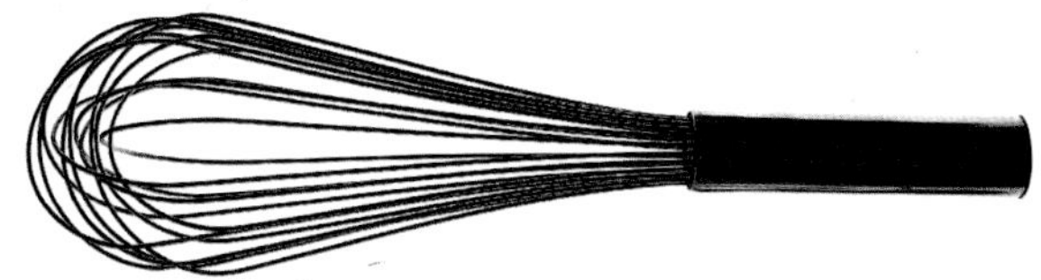

LUNCH, TENTATIVELY OUTSIDE, FOR 8

Crab and saffron tart

Parsley salad

Baked caramel apples

In the heat of the summer you don't want, I think, a rich and odoriferous crab tart. But in those first early days, when it is more hope than convenience that takes you outside, or when the sun is growing weaker but still invites, towards the end of September, this is the perfect lunch: not too filling and not a parody of a picnic to be eaten under those cloudless pre-First World War skies of nostalgic collective memory.

If you think you can't manage the pastry, buy it, but making the rich shortcrust below is not a big deal, I promise you. I tend to make the pastry the night before and leave it in a disc, wrapped in clingfilm, in the fridge to be rolled out the next morning. If I've got time to start it slightly earlier in the evening, I make the pastry, let it rest, then bring it out and roll it, line the flan dish with it and put it back in the fridge, covered with clingfilm again. Then, the next day, all I've got to do is bake it blind (see below and page 44) and then get the filling together, which is not a strenuous exercise.

CRAB AND SAFFRON TART

This recipe is adapted from Simon Hopkinson's *Roast Chicken and Other Stories*. Normally I don't like tomatoes with fish, but here everything melds so harmoniously, seductively together that I forget my usual gripes. With it I'd serve the salad of parsley – flat-leaved, unchopped – capers and red onion that is copied from the salad served with bone marrow at St John's and already mentioned on page 244. The rich and fragrant creaminess of the tart is offset particularly well by it.

PARSLEY SALAD

Don't buy frozen or tinned crabmeat: go to a fishmonger and tell him what you need. He will then do the necessary to the crab. The remainder of the brown meat can be eaten smeared on white bread or brown toast. And it freezes, so you can save it up for when you're in by yourself one night.

for the pastry

150g plain flour, preferably Italian 00

75g butter, chilled and in small dice

1 egg yolk

approx. 4 tablespoons iced water

for the filling

400g tin plum tomatoes, chopped

2 fat garlic cloves

1 bay leaf

1 sprig thyme

300ml double cream

1/2 teaspoon saffron threads

4 egg yolks

white meat from a 1 1/4kg crab (yield should be about 150g) and 2 tablespoons brown meat

First make the pastry following instructions on page 42. You will need to add salted, iced water to form this dough, but go slowly, adding 1 tablespoon at a time. About 4 tablespoons should do it, but you may need more. The weather, the flour, the egg will all make a difference. When the dough coheres into an unsticky ball, press it into a fat disc and cover with clingfilm or greaseproof and put into the fridge for about 20 minutes, more if it's a hot day, or leave overnight.

When you get to the stage of making the tart, preheat the oven to gas mark 6/200°C. Then roll out the pastry to fit a flan or quiche ring about 24–25cm in diameter (measured at the top not the base) and 5cm deep. Bake blind (and see page 44).

Remove from the oven, turn the heat down to gas mark 4/180°C and get on with the sauce (or if you prefer, do the sauce while the pastry cooks). Put the tomatoes, garlic, herbs, salt and pepper in a saucepan and reduce to a thickish sauce. Cool, remove the herbs and spread the sauce in the bottom of the pastry case. Warm together 3 tablespoons cream with the saffron and allow to steep for a few minutes. Beat together the egg yolks and the rest of the cream and add the saffron cream. Season. Loosely fold the crab meat into the custard and carefully pour into the tart case. I think it's easier to pour it in while the pastry case is sitting on its (slightly pulled out) oven rack.

Bake in the oven for 30–40 minutes or until set and pale golden brown on top, but with a hint of runny wobble within. Serve neither hot nor cold but warm: this is at its paradisal, slightly baveuse best about 50 minutes to an hour after it comes out of the oven. And I have found that you can bring any fridge-cold leftover wedges back to optimum, faintly runny room temperature in a low microwave. Strange but true. And if you do have any left over, it is worth cutting into individual fat slices and freezing like that, only to resuscitate them for a perfect, gloriously luxurious dinner for yourself in evenings ahead.

BAKED CARAMEL APPLES

Again, these apples are best eaten not hot but warm. If you put them in the oven just as you take out the crab tart, then they in turn will be ready to be taken out just as you sit down for lunch. Transfer the apples to a large plate or couple of plates, and pour the juices into a saucepan. Then all you need to do at the last minute is come back to the stove to reduce and add cream to the buttery sour-sweet liquor in the saucepan before pouring it thickly over the softly cooling, glossy and bulging apples on the plates. These are my favourite baked apples of all time and I wouldn't change a thing. If, however, you want the sauce clear and toffee-ish rather than dense and fudgelike, then omit the cream.

8 cooking apples
150g butter
150g light muscovado sugar
250ml Calvados
juice of 1 lemon
8 tablespoons single cream (or to fill an American half-cup measure)

Preheat to or keep the oven at gas mark 4/180°C. Core the apples and, with a sharp knife, cut a line round as if circling the equator. Put them in a roasting tin. Press in butter and sugar, alternately, in the holes and press any excess on top. Pour the Calvados and lemon juice into the tin. Put them into the oven and cook for about 50 minutes.

Then take the tin out of the oven, remove apples to a plate or dish and pour the cooking juices and liquid into a saucepan. (I've left them to cool for about an hour and a half and they've still tasted perfect.) When you want to eat pudding, nip back inside and put the saucepan on a high heat on the hob. Let bubble till reduced and thickened; it should be like a gooey sticky syrup. Stir in the cream and let bubble again for a few minutes; pour this fudgy sauce over the apples. Serve straight away, as they are: you don't need to eat anything else alongside or dolloped on top.

SPRING LUNCH TO LIFT THE SPIRITS, FOR 6

Lemon linguine
Green salad
Irish tarte tatin

According to my paternal grandmother, spring no longer exists, though her lament was as much sartorial as environmental: no more spring coats, you see, because no more spring weather. Actually, I suspect the change is in us rather than in the climate: our failure to recognise, let alone celebrate, the advent of spring owes rather more to the fact that we now live in centrally heated homes. The meagre upturn in the weather cannot have quite the impact it must once have had. But I do think there is an idea of spring, culinarily speaking. Of course, seasonal produce has something to do with it, but not everything: for me, that idea is instantly conveyed by this lemony, creamy tangle of linguine which actually you could cook at anytime of the year. It is the easiest thing you could imagine: the sauce requires no cooking, just stirring (and limply at that) and it produces food that is both comforting and uplifting. There must be something about the smell of lemons, so fresh, so hopeful, which makes this instant good-mood food. But it isn't so jaunty and astringent that you need to brace yourself to dive in.

As for the Irish tarte tatin: this is Roscommon Rhubarb Pie as chronicled by Darina Allen in *Irish Traditional Cooking*. The rhubarb and sugar are piled on the bottom of the tin, the scone mixture on top, and the whole turned out later in the manner of a tarte tatin. The upended pie with its bronzy pink crown of rhubarb looks beautiful and it is fabulously easy. For this, you're just mixing stuff around in a bowl, idly and imprecisely rolling it out, and then tucking the large disc of scone like a blanket over the simply chopped and sugar-sprinkled fruit.

Perhaps pastry after pasta sounds stodgy, but it won't taste like that, I promise. And the scent of lemons followed by the sharp-sweet breath of red and early rhubarb conveys the brisk but tender air of early, still faintly wintry, spring.

LEMON LINGUINE

750g linguine
2 egg yolks
10 tablespoons (150ml) double cream
10 tablespoons (about 50g) freshly grated parmesan
zest and juice of 1 unwaxed lemon
15g butter
fresh flat-leaf parsley

Fill just about the biggest pot you can hold with water and bring to the boil. When you have friends coming for lunch, get the water heated to boiling point before they arrive, otherwise you end up nervously hanging around waiting for a watched pot to boil while your supposedly quick lunch gets later and later. Bring the water to the boil, cover and turn off the hob.

I tend to leave the addition of salt until the water's come to the boil a second time. But whichever way you do it, add quite a bit of salt – Italians say the water in which pasta cooks should be as salty as the Mediterranean. When the bubbling's encouragingly fierce, tip in the pasta. I often put the lid on for a moment or so just to let the pasta get back to the boil, but don't turn your back on it, and give it a good stir with a pasta fork or whatever to avoid even the suspicion of clagginess, once you've removed the lid.

Then get on with the sauce, making sure you've set your timer for about a minute or so less than the time specified on the packet of pasta.

In a bowl, put the yolks, cream, grated parmesan, zest of the whole lemon and juice of half of it, a pinch of salt and good grating of pepper and beat with a fork. You don't want it fluffy, just combined. Taste. If you want it more lemony, then of course add more juice.

When the timer goes off, taste to judge how near the pasta is to being ready. I recommend that you hover by the stove so you don't miss that point. Don't be too hasty, though. Everyone is so keen to cook their pasta properly al dente that sometimes the pasta is actually not cooked enough. You want absolutely no chalkiness here. And linguine (or at least I find them so) tend not to run over into soggy overcookedness quite as quickly as other long pasta. This makes sense, of course, since the strands of 'little tongues' are denser than the flat ribbon shapes. But I made this sauce with a very fine pasta, some sort of egg tagliarini, once and regretted it. You need the sturdier, but still satiny, resistance offered up by the linguine, which is why I stipulated this very pasta. Good spaghetti or tagliatelle would do if linguine are not to be found. Since the sauce is the sort of thing you can throw together after a quick rummage through the shelves of the corner shop, it would be unhelpful to be too sternly dictatorial about a pasta shape that is not universally carried.

Anyway, as soon as the pasta looks ready, hive off a mugful of the cooking liquid, drain the pasta and then, off the heat, toss it back in the pan or put it in an efficiently preheated bowl, throw in the butter and stir and swirl about to make sure the butter's melted and the pasta covered by it all over. Each strand will be only mutely gleaming, since there's not much butter and quite a bit of pasta. If you want to add more, then do: good butter is the best flavouring, best texture, best mood enhancer there is.

When you're satisfied the pasta's covered with its soft slip of butter, then stir in the egg, cream, cheese and lemon mix and turn the pasta well in it, adding some of the cooking liquid if it looks a bit dry (only 2 tablespoons or so, you don't want a wet mess, and only after you think the sauce is incorporated). Sprinkle over some just-chopped parsley and serve now, now, now.

As for the green salad: buy a packet of the ready washed and chopped stuff or assemble your own as you wish. But keep it green: by all means add raw sugar-snap peas if you like (a good idea, indeed) and some whole, tender basil leaves (equally so), but remember the idea is to provide something clear and refreshing between the pasta and the pie. Don't let sorry memories rule out the much-maligned soft, round, pale green English lettuce: nothing else, just that, in a plain vinaigrette, no interesting oils.

IRISH TARTE TATIN

Bright-hued, early spring rhubarb is indicated here, but I've used the later stuff with good results. But be stern when inspecting it before buying: there's no point in making this pudding if the fruit's woody and acrid. If it looks as if it's rusting and wilting, then don't bother.

Darina Allen specifies a 23cm x 5cm round tin, and remarks that she uses a heavy stainless-steel sauté pan. I use my regular stainless-steel pie dish. It's about 20cm in diameter, 5cm in depth, has sloping sides and a capacity of about 1¼ litres. Because of the sloping sides, the pie, when turned out, looks rather celebratory, as if it were holding up the rhubarb as an offering.

900g rhubarb (see above)
255–285g granulated sugar

for the scone dough
310g plain flour
20g caster sugar
1 heaped teaspoon baking powder
55g butter
1 egg
about 175ml full-fat milk
beaten egg to glaze
granulated sugar for sprinkling

Preheat the oven to gas mark 8/220°C. Trim the rhubarb, wipe with a damp cloth and cut into pieces about 2½cm in length. Put into the base of a tin or a sauté pan and sprinkle with the sugar. Taste the rhubarb to see how much sugar you'd like.

Into a bowl sieve all the dry ingredients for the scone dough, adding a pinch of salt. Cut the butter into cubes and rub into the flour until the mixture resembles coarse breadcrumbs. (Not hard to do by hand, but I tend to use my KitchenAid free-standing mixer.) Whisk the egg with the milk. Make a well in the centre of the dry ingredients, pour in the liquid all at once and mix to a soft dough. Turn out onto a floured board and roll into a 23cm round (or the size of the pan you're using) about 2½cm thick. Place this fat disc on top of the rhubarb and tuck in the edges neatly. Brush with a little beaten egg and sprinkle generously with granulated sugar.

Bake in the preheated oven for 15 minutes, then reduce the temperature to gas mark 4/180°C for about a further 30 minutes, or until the top is crusty and golden and the rhubarb soft and juicy.

Remove the pan from the oven and allow to sit for a few minutes. Put a warm plate over the top of the pan and turn it upside-down so that the pie comes out on the plate. It is almost impossible (or I, naturally impatient and clumsy, find it so) not to burn yourself with some of the escaping hot liquid. The trick is to find a dish which is flat at the bottom with slightly upturned edges. I'm working on it.

Serve warm with, Darina Allen recommends, soft brown sugar and cream. I can think of nothing nicer. For those who cannot contemplate rhubarb without custard, a good cold dollop of the stuff would be an obvious, but rewarding, choice.

ANOTHER SPRING LUNCH FOR 6–8

Prosciutto, mozzarella and basil, or fresh ricotta

Grilled courgettes or roast asparagus

Salad and bread

Rhubarb meringue pie

I love rhubarb: a quick glance at the entry for it in the Index will suggest how much. But my real passion goes deeper; at home I use it whenever I can get away with it. Maybe it's the relatively short season (although I find I can go from the early forced stuff to the hardy outdoors-reared stalks with hardly a hiccup) that makes it so attractive, but if it's in the shops, I want to cook with it. I make rhubarb fool (divine used to wedge together the two vanilla-scented halves of a Victoria sponge); rhubarb and raspberry crumble (the rhubarb February-fresh, the raspberries always used to be from the freezer cabinet, but more recently they're fresh too, flown in at great expense from Chile); plain stewed rhubarb; rhubarb custard pie; the pie, indeed, above; all the other rhubarb-rich recipes in this book; and my absolute tear-inducingly comforting favourite, rhubarb meringue pie.

It isn't nostalgia that drives me – such puddings, such ingredients, were not a part of my childhood – or a kitsch longing for the retro-culinary repertoire. It's the taste, the smell, the soft, fragrant, bulky stickiness of this that seduces. I cannot pretend any form of meringue pie is easy and because it takes a bit of effort, I have suggested a picnic before it.

For eight people, I get 500g prosciutto (San Daniele or Parma), sliced thin, thin, thin and draped over a big plate like rumpled silk lining. If you can find it, buy a mound of fresh ricotta, but if you can't, then provide fresh mozzarella di bufalo drizzled with basil oil (see recipe below) or just milkily plain and barely sprinkled with salt and pepper and olive oil. Make a salad of lamb's lettuce and little gem with a light but astringent dressing; if it's in season, lay on some asparagus just rolled in oil and coarse sea salt and spread out on a baking sheet in the hottest oven you can muster, for about 5–10 minutes a side, and then left to cool to room temperature or just above and put on a plate with either some lemon wedges bundled alongside or just a sprinkling of good balsamic vinegar over. If asparagus isn't around, then get some courgettes (about 5 courgettes should do for 8 people), slice them thinly lengthways, brush them lightly with oil and cook on a hot griddle, till blistered brown. As they cook, remove them to a large plate, and pour over glass-green oil, a good squirt of lemon juice and a carpeting of just-chopped herbs – parsley, mint, marjoram, basil, some or all. Make sure there's lots of bread and you might, as well, leave some tomatoes whole in a bowl on the table, so that people can take them as they like.

PROSCIUTTO

FRESH RICOTTA

MOZZARELLA DI BUFALO

ASPARAGUS

COURGETTES

BASIL OIL

Sometimes when I've gone out for dinner and get back when the shops are still open in the States, I phone Kitchen Arts & Letters in New York and ask what interesting books they've got in at the moment. My alcohol-induced long-distance phone call becomes very expensive: the mere recital of the credit card number and boxloads of books arrive – the memory suppressed, a surprise – some weeks later. The book from which this recipe comes was in one such batch.

And this book, *Recipes 1-2-3* by Rozanne Gold, is a clever idea: all recipes contain just three ingredients, though further ones in the form of suggested 'add-ons' are posited. It's now published in Britain by Grub Street: so you don't have to stay out too late, drink too much and phone your order to America.

1 very large bunch basil

6–10 tablespoons extra virgin olive oil

Blanch the stemmed basil leaves in boiling water for 30 seconds and then refresh by plunging immediately into iced water. Squeeze out as much moisture as you can and then put in a mini chopper or the small bowl of a processor and whizz with the oil until you have a thickish green purée, like liquid snooker baize. That's it.

This makes enough for 3 balls of mozzarella.

Slice the mozzarella thickly and dribble the basil oil over it. You could equally use the basil oil over sliced tomatoes, pasta, soup, anything.

RHUBARB MERINGUE PIE

for Horatia

I don't go in for flavoured mash, flavoured pasta, or flavoured pastry. I think that mash, pasta and pastry are meant to be the base line, the comforting neutral blanket against which other more sprightly tastes can be set. But orange, in pastry, does work, and subtly. Orange, famously, sets off rhubarb – and it is used also to bind the fruits beneath the meringue topping.

Because I quite often make rhubarb jelly, I tend to have pulpy bags of frozen, poached, sweetened fruit in the freezer. For a 21cm flan dish about 300g of cooked fruit should be fine. And if the purée is already sweetened, you'll need only 1–2 tablespoons of extra sugar rather than the 150g specified.

If you're using raw fruit, proceed as below.

for the pastry

140g plain flour, preferably 00

70g cold unsalted butter, cut in small cubes, or 1/2 lard and 1/2 butter

juice of 1/2 orange

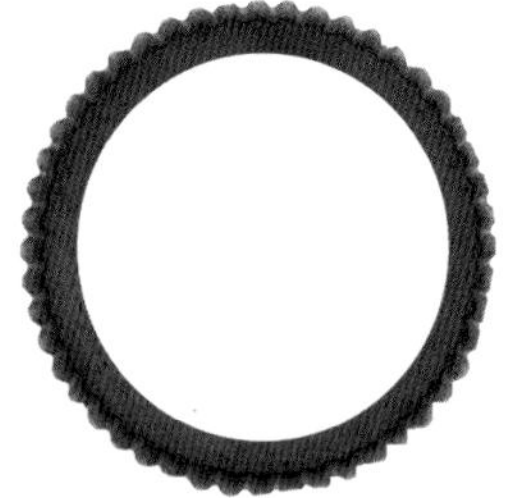

Make the pastry by following the instructions on page 41, freezing the flour and butter for 10 minutes and chilling the orange juice (with a pinch of salt) which you will use later to make the floury, buttery breadcrumby mixture cohere. Go slowly, adding iced water if needed. (Remember you will be using the other half of the orange's juice for the filling, so keep it.) When the dough can be formed into a ball, stop, roll it into a ball in your hands and then press it into a disc, wrap with clingfilm and put in the fridge for 20–30 minutes. Roll it out and line a deep flan/quiche tin of 21cm diameter. Put back in the fridge if possible for about another 20 minutes and preheat the oven to gas mark 6/200°C.

Bake blind (see page 44) until the pastry looks cooked but not brown. Remove from the oven; you don't want the pastry hot when you put all the other ingredients in it.

for the rhubarb
800g rhubarb, untrimmed weight
juice of 1/2 orange
2 eggs, separated
150g plus 120g caster sugar
2 tablespoons plain flour
30g melted butter
1/4 teaspoon cream of tartar

Trim the rhubarb and chop it into roughly 1cm slices; if the stalks are very wide and chunky then cut them in half lengthways, too. Put them in a saucepan with the orange juice and heat briefly, just until the rawness is taken off them. Remove and drain (but keep the liquid).

If you haven't done so already, separate the eggs, putting the whites aside for the meringue later and beat the egg yolks in a bowl. In another bowl, mix 150g sugar with the flour and the melted butter. Then add the eggs, and enough of the orangey-rhubarb liquid which came off the rhubarb in the pan earlier to make a smooth and runny paste. Squeeze in more orange if you need more. Put the rhubarb in the blind-baked pastry case and pour the sugary, eggy mixture over it. Put in the oven and bake until just set, about 20–30 minutes.

Meanwhile beat the egg whites until they form soft peaks, add 1/2 the remaining sugar (i.e. 60g) and continue to beat until glossy. I use my mixer until this point. I then change to a metal spoon and fold in the remaining sugar and the cream of tartar. Spoon this over the hot cooked rhubarb in the flan case, making sure it is completely covered and there is no place, no gap where some rhubarb can bubble up through and over the meringue. Use the spoon to bring some of the meringue into little pointy peaks if you like (I do), but this is an aesthetic diktat not a practical-culinary one. Sprinkle with about 1 teaspoon caster sugar and put back in the oven for about 15 minutes until the peaks are bronzy and brown topped.

I like this cold. But for most tastes, eat it 10–12 minutes after it's been taken out of the oven.

HIGH SUMMER AL FRESCO LUNCH FOR 8

To eat outside, you don't necessarily have to cook a lot, but you've got a lot to think about. I'm talking here about a table-borne lunch outside in the garden. Choose nothing fussy, nothing that will grow waxy or dry in the heat and nothing that will sit too heavily on the digestion. Lots of meat, quivering pots of mayonnaise in the sun's glare, bread already cut – much traditional picnic fare is ruled out. Certainly a hunk of bread, a wedge of cheese and a peppery salame will do on cooler days, but in even moderate heat bread gets stale in a matter of minutes. Cheese and meat quickly grow a patina of rancid sweatiness.

Pitta is better – unsurprisingly – at withstanding heat; it does harden to cardboardy unpliableness if left out too brazenly, but covered with a napkin or toasted to order on a nearby barbecue it will hold up better than ciabatta, baguette or bloomer. Don't bother cooking a pudding. You could go for the Greek yoghurt with honey and passion fruit on page 232; otherwise serve grapes and plums *all'Italiana* – bobbing about in water- and ice-cube-filled bowls – or any amount of fruit cut up with as much dexterity as you can muster (in my case not much), Japanese style. Tropical fruits obviously do well in the heat. Cut pawpaws in half, remove the black stony pips, and squirt with lime or fill the cavities, avocado-style, with strawberries that have been chopped and macerated with a sprinkling of balsamic vinegar or with plain, unadorned raspberries. If you can get the wonderful fibreless Indian or Alfonse mangoes, do buy one, but eat one yourself to test for stringiness before you consider introducing them into polite society.

GRAPES AND PLUMS

PAWPAWS

MANGOES

Food that suits hot weather is – it stands to reason – food that's customarily eaten in hot countries. I tend to go for the food of the eastern Mediterranean. I am not pretending to set up a taverna in my backyard; but when it's hot I want tabbouleh, hummus, garlic chicken, mint-sprinkled slices of aubergine and the balm of juicy, cold, jade-coloured wedges of cucumber.

TABBOULEH

I love this salad of cracked wheat, mint and parsley to be very green and very sharp, but if you want it to be grainier and oilier then adapt it as you wish. In many recipes you will find cucumber stipulated as well: by all means add this if you want, but I tend not to as after a while it makes the salad go wet and watery. I keep leftovers in the fridge to be squished into pitta or a baked potato for the next day's lunch, and indeed eaten whenever the desire overcomes me. Tomatoes seem to hold up pretty well, although I always add them just before serving the tabbouleh the first time; perhaps it's just that I don't mind the pinkly-stained sogginess so much on my own account when it's brought out for the second. Red onions, if they're not mild, can make this very intensely oniony, so taste a bit of the onion (and the spring onions: they too can vary) before you judge how much to add. Tabbouleh, surprisingly, works very well too with cold – poached or baked – salmon for a different, unEnglish take on a traditional summer food. Warm, pink, sweet lamb – noisettes seared on a griddle until medium-rare, let to stand for 5–10 minutes, then sliced thinly on the diagonal, heaped on a near-by plate and sprinkled with some salt, chopped mint and marjoram – is terrific with tabbouleh, too. Like a lot of foods with bite, once you eat this you hanker after it again.

150g burghal
2 bunches flat-leaf parsley
2 bunches mint
12 spring onions or 1 large or 2 small red onions
6 flavoursome tomatoes
10–12 tablespoons olive oil
juice of 2–3 lemons

If you are using fine burghal or bulgar wheat, whatever you like to call it, put it in a bowl, cover with cold water and leave to soak for 30 minutes. If you can find only coarse burghal, then put it in a bowl and cover it with boiling water and leave to soak for 30 minutes. Whichever you are using, at the end of the half-hour drain the burghal in a sieve, getting rid of as much water as possible.

Put the burghal in a serving dish and pour over the lemon juice, 10 tablespoons olive oil and a good sprinkling of salt and pepper. Meanwhile, finely chop the parsley and the mint. Be very wary of using a food processor for this. It does have a tendency not so much to chop herbs as to reduce them to a wet mush. But when you are chopping this quantity the danger can be avoided more easily: just pulse on and off quickly and (after checking) repeatedly so that the herbs don't get pulverised before you've had a chance to intervene. Leave the leaves relatively large, too: after all, the parsley and mint are the major part of the salad itself, not flavouring in it.

Throw the cautiously chopped herbs into the dressed burghal. Slice the spring onions or finely chop the red onion and stir in. Put the tomatoes in a bowl and pour over boiling water from the kettle to cover. Leave for a few minutes, then remove, peel the tomatoes, cut in half and take out seeds. Dice the tomatoes and stir into the herbs and cracked wheat. Taste and add more salt, lemon juice and the remaining tablespoons (or more) of oil if it needs it.

HUMMUS WITH SEARED LAMB AND TOASTED PINE NUTS

This isn't an obvious pairing, but I think it's an authentic one. That's to say, although I've never seen mention of it in cookery books, I've eaten it – in both Turkish and Lebanese restaurants. And I love this combination of cold, thickly nutty, buff-coloured paste and hot, lemony-sweet shards of meat, and the waxy, resiny nuts: it instantly elevates the hummus from its familiar deli-counter incarnation. You could use good bought hummus – but just dribble a little good olive oil on top, and round the edges, before topping with the nuts and lamb.

And as far as authenticity goes, I don't make any claims for my hummus recipe: for I add Greek yoghurt. Nor do I apologise for my innovation. Home-made hummus can be stodgy and claggy, and I love the tender whippedness that you get in restaurant versions (which, come to think of it, are probably bought in). If you leave out the Greek yoghurt, you may have to add a little more of the chick-pea cooking liquid. Don't be afraid of making this too liquid; it'll most likely stiffen on keeping anyway. With the yoghurt, I find I can still use up to 200ml cooking liquid when puréeing the chick peas.

I buy noisettes of lamb here, because I know that, once I've stripped off the encircling fat, they'll be lean but still satiny within. If pressed, I suppose you could buy those little rags of meat carved ready for stir-frying from the supermarket – just make sure you cut each little piece in half again. Think of lardons, then imagine them cut in half horizontally: that's the size of meat strip you're aiming for.

300g dried chick peas
1 onion, whole but peeled
2 bay leaves
3 cloves garlic, unpeeled, plus 4 cloves garlic, peeled
3 tablespoons olive oil
9 tablespoons tahina
2–3 lemons
fat pinch cumin
3–5 tablespoons Greek yoghurt
75g pine nuts
325g lean, tender lamb
3 tablespoons garlic-infused or plain olive oil
flat-leaf parsley

Soak and cook the chick peas following the instructions on page 88, throwing the onion, bay leaves and 3 unpeeled cloves of garlic into the pot, too. It is imperative you taste the chick peas to test they are truly cooked enough before draining them: undercooked chick peas make for an unsatisfactorily grainy texture; you want a voluptuous velvetiness here, no hard surfaces. When you're satisfied the chick peas are buttery and tender, dunk a mug in to catch a good 350ml of the cooking liquid, and then you can drain the chick peas with a clear conscience.

In the bowl of the food processor fitted with the double-bladed knife, add the peeled cloves of garlic, roughly chopped, a teaspoon of salt, 100ml of the cooking liquid, olive oil, tahina, juice of 1 lemon and cumin. Blitz till well and truly puréed. Taste, adding more liquid as you feel you need to slacken and soften the mixture. Process again, then grind in some pepper, add 3 dolloping tablespoons of Greek yoghurt and give another whizz. Taste to see whether you want to add any more lemon juice (and you could want double) or Greek yoghurt, or indeed oil or seasoning. When you have a smooth yet dense purée with the intensity you like, scrape out into a bowl, cover and keep in the fridge until about an hour before you want to eat it.

You can toast the pine nuts before then, but the lamb must be done at the last minute. To be frank, then, you may as well do them both together. Cut the lamb into tiny, thin shreds – little rags and tatters of meat – and decant the hummus into a shallow round or oval bowl, and put both to one side for a moment.

Put a heavy-based frying pan on the hob over medium heat, add the pine nuts and shake every so often until they begin to take on a deep golden colour and their resiny fragrance rises from the pan. Pour onto a plate or into a bowl, and then add the oil to the pan. I often use garlic-infused oil here because I like it when the lamb has a garlicky taste, but I don't want burnt shards of garlic mixed up with it. Marinating with a few cloves of crushed garlic can work, but then the lamb doesn't sear as well. But ordinary olive oil works well too, and because the hummus itself is garlicky, you hardly risk blandness by omitting the garlic with the lamb.

When whichever oil you're using is hot in the pan, toss in the lamb and stir furiously until it begins to crisp and brown at the edges. Hold half a lemon over the pan and give a good hard squeeze. Push the meat about once more and empty the contents of the pan evenly over the hummus, lemony oil juices and all. Sprinkle with, preferably, coarse salt, grind over pepper and scatter with toasted pine nuts. Add some freshly chopped parsley, then serve immediately and with lots of oven-warmed pitta.

TARAMASALATA

I wouldn't eat taramasalata with the lamb-heavy version of hummus here, but it's a bit like giving a present to one child: you just can't give the one recipe and

into roasting tin. Preheat the oven to gas mark 7/210°C. Then cook, basting occasionally, for 45 minutes to an hour until they are very well done, crisp and burnished brown (I like to use butcher's chicken wings which are a good deal fleshier than the supermarket-packaged ones, which will take less time to cook, evidently). Remove from the oven, arrange on a large plate and sprinkle generously with coarse salt.

AUBERGINE SLICES WITH POMEGRANATE JUICE AND MINT

I suppose pomegranates – that Carpaccio-red juice, those glassy beads – always seem exotic to us, and that's partly why I like them. There is something both biblical and almost belle époque about them: both ancient and vulgar. And curiously, I feel rather nostalgically inclined towards them, too: I remember digging them out of Christmas stockings, then sitting for hours with a yellow-mazed half in front of me, winkling the bitter-cased seeds out with a pin.

But they fit best in the time-stamped, opulent Middle-Eastern tradition, as here, with the juice sousing pinkly a plate of aubergine slices fried in olive oil, the seeds like jewels glinting out from behind the aromatic leafiness of thickly sprinkled mint. You can fry the aubergines in advance, but don't do anything with the pomegranate and mint until about half an hour before you eat. After 20 minutes' sousing, the aubergine is at its heady best.

If you like, you can substitute charred, skinned red peppers for the aubergine.

2 aubergines
olive oil for frying – quite a lot
2 pomegranates
handful fresh mint

Slice the aubergine into circles about ½cm thick or cut lengthways to form swelling, pear-shaped slices: the bulging lengths look more beautiful, the discs are easier to eat.

I don't, as I've mentioned elsewhere, salt and soak aubergines: if you buy ones that are taut and glossy and feel light for their size, you shouldn't find them bitter. Once sliced, start frying. If you've got a ridged cast-iron griddle, use that, only brush the aubergine slices as well as the griddle with olive oil before you start. But if you're using a frying pan, just pour oil to a depth of about ½cm in the pan (and be prepared to top up as you put fresh batches in to fry) and leave the slices as they are. Whichever way, cook briskly until the surface crisps and the interior is soft, then remove to plates lined thickly with pieces of kitchen towel and drape some more paper over the resting slices so that the paper absorbs as much oil as possible, and the aubergine is as dry as possible. You can proceed straight away, eating them warm or, if it makes life easier, just leave them to get cold.

EXTRACTING POMEGRANATE SEEDS

Cut 1 pomegranate in half and dig out some seeds: just enough to sprinkle over the slices, about 2 tablespoons should do it. The easiest way to make the seeds drop out is to hold with one hand a halved pomegranate, cut side down, over a bowl; with the other hand take a wooden spoon and thwack the pomegranates. After the third thwack, you will have rubies raining down. Put those aside and squeeze the juice out of the remaining fruit. I find an electric citrus juicer the easiest way to do this, but an ordinary, old-fashioned, manual one will do. (You might, though, need to get more of the fruit if juicing by hand.) Finely chop the mint. Arrange the aubergine slices on a large plate, sprinkle over a little salt, then pour over the pomegranate juice. If you feel you haven't got enough then cut open the second one and juice some of that. Now sprinkle over the mint and then scatter over the pomegranate seeds, but go steady. Of course, you can add more if you think you need some, but this is one of those time when less is more.

On the table with this I'd put a plate of cucumbers, cut into 5cm lengths and then each chunk cut into quarters lengthways. Add a plate of tomatoes, another of raw, scrubbed and peeled carrots, in chunks like the cucumber, and consider decanting a jar of pickled peppers.

A COMFORTING LUNCH FOR 4

Fish and porcini pie

Ice-cream, cherries, flaked almonds and chocolate sauce

Fish pie is not particularly labour-intensive to cook, but it's hard to get right: if the flour/butter/milk balance is off, the sauce bubbling beneath the blanket of nutmeggy mashed potato can be too runny or too solid. Don't let nervousness make you scrimp on the milk: it's better runny than stodgy and even an imperfect fish pie is a delicious one. What's important is not to make the sauce taste too floury (using 00 flour sees to that) and not to let your desire for something comforting blunt your appetite for seasoning. I added porcini because I'd been given some by my Austrian Aunt Frieda, who was coming for lunch. Perhaps it would be more correct to say *Great* Aunt; the title is honorific but she's the generation, was the companion, of my grandmother. She was the matron at my mother and aunts' boarding school and my grandmother, not I think extraordinarily maternal, was so dreading the school holidays that she asked Matron to stay during them. Over forty years later, she's still here, an important figure in all our lives. I wanted to use the mushrooms because she'd given them to me. But I also thought they'd add a creaturely muskiness, a depth of tone, to the milkily-sweet fish-scented sauce. They did.

This is how I made it. You can change the fish as you want.

FISH AND PORCINI PIE

10g dried porcini
300ml fish stock (I used a tub of Joubère fish stock)
175g skinned cod
175g skinned smoked haddock
175g skinned salmon
250ml full-fat milk
3 bay leaves
60g butter
60g plain, preferably 00, flour
1.25kg floury potatoes
150ml double cream (or 150ml milk, with 60g butter, melted)
freshly grated nutmeg

Cover the dried porcini with very hot water and leave for 20 minutes or so. Then drain the mushrooms and strain the soaking liquid into the stock. Choose the dish in which you will cook (and serve) the fish pie and butter it. I use an old, very battered, oval, enamel cast-iron dish of my mother's, which has a capacity of about 2 litres. Put the fish in a wide, thick-bottomed pan – I use a frying pan, but anything that'll take them in one layer would do – and cover with milk, the stock with its mushroom liquid and the bay leaves. Bring to a simmer and poach for about 3 minutes. Remove fish to the buttered dish, and fork into chunks. Sieve the cooking liquid into a jug, reserving bay leaves.

Melt the butter in a saucepan and add the dried soaked mushrooms, very finely chopped and any grit removed. Fry gently for 2 minutes, stir in the flour and fry gently for another 2 minutes. Off the heat, very slowly add the liquid from the jug, stirring with a wooden spoon or beating with a whisk (whichever suits) as you go. When all is incorporated, put back on the heat. Add the bay leaves and stir gently until thickened. If you're going to eat it straight away, pour over the fish in the casserole. Otherwise, remove from heat and cover with butter paper (the foil paper that the butter is wrapped in), buttered greaseproof, waxed paper or a film of melted butter.

You can boil and mash the potatoes with the cream and seasoning now (you want lots of salt and pepper), or you may have done them in advance. When you're ready to roll, preheat the oven to gas mark 4/180°C. The fish and mushroomy white sauce should be in the casserole, the potato on top, with more nutmeg, pepper and butter (little dots of it here and there) added just before it goes into the oven. Depending on how hot it all is before it goes in the oven, the fish pie should need about 20–40 minutes. Test as you go: this isn't an untouchable work of art you're creating; dig a hole, taste and then patch up with potato.

ICE-CREAM

For pudding, buy the best ice-cream, vanilla if you can, or make your own (see page 38). Buy a ruby-glinting jar of bottled, sourish cherries and some flaked or slithered almonds, to go with it and make a glossily dark chocolate sauce, the recipe for which I've given above (see page 245).

SERIOUS SATURDAY LUNCH FOR 8 – NO HOSTAGES

Choucroute garnie

Quince syllabub

In our enthusiasm for all things Mediterranean, some more northerly specialities have got lost. I love Scandinavian food, perhaps because I spent a lot of time in Norway as a child (taken by an adored au pair, Sissel), but I love too those robust, spicily sour Germanic constructs: Pflaumenpfannekuchen, great solid pancakes bolstered with plums and weighed down with a thick layer of granulated sugar; plum tart made with shiny dark Quetschen, sliced, and cooked till a reddy, coppery cinnamon on thick banks of Hefeteig; a long-soused Sauerbraten; stuffed cabbage; Wurst mit Senf; and – we're getting there – an astringent, tangled heap of sauerkraut with boiled potatoes, juniper berries, frankfurters, the works. The choucroute garnie of the title makes this sound Alsatian rather than uncompromisingly German. But, whatever, we're talking about the same, hangover-salving thing.

CHOUCROUTE GARNIE

1 bouquet garni made of 1 bay leaf, 8 juniper berries, 2 cloves, 3 sprigs thyme
150g goose fat
2 medium onions, finely sliced
3 smoked gammon knuckles
3 carrots, peeled and halved
1.4kg sauerkraut
750ml dry Riesling
8 Toulouse sausages or bratwurst
8 frankfurters

First cobble together your bouquet garni. This is not as fiddly as it sounds, or not the way I make it, which is by stuffing the bay leaf, juniper berries, cloves and sprigs of thyme into a popsock and tying a knot in it.

Melt 100g of the goose fat in a heavy casserole – I use a large cast-iron rectangular one which fits over a couple of hobs – and cook the onion in it over medium heat, uncovered, for about 10 minutes or until soft. Add the smoked gammon knuckles, the carrots and bouquet garni and stir. Then add the sauerkraut, a good grinding of pepper and mix well around so that all is combined and the gammon is blanketed by the sauerkraut.

Pour over the Riesling and bring to the boil. Add the remaining 50g goose fat in teaspoon-sized dollops over the top of the sauerkraut. Put the lid on, turn the heat down to very low and simmer for 2½ hours.

Grill the Toulouse sausages or bratwurst and set aside till needed. When the gammon knuckles are cooked, remove, let cool a little, then carve and slice into chunks (neither delicacy nor finesse are exactly required) getting rid of the bones (or keeping them to flavour soup) and return to the casserole along with the grilled Toulouse sausages or bratwurst, and the frankfurters. You can leave all the sausages whole, or halve or cut them into chunks as you like. If you are going to cut them, you can reduce the amount you get: you just need everyone to be able to take some of each. Either way, put back on the heat, covered, and let simmer for 20 minutes till all's heated through.

You can serve straight from the casserole or decant everything to a vast oval plate. With this, I like plain, that's to say unbuttered, boiled floury potatoes with some juniper berries bashed and sprinkled over on serving.

If I have leftovers, I put everything back in the casserole, stash it in the fridge and reheat it up to 3 days later: a little something for the week.

QUINCE SYLLABUB

You cannot want much of a pudding after this: but the syllabub will seep comfortably into whatever small space is left. Turn to page 126 for the recipe, adjusting quantities as necessary.

If this sounds like too much hard work, then bring out a vast tub of Greek yoghurt, the thick, smooth, satiny kind, a jar of, preferably, Greek honey and some flaked almonds you've toasted in a fatless pan over medium heat.

FINALLY, THE BASIC ALWAYS WELCOME SATURDAY LUNCH FOR 8

Sausages and mash with red wine, cumin and onion gravy

Seville orange curd tart, or lemon cream with shortbread

Sausages and mash have to be the most gratefully received lunch ever. For the mash, work on 200g potato per person adding lots of butter, lots of cream, lots of pepper; as for the sausages, I exhort you not to be seduced by interesting-sounding combinations. I always regret falling for the wild boar and ginger, the venison and mint sausages: sausages should be just sausages. I do, though, buy my butcher's Cumberland sausages, now that he makes individual ones, not just the yard-long spiralled link. A reliable choice is something that goes by the name of breakfast sausage, English pork sausage or farmhouse sausage. In the supermarket, look for Porkinson's.

I always cook my sausages in the oven, set at gas mark 6/200°C. Use a roasting tin with a little bit of dripping and prick the sausages before cheerfully shunting them into the oven and forgetting about them. Turn them over after 20 minutes. They should be done after 40.

With the sausages and mash, though, an onion gravy makes all the difference: I make mine spicy and wine-dark here, rather than the more traditional one that accompanies my roast beef (see page 280). If you've got some meat stock on hand, do use it, but I have no qualms about bringing out one of my Italian Knorr cubes in *gusto classico*.

For pudding I give the recipe for lemon cream as well as the Seville orange tart in part to make this do-able whatever the season, but also because it's incredibly easy and incredibly delicious.

RED WINE, CUMIN AND ONION GRAVY

30g beef dripping, or oil
225g onions
1 teaspoon ground cumin
scant tablespoon sugar
2 scant tablespoons flour
500ml meat stock
150ml red wine

Peel the onions and slice them, very, very thinly: I use the food processor for this. Melt the dripping in a thick-bottomed, fairly wide saucepan and add the onions. Turn down the heat to low and cook the onions for about 10 minutes until soft, stirring occasionally to push them around the pot and make sure they're not burning. Stir in the ground cumin and cook for another 5 or so minutes. Turn the heat up and add the sugar: let the onions caramelise slightly by stirring over a medium-high flame for 3 minutes and then, still stirring, add the flour. Stir over the heat for 2 more minutes and then add the stock and wine and keep stirring – or stir now and again but with some concentration – while the gravy comes to the boil. When it does so, turn down and simmer very gently for 30 minutes, stirring occasionally.

You can make this in advance and reheat later; you might need to add some water when you do.

SEVILLE ORANGE CURD TART

I ate this at Alastair Little's Lancaster Road restaurant, just after it opened, one February when the Seville oranges were in the shops, and couldn't believe how transcendentally good it was. The recipe is from Francesca Melman, who was the sous-chef there and, at time of writing, is chef at Tom Conran's pub-restaurant, The Cow, in Westbourne Grove. She describes it as a mixture of Adam Robinson's Seville orange curd from the Brackenbury (served, I think, with shortbread, and you could do the same here, forgoing the pastry case, but then to have enough you'd have to double quantities) and the lemon tart from the River Café. I have introduced some muscovado sugar, which gives off a pleasurable hint of toffee-ish marmalade. I sometimes make a sweet pastry, sometimes a plain shortcrust case for this. The sweet pastry is more delicate somehow, but there really is something to be said for using a plain, unfancy, non-sweet pastry the better to set off the deeply toned curd.

Pastry case, baked blind and cooked through, in a shallow 23cm or deep 20cm flan ring – whichever pastry you want and **see pages 41 and 42** **for recipes – which calls for 120g flour**
3 whole eggs
2 egg yolks
100g caster sugar
75g muscovado sugar
zest and juice of 4 Seville oranges
150g unsalted butter, cut into 1cm cubes

In a thick-bottomed saucepan whisk together the eggs and sugar until amalgamated. Make sure to stir in and scrape up the sugar at the edges or it will burn when it's on the hob. Add juice and zest of oranges and the cubes of butter. Put the saucepan over medium heat and cook, stirring constantly. Again, take care to stir edges as well as middle, otherwise it will catch. The mixture will thicken and then boil. Let it bubble for no more than a minute, then remove from heat and pour directly into the cooled, baked tart shell.

If you're not making a tart, but serving the curd to be eaten with shortbread, then pour into individual glasses when it is cool enough not to splinter the glass. There is a recipe for shortbread below. Or buy really good plain chocolate biscuits of a delicate nature.

LEMON CREAM

I made this by accident when I had some mixture left over from a tarte au citron which I poured into ramekins and baked (in a bain-marie) along with the tart. I loved the lemon cream, and it's easier than pastry and less commonplace than tarte au citron.

It really does make a difference to the intense, satiny lemoniness if you leave it to steep in the fridge for 2 or 3 days before baking it. You could always use Seville oranges, too, in place of the lemons.

3 juicy lemons, preferably unwaxed
275g caster sugar
6 eggs
300ml double cream

Grate the lemon zest into a bowl. Add the lemon juice, sugar and eggs and whisk until well incorporated. Then combine the cream with the lemon mixture and pour into a jug. Cover with clingfilm and refrigerate it until required, but preferably for at least 2 days.

When ready to bake, preheat the oven to gas mark 2/150°C. Boil a kettle. Put 8 ramekins of 150ml capacity into a roasting tin and pour in the lemon cream mixture. Pour hot, not boiling, water into the roasting dish to come about halfway up the ramekins and bake for about 20–30 minutes. They should be just set but still with some wobble:

they will set more as they cool, but there should always be a slight and desirable runniness about them. Remove and cool. If you're eating them soon, don't put them in the fridge and if you're making them in advance and therefore need to refrigerate them, make sure you take them out to get them to room temperature for a good hour before eating.

SHORTBREAD

You do need biscuits with the lemon cream: make these. There is no one way of going about shortbread: ask any Scot; this version is buttery and short, but with a certain gritty density. I find the way of shaping then baking the biscuits as specified below the easiest way to go about it, but you can press into a traditional mould, or push into a swiss-roll tin and segment when fresh out of the oven if you prefer a more orthodox approach. Obviously, too, you can make these by hand if you don't like or don't have the machine.

100g butter, very soft
50g icing sugar
100g plain flour, preferably Italian 00
50g cornflour

Cream the butter and sugar in the food processor; you may need to stop and push down the buttery bits if the mixture's not combining properly. Add the flours and a pinch of salt, and process to combine again; again, you may need to push the mixture down if it goes up the sides of the bowl.

Remove and knead into a cylinder shape. Cover with clingfilm and chill in the fridge. (At the same time, preheat the oven to gas mark 3/160°C.) After about 20 minutes, when this buttery cylinder feels hard to the touch, slice into half-centimetre-thick disks – or thinner if you want and can – put onto a greased or lined baking tray, dredge with caster sugar if you want a sweet, crunchy edge, and bake for 20–30 minutes. Remember, like all biscuits, they'll crisp up when they're cold; just check the top's dry and that the base is no longer doughy at all.

Remove with a spatula and cool on a wire rack.

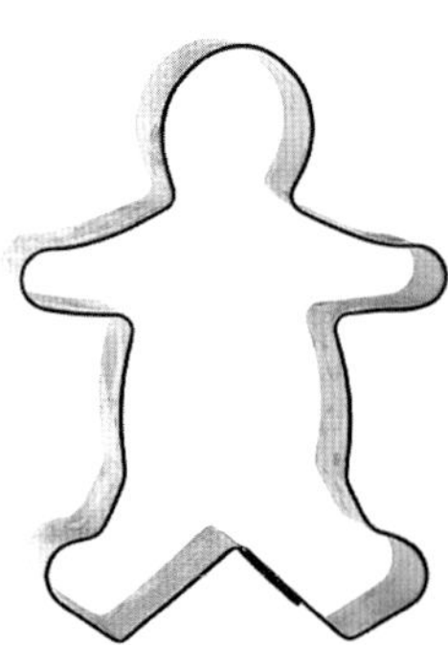

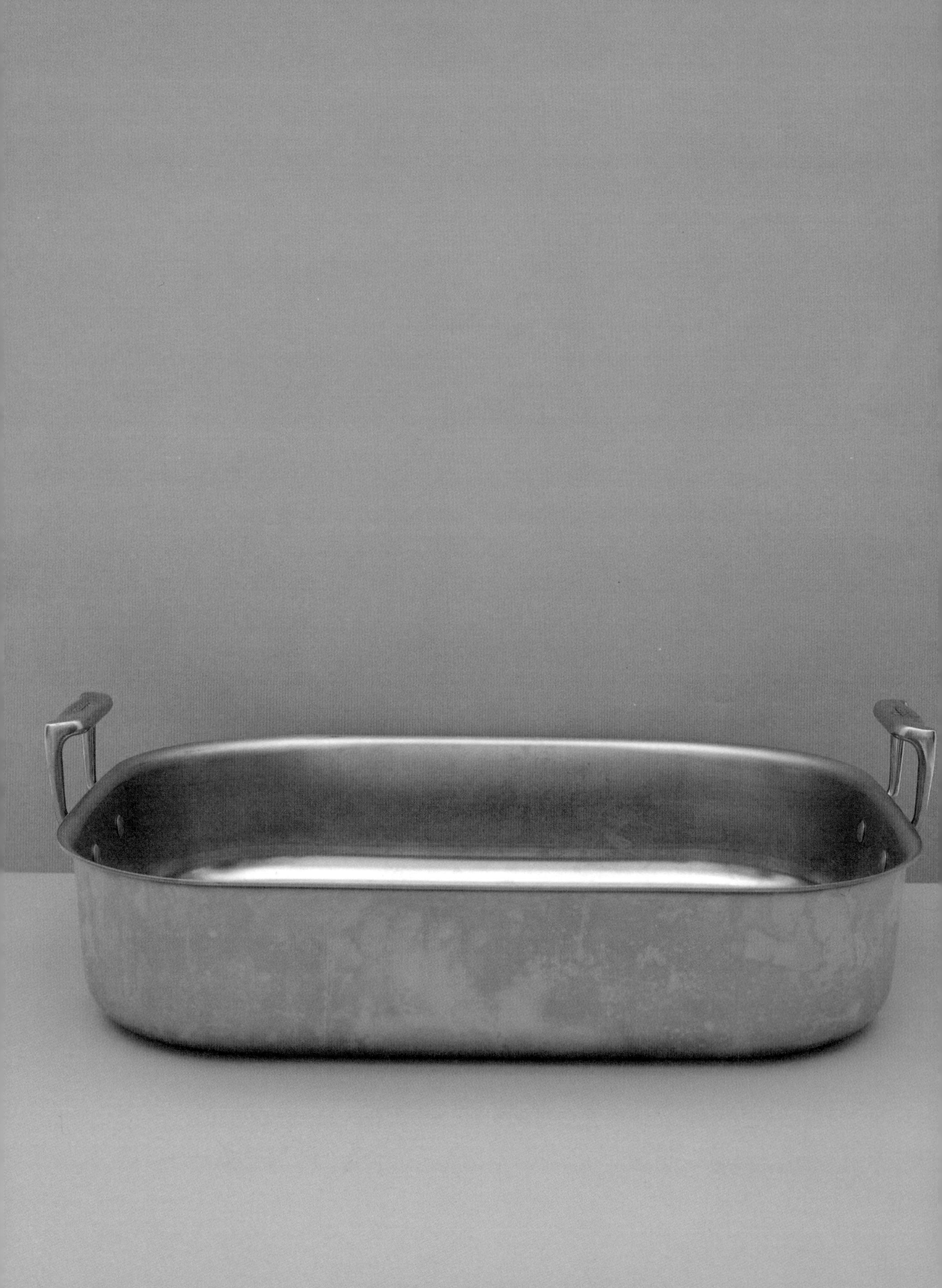

SUNDAY LUNCH

Proper Sunday lunch is everything contemporary cooking is not. Meat-heavy, hostile to innovation, resolutely formalised, it is as much ritual as meal, and an almost extinct ritual at that. Contemporary trends, it is true, have hastened a reappraisal of traditional cooking. But neither nostalgia for nursery foods nor an interest in ponderous culinary Victoriana is what Sunday lunch – Sunday dinner – is all about. It doesn't change, is impervious to considerations of health or fashion; it is about solidity, the family, the home.

One of the silent, inner promises I made myself on having children was to provide a home that made a reassuring, all-comers-welcome tradition of Sunday lunch. It hasn't materialised quite yet, but few of my generation lead meat-and-two-veg lives any more. We are generally more mobile, the weekend is no longer home-bound. Nor do we want to be kitchen-bound (and those with small children hardly have the time on their hands for involved cooking). The fact is that Sunday lunch is impossible to pull off without putting in at least a couple of hours by the sink and the stove. And it is far from being the sort of cooking anyway that finds favour now: the relaxed, let's throw this with that and come up with something simple and picturesquely rustic approach will not put a joint, Yorkshire pudding and roast potatoes on the table. To cook a decent Sunday lunch needs discipline and strict timekeeping.

But with modest organisation, there can be something strangely reassuring about cooking a traditional meal. It is about choreography, about timetabling, and has its own pleasures. We are so accustomed to being invited to consider cooking an art that we forget just how rewarding and satisfying it is as pure craft. My Latin teacher, Miss Plummer, who had the misfortune to teach at one of the less academic schools I frequented, used, with a sort of elegiac condescension, to remark that none of us could know the simple yet substantial pleasures of the carpenter in making a chair. But cooking does give that pleasure, and there are particular satisfactions peculiar to the making of Sunday lunch.

I love the solidity of it all: I don't mean by that the robust nature of the food alone, so much as the weighty texture of hospitality, of plain food warmly given. But it would be wrong to dwell too much on some notional and universally shared longing for a family group assembled around a big table, sharing food. There is that, maybe, but I think people tend to be frightened of cooking Sunday lunch themselves because of a fear or dread that is, frankly, family-induced. The still-remembered tensions of Sunday lunches of the past must be the underlying deterrent, rather than the cooking itself, in the present.

But it is possible to have a family lunch which dispenses, in any literal sense, with family (not that this is necessarily desirable). In the past, connections were familial; the boundaries were of blood. Today, people get their sense of extended family from their friends. I tend to find myself surrounded by people with small children. Others are differently bound.

Now there is no reason on earth why you should feel it incumbent on yourself to get into a frenzy of batter-making and parsnip-peeling just because it is Sunday. And it's true that I might well have people over for Sunday lunch and give them pasta. The rule – if rule there can ever be – is the same rule that applies in any form of cooking: be honest; cook what you want to eat, not what you want to be seen eating.

Of course, what you eat for Sunday lunch doesn't have to confine itself just to the pages of this section: it is simply that in writing this I have been thinking of the food I like eating and cooking for Sunday lunch. Equally, many of these recipes, these ideas, fit just as easily at other times.

Whenever I cook for people I find it easier to have scribbled down in front of me the times at which I'm meant to do any key thing – put things in the oven, take them out – just because once I start talking or drinking I tend to lose track. I haven't suggested this alongside the dinner party menus or elsewhere because I can't know what time you'll be eating and anyway have tried not to be too bossy. With full-on Sunday lunch, I have no such compunction. It has to be planned as efficiently as a military campaign.

Traditional Sunday lunch does, of course, mean beef. So this is the place to bring up BSE. I suggest clearing it first with those you're thinking of inviting. I don't mean asking permission, but merely airing the suggestion. There's no point going to all this expense if everyone's going to turn their noses up at it. It is essential to get good beef from a butcher you trust. I go to Mr Lidgate in west London and I know that the beef I get from him comes from organic and suckler herds (in other words, the calves have been suckled by their mothers and remain in the herd throughout their lives, so that there is complete traceability) and have never been fed any animal proteins. No BSE has ever been found in animals born and reared in organic herds. And, apart from anything else, no good butcher would give you beef from a dairy herd: you shouldn't be eating cow in the first place.

As for cuts: it helps here as well to go to a butcher rather than the supermarket. You can explain what you want, or ask what you think you should want, for how many people, how you want to carve it and so on. Rib of beef gives the best flavour, but it is very difficult to carve and it is, at time of writing, illegal to sell it. But I am, anyway, a hopeless carver and believe that in cooking especially, though in everything really, it is better to play to your strengths than your weaknesses. Besides, if you can't do much more than hack at it, it's a waste. I am resigned to buying a boned joint. I have recently become very extravagant and gone for contrefilet; a boned sirloin would be good, too, though.

I have always found gravy problematic, but for beef I don't think you can casually deglaze the roasting dish with some red wine and hope it'll be all right. Nor does that mean the opposite extreme: the thick, floury, school gloop. Banish instant gravy powders and granules from your thoughts and your store cupboards. Instead, start caramelising your onions early, and cook them slowly. This may be difficult when you're trying to orchestrate everything else for lunch, but you can easily do the gravy the day before and then just reheat and add meat juices at the last minute.

Roast potatoes are another fraught area. I have, in the past, got frantic with despair as the time for the meat to be ready drew closer and the potatoes were still blond and untroubled in their roasting pan. The key here is to get the fat hotter than you would believe necessary before you start and to continue to cook the potatoes at a higher heat and for longer than you might believe possible. And you must roughen them up after parboiling.

The heat of the fat is again the crucial element in making a Yorkshire pudding rise. There's no doubt this is easier if you have two ovens (one for the beef, one for the Yorkshire pudding), but the beef can either be cooked at a very high temperature for a quick blast and then at a moderate one for a while or at a highish one all the time. You can always blast the Yorkshire pudding on a high heat while the beef is resting on its carving board.

Roast root vegetables are traditional, but I tend not to bother. With the roast potatoes and Yorkshire pudding, you hardly need more starch, though if I'm cooking roast pork, or roast beef without the Yorkshire pudding, or the usual roast chicken, I might do parsnips, either roasted alongside the potatoes, or in another pan anointed with honey and put in the oven to grow sweet and burnished.

As for other vegetables, I think you need two sorts. This can make life difficult, but not insurmountably so. It's just a matter, again, of time management: the important thing is not suddenly to need about 6 pans on a 4-hob stove. And there doesn't need to be too much chopping. Choose, for example, frozen peas and something to provide fresh, green crunch: beans, Savoy cabbage, pak choi. I love broccoli, but it is very sweet, and with the peas you don't really need any more sweetness. It's unconventional, but I do rather like a tomato salad somewhere too, especially if it's still warm outside.

I don't often make my own horseradish sauce (though see page 294 for a recipe) – I buy a good bottled one and add a bit of crème fraîche, ordinary cream or Greek yoghurt – but mustard must, for me, be English and made up at the last minute. I don't mind having other mustards on the table, but for me the whole meal is ruined without proper English mustard.

Traditionalists will insist on a sturdy pie or crumble for pudding, but really, after all that carbohydrate, have you got room? I am immensely greedy, but I don't like that invasive and uncomfortable feeling of bloatedness that can make you regret eating much more than a hangover can ever make you regret drinking.

Now that you seem to be able to get blueberries all the year round, I often serve them with a large, shallow bowl of Barbados cream. This – yoghurt and double cream stirred together, fudgy brown sugar sprinkled on top – has the advantage of having to be done the day before (see page 131). I love lemon ice-cream after this (and it's good with blueberries, or indeed any berries, too) and I sometimes make one that doesn't need fiddling about with while freezing – you just bung it in the freezer (see page 282). Nothing is quite as good as proper ice-cream, made with a custard base and then churned until solid, but home cooking is based on compromises, and a simple pudding is a compromise I am often grateful to make. You could consider a crumble (see page 45 for a recipe and adjust quantities as necessary) if only because the crumble mixture can be made up earlier and just sprinkled on the fruit as you sit down and cooked while you eat the beef. Remember: you are not trying to produce the definitive Sunday lunch to end all Sunday lunches. Nor are you a performance artist. The idea is to make a lunch which you want to eat and can imagine sitting down to do so without bursting into tears.

TIMETABLE

I'm sorry to sound bossy, but Sunday lunch, as I've said, has to be run like a military campaign. I find it easier to decide when I want to eat and then work backwards, writing every move down on a pad which I keep in a fixed place in the kitchen. This timetable is engineered towards having lunch ready to eat at 2pm exactly. I take it for granted that pudding's been made already.

All quantities and timings have in mind a lunch for about 6 adults and perhaps some children and are based on having a 2¼kg joint to cook.

11.20	Start gravy
11.30	Take beef out of fridge
11.50	Peel potatoes
12.05	Put the potatoes in their water in the pan, bring to the boil and parboil. Preheat oven to gas mark 7/210°C
12.15	Put roasting pan in oven with a knob of dripping for beef
12.20	Put beef in
12.35	Prepare any veg that need chopping or cleaning, etc.
12.40	Put pan with dripping for potatoes in oven
12.50	Make Yorkshire pudding
1.00	Put potatoes in
1.05	Prepare veg. Turn on plate warmer or hot cupboard
1.25	Put veg water on
1.35	Put pan with dripping for Yorkshire pudding in oven
1.40	Take out beef and put in Yorkshire pudding, turning oven up to gas mark 8/230°C as you do so. Let beef stand
1.45	Cook vegetables
2.00	Take out Yorkshire pudding and potatoes

THE ROAST BEEF

I think many people underplay how much meat you need. For 6 people, I wouldn't consider getting under 2¼kg (or 5lb), which, in other words, is about 375g per person. A joint is a sad prospect without the possibility of leftovers. For a rib you should add on about 1kg extra here.

For rare meat you can either cook the beef at the highest possible temperature for 15 minutes and then turn it down to gas mark 4/180°C and cook for 15 minutes per lb (I still find it easier to calculate the cooking time per lb) or at gas mark 7/210°C throughout for 15 minutes per lb, which is what I did here. Think of 15 minutes per lb as about 33 minutes per kg. I usually do 15 minutes per lb and then add on an extra 5 minutes so that those who don't like rare meat have a bit of slightly more cooked beef from the ends. Those who don't like blood don't have to get it: the rest of us gratifyingly do.

All I do to the beef is to massage it with dry mustard powder after I've taken it out of the fridge. I use a knob of dripping for the pan, but you could use whatever fat you have to hand.

THE GRAVY

Gravy is one of my weaknesses, which is to say I find it hard to make a convincing light and thin juice. To overcome my deficiencies I took to following Jane Grigson's recipe for onion gravy (indeed most of my Sunday is Grigson-based), adding a drop of Marsala to it. You don't need to – you could use some Madeira or even some sweet sherry or just add a little bit more sugar – but the Marsala brings a wonderful aromatic muskiness to the gravy. If I don't have any real beef stock, I use a tub of Joubère beef stock (see page 506). You can use a stock cube (try an Italian one), in which case use it well diluted and taste before putting in any more salt.

You can start the gravy the day before if you want, just reheating and adding meat juices at the last minute.

15g butter or dripping, and a dribble of oil
1 onion, sliced very thinly in the food processor
pinch brown sugar
1 teaspoon flour
300ml beef stock
2 tablespoons Marsala

Melt the butter (with the oil to stop it burning) or dripping in a saucepan and cook the onion in it at a very low temperature, stirring often. When the onion is soft add the sugar and Marsala and let it caramelise. Cover with foil, putting the foil as near to the bottom of the pan as possible and continue to cook, still on a very low flame, for about 10 minutes. Then stir in the flour and cook, stirring, for about 2 minutes. Stir in the stock, bring to the boil (you can turn the heat up here) then reduce the heat to very low again and simmer gently for about 20 minutes. Purée in the food processor (or you can strain it, pushing the soft onion through the sieve). Pour back into the saucepan. At the last minute, reheat and add meat juices from roasting pan. This gravy is wonderfully stress-free, since you don't have to be doing furious deglazing at the last minute.

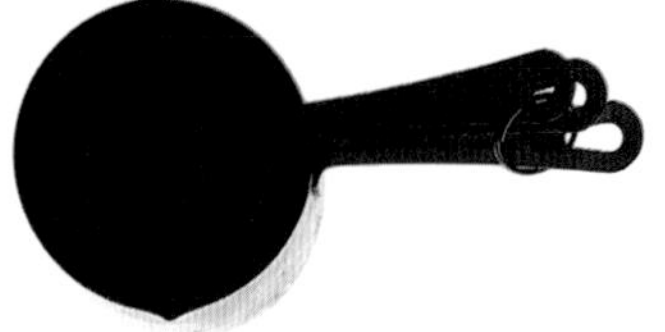

THE ROAST POTATOES

I like roast potatoes fairly small, so I cut a medium-to-large one into about 3. For 6 people, I suppose, that's about 1¾kg. Well, that may be over-generous, but nothing is worse than too few.

Peel the potatoes and cut them into large chunks. Put them in cold salted water, bring to the boil and parboil for 4–5 minutes. Drain, put back in the saucepan, put on the lid and bang the whole thing about a bit so that the edges of the potatoes get blurred: the rough edges help them catch in the fat and so get crisp. Add 1 tablespoon or so of semolina and give the pan, with its lid on, another good shake. The semolina gives the potatoes a divinely sweet edge: not at all cloying or inappropriate, just an intensified caughtness, as it were. When my mother and aunts were young, they had an Italian au pair, Antonia, who, when required to make a British Sunday lunch (having never cooked anything other than Italian food), adopted, or rather invented, this practice. If you're unconvinced, or don't have any semolina to hand, just use flour and shake the warm potatoes around in it. The flour doesn't give the same honey-toned depth as semolina, but helps the potatoes catch and brown wonderfully.

It's essential that the fat's hot before the potatoes go in. I use 2 tablespoon-sized lumps of goose fat or some truly superb grass-fed beef dripping. If you can lay your hands on neither, of course you can use oil or even vegetable fat. The potatoes must not be taken out of the oven until you are absolutely ready to eat them. They will take approximately an hour to cook.

THE YORKSHIRE PUDDING

I always use Jane Grigson's *English Food* for the Chinese Yorkshire pudding recipe, which is not as odd as it sounds. The story is that when a big competition was held in Leeds for the best Yorkshire pudding, the winner was a Chinese cook called Tin Sung Yang. For years it was held to have a mystery ingredient – tai luk sauce – until, Jane Grigson reports, a niece of hers found that this was a Chinese joke. Nevertheless, the recipe is different from normal: it works backwards. That's to say, you mix the eggs and milk and then stir in the flour, rather than making a well in the flour and adding the eggs and milk: and it works triumphantly; it billows up into a gloriously copper crown of a cushion. I am able to cook this for the most die-hard, pudding-proud northerners without inhibition or anxiety. I prefer Yorkshire pudding to be in one dish rather than in those depressing, canteen-style individual portions, so for this amount, I use an enamel dish about 30cm by 19cm and 7cm deep. Cook it on the top shelf of the oven but make sure the shelf isn't too high up as the Yorkshire pudding really does rise. I have had to prise it off the ceiling of the oven, which slightly dented its magnificence and my glory.

300ml milk
4 eggs
250g plain flour, sifted

Mix all the ingredients, except the flour, with pepper and a scant ½ teaspoon of salt, beating them well together. I use my free-standing mixer, the fabulous American KitchenAid, but anything – hand-held electric mixer, rotary or balloon whisk – would do. Let these ingredients stand for 15 minutes and then whisk in the flour. Meanwhile put the pan with 1 tablespoon or so of dripping or whatever other fat you're using in a very high oven. Into this intensely hot pan you should pour the batter, when you're ready for it, and cook for 20 minutes. Bring it, triumphant, to the table.

THE PUDDING

The recipe for Barbados cream is on page 131.

Recipes for crumble are on pages 45 and 174; custard to go with is on page 36.

LEMON ICE-CREAM

Years ago, when I bought my enormously expensive ice-cream maker, a friend of mine brought round her copy of Shona Crawford Poole's *Iced Delights* for me to play with. Naturally, the recipe I fell upon was one that didn't need an ice-cream maker. I include it here out of fondness – my sister Thomasina loved it and often made it herself.

It's very quick and easy to make. Even though I have doubts about non-custard-based ices (they freeze very hard and then melt back into a runny creaminess so you have to be very careful about ripening them in the fridge for a good 40 minutes before eating them, rather than letting them thaw in the kitchen, and thus start dripping), it's worth having this one under your belt as it is good by itself and wonderful as an accompaniment to a tarte au citron (bought or made, but especially useful to zhuzz up a bought one), rhubarb pie, a plate of stewed rhubarb, wine-candied quinces (page 366) or any assortment of berries.

3 juicy lemons, preferably unwaxed

170g icing sugar

420ml double cream

Grate the zest from 2 of the lemons. Squeeze the juice of all 3 and pour into a bowl with the zest and sugar, stir to combine and leave for 30 minutes, if you can, to let the flavour deepen.

Whip the cream with 3 tablespoons iced water until it holds soft peaks, then whisk in the sweetened lemon juice. Turn into a shallow container, cover and freeze – no stirring, crystal-breaking-up, mixing or anything needed – until firm. Bear in mind my comments about thawing and melting, above, when you want to eat it.

LEMON MERINGUE ICE-CREAM

This is an ice-cream along much the same lines. I saw this recipe of Jane and Elizabeth Pelly's in *The Women Chefs of Great Britain*, though I've changed it slightly here. The original version specified home-made meringues and home-made lemon curd, but I brazened it out with the bought stuff, and suggest, for ease, that you do too. If you are using shop meringues and curd you may have to add more lemon juice and zest or it will be too sweet. Taste to see: it needs an edge to it.

600ml whipping cream

225g Greek yoghurt

320g lemon curd

juice and zest of 2 lemons

6 meringue nests (see above)

Whip the cream until fairly stiff and fold in the yoghurt. Add the lemon curd, lemon juice and zest (you will find it easier to stir in the curd if you add the lemon juice to it first) and the meringues, broken up into small pieces, but not so small that they'll dissolve into dust.

Put into a container – it should really be a shallow rather than tall one – and freeze. And that's all there is to it. Ripen in the fridge for 40 minutes before you want to eat it. You could dribble over it either some clear honey or some more lemon curd diluted to runniness with lemon juice.

A SUMMER LEMON MERINGUE PIE

A propos of this, one year I made a summer version of lemon meringue pie, or maybe it would be better to describe it as a cross between lemon meringue pie and pavlova: make a pavlova base – see page 373 – smear it with some thickly whipped double cream, as if one were spreading some butter on bread, then thickly cover that with lemon curd, then even more thickly with more whipped double cream and then dot with some raspberries.

LATE-SUMMER ROAST BEEF AND YORKSHIRE PUDDING FOR 8

Cold roast fillet of beef

Rosemary and anchovy mayonnaise

Warm cannellini or borlotti beans with garlic and sage

Tomato salad

Yorkshire pudding with syrup and cream

This, I think, is one of my favourite Sunday lunches, and you can get away with it at any time the sun is warm enough to make a cold roast fillet of beef seem a treat. It's certainly too expensive to produce if you believe people will think cold food a disappointment or an easy option.

Most of this lunch can be made in advance: you can cook the beef the day before, and boil some beans in readiness for a quick sousing in sage and olive oil just before you eat. Make the mayonnaise on Sunday morning and all that will need doing around lunchtime is a tomato salad or green salad to go with it. I don't think you need potatoes. You do, you see, have Yorkshire pudding coming too, not with the beef but after, as pudding, served searingly hot with golden syrup poured over and thick whipped or, even better, clotted cream with. This is heaven. When I was young there was, tucked behind Fulham Road, a restaurant called the Hungry Horse where it was considered frightfully fashionable to go for Sunday lunch. One of the highpoints of its menu was Yorkshire pudding for every course.

COLD ROAST FILLET OF BEEF

I think people tend not to eat as much fillet as other cuts of beef, but I would still make a more generous allocation than the normal reckoning of 200g per person: so instead of getting a 1¾kg or 4lb fillet I'd get one large fillet of 2¼kg or 5lb. In fact, I'd probably take fright at the idea of skimpy portions once I was in the butcher's and then nervously settle on the heavier weight. Anyway, who's going to complain about leftover fillet sliced into cool thick slabs, smeared with mustard and eaten with warm pebbly new potatoes and alligator-skinned cornichons or an astringent salsa verde (see page 200) or with thickly sliced boiled potatoes (in this instance the floury maincrop sort) fried till crisp and blistered without, steamed creamily sweet within.

I would give it 10 minutes per 500g plus 10 minutes, in a pretty hot but not searing oven (gas mark 7/210°C). Remember that the beef will carry on cooking as it cools, and you do want it rare (or I do; adapt to please yourself). You really don't need to do much to the beef. Just anoint it with some oil. And I would use oil, not dripping or goose fat, since you're going to eat it cold. I have some olive oil which has been infused with bay and rosemary and this is what I'd use here. Normal olive oil, with no other seasoning, will be fine enough though, or you could make your own rosemary oil, see below. I sometimes add some mashed anchovies to the herbed or herbless oil, which I then apply as the meat-massaging unguent. The meat tastes good, too, simply wiped down with mustard to which you've added 2 teaspoons of oil.

So: you anoint the fillet, roast it, let it cool, wrap it in tinfoil and put it in the fridge. What you absolutely must remember to do is take it out of the fridge a good 2 hours before lunch. Yes, it should be cold, but it should not have the merest smack of the refrigerator's chill about it. Alternatively, you could cook the fillet early on Sunday morning and let it cool in the kitchen to room temperature, even slightly above, so that you eat it not cold but not hot either. Always a pleasurable possibility.

If you think the fillet looks too spooky or too brown as it sits ready to be sliced, then do sprinkle with freshly chopped parsley or chives, not too many, just enough to lift it, or just carve it in readiness. You should, too, sprinkle with salt, unless of course you've mashed anchovies into it before roasting.

ROSEMARY AND ANCHOVY MAYONNAISE

Anchovy really does give something to meat (though this mayonnaise is also wonderful with crabcakes or indeed any fishcakes).

You can use bought rosemary-infused oil, or make your own, or leave the rosemary out and let the anchovies speak eloquently for themselves.

9 anchovy fillets in olive oil, drained and finely chopped
1/2 clove garlic, peeled and minced
3 egg yolks
approx. 325ml groundnut or sunflower oil
few squeezes lemon juice
approx. 75ml or 8 scant tablespoons rosemary oil or olive oil infused with rosemary, see below

Mash the anchovies and garlic to form a paste and then whisk together with the egg yolks in a large bowl. The egg yolks should be at room temperature. You can use an electric hand-held mixer (or indeed a free-standing one) but what you can't use, and I'm sorry to be a bore about this, is the food processor. Drip by slow drop, pour in the sunflower or groundnut oil, whisking all the while. The mayonnaise should slowly emulsify. Squeeze in some lemon, going carefully. Don't worry if it still doesn't taste lemony enough now. Keep whisking and now add the rosemary oil, still pouring slowly. Taste and add freshly ground pepper, some salt – if, after the anchovies, you need it – and more lemon juice as wished. Cover with clingfilm.

It's best not to keep mayonnaise in the fridge, but rather in a cool place. If the mayonnaise develops a greasy, glassy top (this tends to happen when it's refrigerated) just skim this off with a spoon before serving.

ROSEMARY-INFUSED OIL

Put about 12 tablespoons olive oil in a saucepan and add 3 tablespoons of rosemary needles. Put on the heat and shake about while warm and then let sizzle for a very short while, about 10 seconds. Pour through the finest mesh sieve. Don't use the rosemary-infused oil in the mayonnaise until it has cooled, though it's fine to massage a few warm tablespoons of it into the meat before roasting. This should give you enough for both.

WARM CANNELLINI OR BORLOTTI BEANS WITH GARLIC AND SAGE

It really doesn't matter whether you use cannellini or borlotti beans here. I tend, more often, to use cannellini, just out of habit I think, but adore the soft pink speckledimess of borlotti, too. I suppose it's just that I associate them more with soups. No matter: choose which you prefer.

500g cannellini or borlotti beans
1 large onion, peeled and halved
1 carrot, peeled and halved
3 sage leaves
7–8 tablespoons olive oil
4 cloves of garlic, minced
4 sage leaves, chopped finely
parsley

Soak the beans overnight in cold water. Drain them, and put them in a thick-bottomed large saucepan along with the onion, carrot and the 3 sage leaves. Cover by about 15cm with cold water, bring to the boil and simmer for 1–1½ hours or until done. How long it actually takes depends on the age of the beans, but start tasting after 50 minutes and keep a beady eye on them as you don't want them to melt into fudgy rubble. When they are tender, drain them (reserving some cooking liquid for later). Stir in 3 tablespoons olive oil and some salt. When they are cool remove the bits of onion and so on. Cover the beans and leave in a cool place or refrigerate.

When you want to eat them, get a heavy-bottomed or, even better, terracotta, dish and pour in the rest of the olive oil. Add the garlic and the very finely chopped sage leaves (no more than 4: you want a vague scent, not – on top of the rosemary on the meat and in the mayonnaise – a herbal conflict), then sprinkle over some salt and cook at a gently sizzling heat, stirring all the while to stop the garlic catching. You don't want it to brown, just soften. Stir in the beans, add some of the reserved cooking liquid and warm through. Pour over some more olive oil and serve, sprinkling with chopped parsley if you like (I always do).

TOMATO SALAD

There is no recipe to follow here: no one needs to be told how to slice tomatoes. But there is an injunction: leave them plain. You can peel them if you are up to it, but it doesn't matter if you don't. Get the best tomatoes you can and make sure they aren't cold before you start (they should never be kept in the fridge, anyway). Slice thinly, arrange on a plate, sprinkle with salt, pepper, sugar if you think they really need it (but even so, just a pinch), some finely chopped spring onions, a drop or two of balsamic or else good red wine vinegar and a drizzle of glass-green olive oil. Small cherry tomatoes should be halved or quartered and tossed with the other ingredients in a shallow bowl.

YORKSHIRE PUDDING WITH SYRUP AND CREAM

Follow precisely the instructions for Yorkshire pudding, above (see page 281), only instead of using dripping, use vegetable oil or shortening.

While the Yorkshire pudding is cooking, pour some golden syrup into one jug and some thick double cream in another or, if you're using clotted cream, just put it in a bowl. The best vanilla ice-cream you can find – which if you're lucky will be Rocombe Farm's – would also be heavenly with the blisteringly hot batter and gooey golden syrup.

Fillet of beef is also useful when you want to make a special Sunday lunch for just a few people. Instead of fillet, you could also buy topside, though you must ask for the corner cut.

THE PERFECT PLAIN SUNDAY LUNCH FOR 3

Corner-cut topside of beef

New potatoes with truffle oil

Peas and mangetouts, or dark leaf salad

Rice pudding

For three, I would buy a joint weighing about 1¼kg or even 1½kg. I love it cold the next day, cut into thick chips and put into a salad, with lettuce, cucumber, sliced gherkin and spring onion, with a mustardy dressing and topped with crumbled, finely chopped hard-boiled egg. And any leftover potatoes can be halved or thickly sliced and profitably thrown in, too.

Preheat the oven to gas mark 7/210°C. While it's heating up, put in the dish in which you're going to roast the beef, then, 5 or so minutes before you want to put the beef in, add a small dollop of dripping or whatever fat you're using. Work out the roasting time for the meat, based on 30 minutes per kg – that's if you like it bloody, see also page xii. Put the meat in the dish and in the oven along with a tomato, cut in half, an onion, ditto, and 2 unpeeled garlic cloves.

When the beef is ready – and taste to see it's how you like it – remove to a carving board or plate and let sit for 10 minutes. Meanwhile, make a thin gravy by putting the roasting dish on the hob, removing tomato, onion and garlic if you can't be bothered to sieve later. Add about 125ml beef stock and the same amount of red wine and let bubble away, adding salt and pepper and maybe a pinch of sugar. Strain into a warmed jug.

NEW POTATOES

The potatoes I choose are those small, buttery, waxy-fleshed, thin-skinned ones, which seem to be available even in darkest winter. New potatoes, unlike maincrop ones, should be put into boiling water, salted and cooked for the 30 minutes or so they need. Drain them and return them to the pan with a fat dollop of unsalted butter. Shake the pan gently so the potatoes are all glossily covered. Grind over some white pepper (though, of course, black pepper wouldn't be a catastrophe) and add a few drops of truffle oil, tiny bottles of which can be bought at delicatessens and supermarkets. You don't need much; if you have too heavy a hand, you will begin to notice a positively farmyard fragrance wafting from the pan. I like these potatoes warm rather than hot, so leave them with the heat turned off but the lid on before decanting them into a warmed bowl.

In winter, I'd make a buttery mixture of peas – good frozen petits pois – and just-cooked mangetouts. In summer, I love a peppery salad with the soft, pink, sweet meat. Any strong dark leaves in more or less any combination, would work: tender spinach, watercress, rocket, mizuna; unchopped, robust flat-leaf parsley. Use oil – stick to olive if you've made the truffle-scented potatoes, or else a nut oil – and lemon juice for the dressing: nothing fancy, but remember to add salt while tossing. I think a salad like this is better on a large flat plate rather than in a normal salad bowl.

RICE PUDDING

Everyone is convinced of the importance of getting a rice pudding absolutely right, but unfortunately no one agrees what that means. Definitely it shouldn't be claggy, though neither should it be watery; the rice shouldn't be too firm, but it shouldn't be mush either. And between those two extremes, there is room for intense disagreement. For me there is indeed such a thing as a too-creamy rice pudding: I like it milk-white and less than Ambrosial; I live with someone who regards an almost butter-yellow, fat-thickened, rice-beaded soup as so much perfection attained. I loathe and detest skin on rice pudding (but rather less than I hate and fear skin on custard): just writing the words makes me shiver; I concede, though, that for most people the skin is almost the best part.

The rice pudding below cannot quite straddle all these oppositions. But, bearing in mind these proportions, you can alter the ingredients, adding cream, single or double, or melted butter, to make it as rich and softly fatty as you like. And if you want to add raisins, do: just don't tell me about it.

45g (3 tablespoons) butter, melted
60g (4 tablespoons) pudding rice
30g (2 tablespoons) vanilla sugar or caster sugar
½ teaspoon pure vanilla extract
500ml full-fat milk
fresh nutmeg

Preheat the oven to gas mark 2/150°C. Use some of the melted butter, about half, to grease an ovenproof dish with a capacity slightly over 1 litre. I like to use an oval cream stoneware dish for this. In this dish put the rice, then the sugar and then pour over the milk and vanilla. Pour the rest of the melted butter on top of this (if you're going to have a skin you may as well have a good skin) and then grate over some nutmeg. Put in the oven and bake for 2½ hours, giving a good stir after the first ½ hour and first hour.

If you angle a wooden spoon in slightly aslant you won't disperse too much of the nutmeg on the top.

It's traditional to eat this with jam, but I prefer golden syrup – with or without a dollop of thick double cream.

The idea of a luncheon party is somehow vulnerably old-fashioned but occasionally you want to invite people to a lunch with a more celebratory feel about it.

LUNCH-PARTY LUNCH FOR 8

Spinach, bacon and raw mushroom salad

Baked sea bass with rosemary

Bakewell tart with fresh raspberries

SPINACH, BACON AND RAW MUSHROOM SALAD

Lazy as I am, I wouldn't consider making this salad if I had to wash, drain and de-stem everything. Instead, I buy spinach in packets. I think I'd get 3 250g packs for this, although a wiser woman might stop at 2, and then 200g or so of those firm but otherwise unexceptional button mushrooms. Wipe them if you must, but otherwise just slice them finely-finely, so that you have masses of wafer-thin mushroom-shaped slices. Get some bacon – about 8 thin rashers of the best (unwatery) streaky – and fry or grill it till ochre-tipped and crisp and then crumble it into the mixture of mushrooms and young spinach leaves. I like a garlicky dressing: peel 2 cloves and fry them gently in about 4 tablespoons good olive oil. Don't let the oil hiss and sizzle and don't let the cloves burn. Take the pan off the heat and leave the oil to cool. Remove the cloves, squeeze some lemon juice into the pan, sprinkle in some salt and grind in some pepper – and that's your dressing.

I sometimes do a version of this salad with whole fried, peeled garlic cloves and/or croûtons, too.

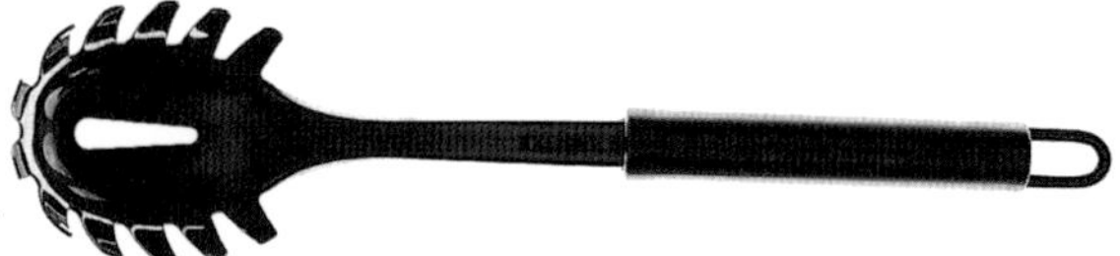

BAKED SEA BASS WITH ROSEMARY

You want food for a lunch party that tastes like a treat, so I suggest here some sea bass. It is expensive, but it is such a wonderful fish and, cooked whole, has inevitably something festive, something important, about it. A sea bass, boned, with fistfuls of rosemary stuffed inside and baked, is easy to cook, looks beautiful and has that perfect simplicity of taste that throws any amount of chi-chi food into a cocked hat. I take it for granted, while talking blithely of how easy it is to do, that you won't be boning it yourself. But, since there's no point buying expensive fish like this unless you can be positive it's the best and freshest possible, you will, anyway, be roping in a fishmonger for this.

The advantage of stuffing a boned, whole fish with herbs (and if you haven't got any rosemary growing in the garden, indeed haven't got a garden, buy a small plant rather than masses of supermarket packets of the stuff) is that although it sounds like more work than just baking fillets, it isn't, because the timing, although still crucial, isn't quite as cut-throat. Also, you can keep the fish waiting in its foil package while you have the first course, whereas single pieces of fish really would be tricky to leave hanging around. And although you can't make this really in advance, you can stuff the fish and wrap in foil a good 1–2 hours before putting it in the oven.

I find it easier to serve 2 smaller rather than 1 larger fish, simply because it can be a tight squeeze fitting a fish over 2kg in my oven. But if you can, do: one enormous bass does look splendid. And if you prefer you can buy small sea bream, using one per person.

2 x 1.3kg sea bass
about 20 10cm sprigs of fresh rosemary
2 tablespoons good, preferably Ligurian, olive oil

Ask your fishmonger to bone the fish entirely for you. Explain that you want the head and tail, but want to serve the fish whole, stuffed, then cut into slices.

Preheat the oven to gas mark 5/190°C.

Oil 2 pieces of foil big enough to wrap each fish in and lay the fish on top. Stuff the cavities with the rosemary, as it is, not chopped or taken off the branches at all, plonk the fish on the foil, dribble some oil over, sprinkle with coarse salt and grind over pepper. Make parcels with the foil, twisting the ends very tightly but keeping the parcels themselves baggy. You can leave in a cool place, or fridge if it's hot, for an hour or so, then put in the oven for 20–25 minutes. Keep in unwrapped foil packages until you've eaten your first course, then remove to 2 oval plates (or one if you can fit them) and serve by slicing with a fish-slice, though you'll have to remove the rosemary to one side first. Spoon over the oily, rosemary-scented juices.

New potatoes, either boiled or roasted, are wonderful with this, as are puy lentils, cooked then tossed in an oil-softened dice of garlic, onion, celery and carrot, and sprinkled with parsley.

BAKEWELL TART WITH FRESH RASPBERRIES

We had bakewell tart, or bakewell pudding, at school: sweet, stodgy, dense and heavy, a rigid disc of pastry smeared with red jam and topped with a sandy paste which itself bore the weight of a hardened pool of greying white icing. It had its charms, but I don't intend to emulate them here. This version is bold with almonds: the traditional frangipane topping is rich with them of course, but here the pastry also has a good couple of tablespoons of them which both lightens the texture and stops it from going soggy. This is important, since this version includes fresh raspberries, which create an altogether less stodgy, more elegant pie, but more seepage. It is fabulous, the sort of pudding people who say 'I don't eat puddings' have second helpings of. Serve with more fresh raspberries and a bowlful of double cream or crème fraîche on the table, alongside.

for the almond pastry

175g flour, preferably 00

30g ground almonds

65g icing sugar

130g butter

1 egg yolk

for the filling

300–350g raspberries

3 tablespoons raspberry jam, optional

3 eggs

125g ground almonds

125g butter, very soft

125g caster sugar

15g flaked almonds

Make the pastry by hand, in the processor or in a free-standing electric mixer as you like. If you're making it by hand, sift the flour, a pinch of salt, the ground almonds and sugar into a mixing bowl. Add the diced butter and cut in the flour mixture using a round-bladed knife or pastry blender or as you do normally. When the butter has been reduced to flakes, use your fingertips to rub it into the flour. And then, when it looks like fine crumbs, stir in the egg yolk to make a soft but not sticky dough. You may need to add a few drops of icy water if some crumbs of pastry remain at the bottom of the bowl. Wrap the disc of dough – as usual – in greaseproof paper or clingfilm or foil and let it rest in the fridge for 15–20 minutes.

After you have rolled out the pastry and used it to line a deep 26cm quiche case, prick it and then put it back in the fridge while you make the filling.

Melt the butter, then put to one side for a moment. Beat the sugar and eggs together and then, still stirring, pour in the melted butter. When all's mixed, stir in the ground almonds. That's all there is to it.

Spread the jam on the base of the flan case, then cover with the raspberries. If you've managed to get really wonderful, sweet and raspberry-tasting raspberries then you can probably do without any jam at all. But I find that the raspberries that are in most shops tend to perform better with about 3 tablespoons of best quality (even sugar-free – that is, additional-sugar-free) jam. Pour the mixture over that and then scatter with the flaked almonds.

Bake in a preheated oven (gas 6/200°C) for 35–45 minutes until the tart looks golden and swollen. Remove and let stand until warm.

ONE MORE BEEF: STEWED, FOR 6

Stewed beef with thyme and anchovies

Fresh horseradish sauce with chives

Baked or mashed potatoes and cornichons

Treacle tart with vanilla ice-cream

Sometimes a stew is just what you want for Sunday lunch. This one is a particularly special one: elegant yet bolstering; and turn to Cooking in Advance, page 112, for the recipe. As suggested there, I like this with baked potatoes and some cornichons, their vinegariness contrasting beautifully with the salty mellowness of the stew.

It may seem odd to suggest giving horseradish sauce with stew, but think of this as a raita, rather. Again, this is about contrasts: the rasp of the horseradish, the cold, sour creaminess of the sauce, provide both foil and balm. And it's heavenly dolloped into the potatoes, too. The recipe for this comes from Arabella Boxer's *Herb Book*: though I have to say when I couldn't get any fromage frais once, I made this with crème fraîche and 0-per-cent-fat Greek yoghurt (well, that's what I had in the fridge), half and half, and it was wonderful, too. If you haven't got oven space for the potatoes, though the treacle tart should leave room, consider mashed instead.

FRESH HORSERADISH SAUCE WITH CHIVES

I don't normally make real horseradish sauce, as I've already confessed, but I give you Arabella Boxer's recipe, which is staggeringly good. Supermarkets have started stocking fresh horseradish root now (and you can stash some in the freezer), but, if you can't find any, use instead bottled grated horseradish that has been preserved in soya bean oil and citric acid; Arabella Boxer warns against the woodiness of the dry-packed grated horseradish.

400ml fromage frais
4 tablespoons grated fresh horseradish
1 teaspoon Dijon mustard
2 teaspoons white wine vinegar
8 tablespoons chopped chives

Beat the fromage frais till smooth, then stir in the freshly grated horseradish, mustard, vinegar and a good pinch of salt. Finally, stir in the chopped chives. Turn into a clean bowl and serve.

TREACLE TART

Treacle tart should be thin and chewily crisp rather than deep and wodgy. It should be warm, too.

Some people will try and persuade you of the superiority for treacle tart of a buttery sweet pastry, the sort the French use for fruit flans and lemon tarts. I am not convinced. I think the intense sweetness of the filling is better served by a plainer crust and that the important thing is to get the pastry as thin as possible. Ordinary shortcrust (see page 41) is really a doddle to make; even I, so undeft as to be embarrassing, can roll it out thinly and drape it silkily over a waiting 20cm flan case. You can use the recipe below, or the one for jam tarts on page 499.

If you don't want to go in for baking, buy a pot of ice-cream and make the butterscotch sauce on page 304.

for the pastry

100g plain flour, preferably Italian 00

25g cold unsalted butter, diced

25g vegetable shortening, diced

few tablespoons iced water

2 tablespoons lemon juice

for the treacle filling

225g golden syrup

60g fresh white breadcrumbs

zest and juice ½ unwaxed lemon minus the 2 tablespoons used for pastry

3 generous tablespoons double cream

Make the pastry according to the instructions on page 41, using the water and lemon juice to bind, and let rest in the fridge. Roll out to line the flan dish and then put back in the fridge for about ½ hour or so. You can do this a day or so ahead. Traditionally a treacle tart is covered by a lattice-work of pastry. I like it plain, but if you want to you can cut out strips from the leftover pastry and make a criss-cross design to cover before putting it in the oven.

Make sure you've made the breadcrumbs in time (see page 24 for method), using 3–4 slices of bread.

Preheat the oven to gas mark 6/200°C and put a baking sheet in to warm up, too.

Put the syrup in a pan on the hob and when warm and runny add breadcrumbs, lemon juice and zest and heat until warm and runny-ish. Leave for 5 minutes, then stir in the cream. I know this isn't traditional but don't be tempted to leave it out: it gives a soft roundedness to the sweet filling and stops it from drying out. Pour or spoon this mixture into the prepared pastry case, place on the baking sheet and cook for about 15 minutes, then turn the oven down to gas mark 4/180°C and cook for another 15–20 minutes. Check to see that the pastry is fully cooked.

I like this best hot, with cold, cold vanilla ice-cream.

ELEGANTLY SUBSTANTIAL TRADITIONAL ENGLISH LUNCH FOR 8

English roast chicken with all the trimmings – plus some

Trifle

When you speak to ladies of a certain generation, you will notice that they use 'meat' to mean 'beef'. Thus 'We only ate meat once a week' doesn't preclude the consumption of vast and daily, or twice daily, platefuls of ham, pork, chicken and lamb. A fine Sunday lunch was roast chicken as it always used to be done, with parsley and thyme stuffing, bread or onion sauce, roast potatoes and sausages and honey-roast parsnips, rather than the modern take (lemon, garlic, onions, olive oil – see page 8) much as I love it.

A traditional English pudding is what you want after: of course any pie or crumble or indeed steamed sponge pudding would be just fine, but a trifle would be perfect.

ENGLISH ROAST CHICKEN WITH ALL THE TRIMMINGS

2 chickens, and to stuff them you need:
60g butter
drop oil
1 onion, finely chopped
6 rashers smoked streaky bacon, derinded and finely chopped
500g button mushrooms, finely chopped
200g fresh breadcrumbs
3 teaspoons dried thyme (or leaves from about 8 sprigs fresh thyme)
6 tablespoons chopped fresh parsley
zest of 1 lemon

Put 30g of the butter, with a drop of oil, in a thick-bottomed pan and when melted add the onion and bacon. Fry together, over medium heat, for about 10 minutes or until onions are soft. Remove the bacon–onion mixture and in the same pan melt the remaining butter and cook the finely chopped mushrooms, covered, with some salt and pepper, for about 5 minutes. Remove to a plate to cool. Put the breadcrumbs in a large bowl and mix in all the other ingredients, seasoning with salt and pepper to taste. If you want the stuffing to be a stiff rather than dense and crumbly mass, add a beaten egg to combine before stuffing the birds. Either way, add 20 minutes to the chickens' cooking time (and see roasting chart on page xii).

As for the sausages: what I do is get about 3–4 little sausages (you don't want vast breakfast ones) a head, then I cook them slightly in advance for 30–40 minutes in a gas mark 6/200°C oven. Then, just about a quarter of an hour or so before eating, I put them back in the oven the chickens have just been taken out of to heat up.

The potatoes really need a hotter oven – and turn to page 281 for method – but if you haven't got a double oven, you will just have to let the chickens stand for a while and turn up the potatoes for the final 20 minutes or so (in which case cover the reheating sausages with foil). If you like living dangerously, you can brown the potatoes by putting them, hot fat, baking tray and all, on the hob. But don't say I didn't warn you.

The recipe for bread sauce can be found on page 66. Onion sauce, however, was what my mother more often cooked to go with roast chicken, whether it was stuffed as above, or just with a squeezed-out lemon half.

ONION SAUCE

Many people like a Frenchified onion sauce, with the onions almost minced and disappearing into a velvety mush. I love this sauce as we ate it at home: the onions boiled, drained, and some of the water added to the milk to make the white sauce.

600ml full-fat milk
2 cloves
1 bay leaf
6 small or medium onions
500ml onion cooking water
90g butter
90g plain flour, preferably Italian 00
100ml double cream
fresh nutmeg

Pour the milk into a saucepan, add the cloves and bay leaf and bring to boiling point. Just before it boils, remove from heat, cover and let steep for 20 minutes or so, while you cook the onions.

Peel and halve the onions, put into a saucepan and cover with cold water. Bring to the boil, add salt and cook, covered, at a gentle but insistent simmer until the onions are soft and cooked: 20 minutes should do it. Onions retain the heat ferociously (which is why an onion, boiled and wrapped in a tea towel, was always used as a remedy for earache, staying warm for hours as it was pressed against a throbbing head). Pour the onions into a sieve or colander suspended over a wide-necked measuring jug or other saucepan. Let them drip in for a good 5 minutes. Then add 500ml of oniony water to the milk. If you haven't got that much, just make up the extra with more milk.

Now make the sauce: put the butter in a saucepan over a low to moderate heat, and when it's melted stir in the flour (I always use Italian 00 flour, see page 506) and cook, stirring while the roux turns nutty, for 2 minutes. Make sure it doesn't brown, though.

Off the heat, slowly pour on the milk and onion water, stirring all the time. I use a plastic whisk for this. Do it gradually, so the liquid is smoothly incorporated into the roux. Put back on a low heat and cook for about 15 minutes until the sauce is cooked: it should be smooth, very thick (the onions and cream will thin it in a minute) and velvety.

Stir in the onions and leave covered with a piece of butter paper or greaseproof until you want to eat it. At which time, reheat and then stir in the cream. Taste for seasoning and add a grating of nutmeg.

Serve not in a gravy boat (it's too thick) but in a bowl with a spoon.

Three things:

I don't bother to fish out the cloves and bay.

If you don't want to add cream, and I often don't, just make the initial milk up to 600ml instead.

Substitute 6 leeks, each cut into 3 logs, for the onions if you like. We nearly always ate leeks cooked like this in white sauce, at home, and they are particularly good, too, with roast pork or ham.

PEAS AND PARSNIPS

I like peas with this as well as the parsnips. Normally I'd allocate a medium-sized parsnip per person but – with so many sausages – it's probably more sensible to work along the lines of 3 parsnips per 2 people. Peel them, cut them into 4 – that's to say, cut them in half crossways and then cut each half lengthways – and parboil them in boiling, salted water for 3–5 minutes. In a baking tray in which they will fit in one layer, melt some fat: good dripping or lard is best; however, if you blanch at the very idea, do use oil. Put in the parsnips, toss well so that they're coated and drizzle about 3 tablespoons runny honey over them. Roast them in the oven for about 30 minutes at gas mark 7/210°C or 40 at gas mark 6/200°C. And give them a blast, the oven turned to very high, at the end of cooking while the chicken is resting. When they're ready they should be tender at the prod of a fork within, but brown and shiny and crisp without. It you can't find room to roast the potatoes and the parsnips separately, then bung them all in together, but you will then have to forget the honey over the parsnips. It's not ideal for the parsnips to be cooked at the high heat the potatoes require (you will end up with perhaps more burnt and crusty exterior than you'd like and rather less sweet and creamy interior), but it's not the end of the world.

GREENS

I think as a third vegetable, if you're willing to go the extra mile, you need something grassy and unsweet, and for that reason I'd choose kale or greens of some sort rather than white cabbage. Spinach is not at all a bad idea either: I am quite equable about the idea of frozen whole leaf spinach; if you do fresh spinach for 8 people you will have to be carting kilos of the stuff back from the shops.

See the recipe in Cooking in Advance, page 123: the proper English trifle is the one I had in mind, but the rhubarb, muscat and mascarpone one has an awful lot going for it here too.

TRIFLE

SPRING-SCENTED LUNCH FOR 8

Tarragon French roast chicken

Leeks, rice, peas and mangetouts

Lemon pie

GERMAN LEEKS AND WINE

With tarragon chicken, I like rice or mashed potato, to mop up the chickeny juices. And I'd adapt Jane Grigson's recipe for German leeks and wine. You cut the clean leeks into logs about 6–9cm long, depending on overall size of leek. (And work on the principle of 3 logs, that's to say probably 1 leek, per person.) Stew these logs slowly in butter in a covered pan for about 5 minutes, turning them occasionally: they should all be buttery. Then, pour in 175–200ml dry white wine (more if the arrangement of the pan seems to demand it) and keep cooking over a low heat, lid on. After about 10 minutes, when the leeks are ready (tender but not squidgy) remove them to a dish and, if there's too much liquid left, boil down the juices. Whisk in a knob of butter and pour over the leeks. Use white not black pepper, or it'll just look as if you haven't cleaned them properly.

TARRAGON FRENCH ROAST CHICKEN

2 large chickens
butter to smear over
small bunch tarragon, chopped
1 scant teaspoon sherry
500ml chicken stock

This should also give you wonderful leftovers for salad or sandwiches. Soften the butter – enough to smear over the breasts of both chickens – and mix well with the chopped tarragon, reserving the tarragon stalks for later. Don't go mad: tarragon is wonderful used with a light hand, suddenly whiffy when thrown in with too much exuberance. A straggly bunch comprising about 10 sprigs should be more than enough, which is about as much as is contained in those irritating see-through plastic envelopes hanging up on their little hooks at the supermarket. Add the sherry and a good grinding of white pepper. Push your fingers underneath the skin of the chicken so that you've got a pocket between breast and skin. Be careful not to break the skin, so proceed slowly. Smear most of the tarragony butter on to the breast, pat the skin back over and dot the rest in the bit between leg and body.

Heat up the chicken stock, either home-made or a well-diluted stock cube (the best you can find). Pour the stock into the bottom half of a roasting pan which has a grid that fits over, on which you can sit the chickens. Add to the hot stock the stalks of the freshly chopped tarragon. Sit the chickens on the grid. If you're not sure about the quality of your chickens, make a domed lid with tinfoil: it should be baggy and roomy over the chickens; tight and firmly fastened around the tin's edges. Keep the tinfoil on for just 1 hour, though. Otherwise, just let the chicken sit on its rack on the hot stock, untended.

Put in a preheated oven gas mark 6/200°C and roast for 20 minutes per 500g plus 30 minutes; remember to get 2 chickens of almost equal weight. If you're cooking a lemon pie at the same time – and the sour-sweet intensity of the lemons, and the old-fashioned comfort of the pie, are just right after the herbal hit of the buttery tarragon – you can have the oven on at gas mark 5/190°C and just make sure the chicken has 15 minutes or so longer in the slightly cooler oven. Alternatively, you can cook the lemon pie in advance (or if you have one, cook it in a double oven).

When the chickens are ready, take them out of the oven and switch it off. Pour off the juices, and either put the chickens in their tin back in the oven to keep them warm or let them wait on their carving board. I don't mind what temperature chicken is when I eat it; and actually, there's a lot to be said for that salmonella-taunting, puffed-breath warmth.

Pour the chicken–tarragon juices into a measuring jug. Pour some off into a small saucepan to boil down into a gravy-ish sauce. Obviously, taste for seasoning, too.

FOOLPROOF RICE

For 8 people, you need 4 American cupfuls (or up to the litre mark on a measuring jug) of basmati rice and 4 cups of water. Pour the measured rice into a large strainer and hold under the cold tap for a while to soak and rinse the rice. Shake well to drain. Melt 3 tablespoons of butter in a heavy-based saucepan (which has a lid that fits) and stir in the rice till all coated. Then add the water, bring to the boil, add a good pinch of salt, then cover and turn down heat to absolute minimum. For preference use a heat-disperser mat. Cook for 30–40 minutes or until all the water is absorbed and the rice is cooked. You can leave it with the lid on but the pan off the heat for 10 minutes or so without harm.

You might consider, too, syphoning off some of the chicken stock from the tray to add to the water and lend flavour to the rice while it's cooking.

All I want else with this are some mangetouts, possibly with some buttery petit pois stirred in.

LEMON PIE

I first came across a recipe for lemon pie (as distinct, very, from lemon meringue pie or lemon tart) in Norma MacMillan's *In a Shaker Kitchen*, a book I curl up with and read in a metaphorical fug of home-baking after another stressed-out urban day. Reading recipes for chicken pot pie and maple wheaten loaves is a wonderful antidote to modern life. The Shaker version of lemon pie takes lemons, slices them, macerates them in sugar and then adds beaten egg yolks to this viscous sherbety mix and cooks it in an old-fashioned double crust. For me, it has the edge on both lemon meringue pie (the least impressive example of the type – and, if you want a meringue-topped pie, please just turn to the rhubarb-filled, meringue-topped, orange-fragrant pastry based version on page 258) and tarte au citron. I noticed when I made it with sliced lemons, most people left pithy piles of politely regurgitated rubble on their plates. So I now cut off the pith after zesting and before slicing them.

In effect what you are making is a nubbly lemon curd, but even when you get rid of the skins, the fruit will hold up enough to create a proper pie filling rather than just goo. But although it's solid enough, it isn't stiff, and you'll need a spoon rather than a cake slice to serve it out.

for the filling

4 unwaxed lemons

425g sugar

4 eggs

2 tablespoons softened butter

for the pastry

280g self-raising flour

70g fridge-cold butter, in small dice

70g fridge-cold vegetable shortening, in small dice

1 egg yolk

Zest the lemons into a large bowl. Then, with a sharp knife, cut the pith off the lemons. I find the easiest way to do this is by standing a lemon on a chopping board and then cutting thin slices off downwards. Don't worry that you're carving the lemons into interesting geometric forms: you can afford to lose some of the flesh along with the pith anyway; and, besides, it doesn't matter what they look like. And don't worry, either, about this being a bit of a sweat: it doesn't take longer than a few clumsy swipes of a knife.

Once the lemons are that pale glacial yellow, rather than stringy white, slice them medium-thick and put them in the bowl. Just try and make sure you don't lose too much juice. I pour the liquid which gathers on the board into the bowl after peeling each lemon and then again after slicing it. Pour over the sugar and turn well (but gently: as much as possible you want the lemon slices to hold their shape) so that all the lemons are coated with sugar. (And don't use anything metal: a wooden spoon or plastic spatula will do fine.) Cover and put the bowl in a cool place (or the fridge) for at least 12 hours or preferably 24.

Make the pastry following the instructions on page 42, adding a pinch of salt and a few tablespoons of iced water to the egg to bind the dough. The self-raising flour will make it a thicker but also lighter crust, although you can of course use plain flour.

Divide the dough into 2 portions, one marginally bigger than the other and then press each into a flattened ball, cover both discs with clingfilm and put in the fridge. The pastry will need to rest in the fridge for at least 20 minutes, but you can leave it in for days as long as you remember to take it out so that it isn't icy-cold when you start rolling.

When you're ready to cook the pie, preheat the oven to gas mark 5/190°C. Roll out the slightly larger disc of pastry and use it to line a pie dish 22cm in diameter and 5cm deep. I have a stainless-steel one of these dimensions which I am very fond of, not least because the pastry never seems to stick to the metal; I am not keen on ceramic pie dishes.

Beat the 4 eggs and stir them, with a wooden spoon or spatula, into the lemon mixture until well combined. Spread the softened butter on the base of the pastry (much as you would butter a slice of bread) then (tasting it first) pour in the lemons and their eggy-sugary juices. Sprinkle with more sugar if you feel they need it. Wet the rims of the bottom crust, roll out the other disc of pastry and place on top. Crimp the edges to seal and cut some slits in the centre to let steam escape.

Cut a strip of tinfoil, enough to cover, loosely, the perimeter of the pie dish, so that the thinner, crimped edges don't burn. I find the pie needs about 1 hour in full, but you should start checking after about 45 minutes. I keep the foil on for about 30 minutes. You can always do it the other way round, if you like: that's to say, leave the pie uncovered for 30 minutes and then put the foil on to stop it burning.

Remove from the oven and put the dish on a wire rack. Sprinkle with sugar and serve from the pie dish, hot, warm or cold.

Even I cannot live by roast chicken alone: so, I move on. I love duck for Sunday lunch, if only because it is made to pick at as you sit around the not-cleared table, lazily finishing up whatever remains. There are drawbacks: it is not easy to carve and it doesn't go very far. Keep it, then, for when there are just 4 of you, along with a child or two, as well. The recipe I use makes the carving point less pertinent: you can almost treat it like crispy Peking duck; what you can carve, carve, and as for the rest, pull it into soft strips and gloriously crispy shreds.

With duck, how can you not have peas? Some will want also plain potatoes, to offer a foil to the rich and unctuous meat.

Don't go berserk over pudding. Yes a sharp and fragrant fruit tart *would* be lovely (and my Seville orange curd tart (see page 271) is an obvious contender here, evoking as it does another traditional culinary conjunction with the duck) but just as good, certainly easier, perhaps even more judicious, would be a heaped mound of tropical fruit salad: get pawpaw, get mango, some headily perfumed melon and, just for the look (there's certainly no taste), slice some star fruit into the bowl, too. The juice of the fruit (cut them over the bowl so you don't lose any) should provide some liquid, which you can supplement with squirts of lime juice and the pulp of a couple of passion fruits. And although it might sound excessive – well, it *is* excessive – I serve with it a jug of warm, even hot, butterscotch sauce. You may not believe me before tasting it, but this is an ecstatically successful culinary combination.

RELATIVELY EASY LUNCH FOR 4

Soft and crisp roast duck

Petits pois à la française and potatoes

Tropical fruit salad with butterscotch sauce

The reason why this is relatively easy, if not just plain simple, is that quite a bit of it can be done in advance. The ducks can be poached in advance, and then all you need to do is roast them. The peas can certainly be done slightly in advance. The fruits must definitely be bought quite a bit in advance. Nearly all fruit is sold before it is anywhere near ripe these days, so unless you're very confident, I wouldn't consider buying fruit to eat on Sunday any later than

Wednesday. And you probably don't need me to say this, but don't keep the fruit in the fridge.

The recipe for the duck is in Cooking in Advance, on page 100; for 4 adults, you will need 2 ducks (and that'll provide enough for a few smallish children, too, who love this) and the recipe for the peas is in the same chapter, too (on page 118). For just 4 of you you need to think of using about 1kg peas, unpodded weight, or about two-thirds of a 500g bag of frozen petits pois.

QUICK STOVE-TOP BUTTERSCOTCH SAUCE

To make a quick stove-top butterscotch-toffee-ish sauce for the tropical fruit, melt 3 tablespoons light muscovado – or other soft brown – sugar, 2 tablespoons caster or granulated sugar, 50g unsalted butter and 150g golden syrup together in a thick-bottomed pan. When smooth and melted, let it bubble away, gently but insistently, for 5 minutes or so. Then, off the heat, beat in 125ml (an American halfcupful) of the single cream and ¼–½ teaspoon good quality vanilla extract. (Or maybe add instead a slug of rum.) You can pour the sauce into a jug, or bowl with ladle, and serve hot, or you can do it in advance and reheat.

Respectful though I am in general of tradition, I don't like English-style roast lamb. Nostalgia makes me forgiving of redcurrant jelly or mint sauce but neither is my first choice. You could consider an amalgam of mint and redcurrant, which works better than either sauce on its own.

MINT, ORANGE AND REDCURRANT JELLY

Decant your jar of bought good redcurrant jelly, grate over the zest of ½–1 unwaxed orange, and add 1 heaped tablespoon (or more, if when you taste it you feel it could do with it) of chopped mint. I use my mother's rusted-up old Moulinex herb mill; I hold it over the bowl of jelly and just turn the handle till I think I've got enough. Hold one of the orange halves over the bowl and give it a squeeze. Stir everything together, and if you made a mess decant into a clean bowl for serving.

Lamb is best, I think, when the sweetness of the meat itself is in relief, rather than rudely overtaken by a less subtle sugariness. This means serving it warm rather than hot; and if eating it cold, at room rather than at fridge temperature. The smoky sweetness of peppers is perfect here: they complement rather than compete with the lamb's almost musky meatiness. Most people give you leg of lamb, but you should try shoulder: the flavour is deeper, more rounded, and the texture is fat-irrigated and plumply velvety. I am an awful carver and end up hacking a shoulder into oblivion. If you can't carve either, but mind chunks, get leg instead.

LATE-SUMMER LUNCH FOR 6

Roast shoulder of lamb with ratatouille

Green salad with green beans

Translucent apple tart

I've called this a late-summer lunch, because this is when it is eaten at its best: the air still warm, the wind beginning to bluster limply; it may be a late, weak August, it may be early September. But, hell, you could eat it any time: even in the depths of winter. Mostly, I hate too much Mediterranean sprightliness when the weather is shoulder-stoopingly brutal, but the soft stewiness of ratatouille (or at least, that's the way I like it) accommodates itself elegantly enough to an alien climate.

The recipe for ratatouille is in Cooking in Advance (see page 115).

ROAST SHOULDER OF LAMB

2kg shoulder of lamb
1 sprig rosemary
3 cloves garlic
1 tablespoon olive oil

Preheat the oven to gas mark 7/210°C.

Peel and mince the garlic and finely chop the rosemary. Put in a bowl with the olive oil and stir and mash together. Get a sharp knife and stab the lamb in several places. Using your fingers, push small amounts of the rosemary–garlic mixture into the cavities and, if there is any left in the bowl, swill it out with a little more olive oil and coat the top of the lamb with it. Sprinkle with coarse sea salt and put in the oven. Roast for 30 minutes per kg plus 20 minutes. Then let stand for a good 10 minutes before carving.

If you're in a hurry, you can stud the lamb just with garlic, in which case cut the garlic lengthways into thin slivers and push them into the cavities. And you could, if you wanted, smear the top with a spoonful of good pesto. I'm not mad about the cheese element, but I have been reduced to this, and it works, which is why I pass it on.

If you want a gravy, just remove as much of the fat as you can, and while the tin is on the hob swill it out with a glass of red wine. Taste to see whether salt or water are needed. You don't need to make much gravy: just enough to drizzle over the carved slices of meat, not so much as to provide a puddle on the plate.

GREEN SALAD WITH GREEN BEANS

You've already got the sweet soft mush of the ratatouille: what you want here is something crisp and fresh and plain. I'd stick to the paler lettuces: 1 soft English round lettuce and 2 little gems, the leaves just separated, not torn into chunks. Get about 100g green beans, top, tail and halve them, so you have a pile of short lengths and cook them in salted boiling water until they're properly cooked. You want them to have bite, but not too much: green beans are horrible undercooked. While they're cooking, fill the sink with cold water and chuck in a few ice cubes. As soon as the beans are cooked (start tasting after 5 minutes) drain them and then plunge them into the sink of icy water. Drain again and dry, either on kitchen towel or in a salad spinner, toss with the lettuces, adding some tender little basil leaves, whole, or some chopped fresh parsley or the tiniest grating of lemon zest. Make the simplest dressing of olive oil, salt and lemon juice or vinegar (using hardly any lemon or vinegar and even less if you've grated in some zest) and maybe a dot of mustard, if you like.

TRANSLUCENT APPLE TART

I came across this tart one Sunday lunch at the house of friends. When I arrived the pastry was being made; in the brief pause between first and second helpings of the main course the apple was grated relaxedly into the butter mixture; and then, at the end, we ate it. And it reminded me how nice it is to see food being prepared, rather than just being presented with the finished product. The lack of anxiety in the cooking inevitably transferred itself and that's a salutary lesson. The recipe is adapted from Jane Grigson's comforting and instructive *Fruit Book*. She, in fact, calls it Apple Cheese Cake or Apple Curd Tart, but she makes the comparison between this and what the southern Americans call a transparent pie, in which the custardy filling made with melted butter in place of cream or milk becomes translucent as it cooks. The word translucent evokes the light and melting delicacy of this tart, and I can't help finding both the idea of cheese and curd a distraction. The only drawback for me is that it needs only one apple, thereby hardly relieving me of the reproachful mound of bramleys in the garden in August and September.

I find it easier to get the pastry made, rested, rolled out and the flan case lined the evening before. Pâte sucrée, Jane Grigson stipulates, but I use my foolproof sweet pastry (page 43) instead. I have made this with bought puff pastry and it's still good; I should think bought shortcrust (or the sweetened version) would do as well. But you must believe me when I tell you how easy my pastry is. You are not baking this blind, so once the pastry is lining its case, you can proceed to fill and bake it.

for the pastry

see Basics, page 43, for the recipe, which is sufficient for the shallow 23cm flan tin needed here.

for the filling

60g lightly salted butter

60g vanilla sugar, or caster sugar and a few drops pure vanilla extract

1 egg

1 cooking apple

Preheat the oven to gas mark 7/210°C.

Melt the butter and sugar together over such a low heat that they become no more than tepid. Remove from the stove and beat in the egg. Quickly peel, core and grate the apple coarsely and stir thoroughly into the butter mixture.

Pour and spread over the pastry-lined flan tin and bake for about 15 minutes, until golden brown. Lower the heat to gas mark 4/180°C and cook for a further 15–20 minutes, until nicely coloured.

As with most puddings, it is best to time this to come out of the oven not long before you're sitting down: it will be warm but will have had time to settle. But this, as Jane Grigson says, is wonderful whether hot, warm or cold.

FRANCO-AMERICAN LUNCH FOR 6

Gigot boulangère

Sliced green beans or green salad

Red slump

I've mentioned that I like lamb as cooked by the French: and a gigot boulangère is particularly glorious: both dignified and comforting.

After the garlicky lamb, do something simple. If you want it to be pudding, rather than plain fruit or ice-cream, then I'd go for red slump, which is a fabulous American term (as is red grunt, which has a synonymous application) for red fruits baked in the oven with little dumplings. This is easy and suits late summer, when the fruit's around, though you can use frozen.

GIGOT BOULANGÈRE

Shoulder, not gigot, of lamb baked over potatoes is probably the origin of this dish; the shoulder would have been boned and so, really, should the leg. But don't worry about it: nor about making this historically authentic. We no longer take the roasting tin or casserole over to the baker's to cook in his oven (hence the name), so we can liberate ourselves from the other connotations of the dish without going into a frenzy of culinary self-doubt. Elizabeth David specifies new potatoes to go underneath the joint, and feel free to do likewise. The French certainly eat waxier potatoes than us. I specify floury maincrop potatoes simply because that's the way I have always eaten this.

3 cloves garlic
1 large leg lamb, approx. 2¼kg, or more if available
100g butter, plus more for greasing pan
1 large onion or 2–3 banana shallots
3 bay leaves
small bunch of 6 or 7 sprigs thyme or 1 teaspoon dried thyme
1½kg potatoes
200ml lamb stock or water

Preheat the oven to gas mark 6/200°C.

Peel the garlic and cut into spikes. Stab the lamb in several places with the point of a sharp knife and insert the garlic. Cut a quarter of the butter off, and put it to one side.

Cut the onion into quarters, crumble the bay leaves and put both in the bowl of a food processor fitted with the steel blade. Reserving a couple of sprigs, hold the rest of the thyme over the bowl and, squeezing each stem by turn, pull downwards so that the leaves fall into the bowl. Turn on until everything is chopped finely. Naturally, you can do this by hand if you prefer.

Butter a deep oven dish large enough to take all the potatoes and the lamb; an ordinary high-sided roasting tin will do, and indeed is what I use. Peel the potatoes and slice them thinly but not transparently so, blanch them for 2–3 minutes in boiling salted water, drain, dry and layer them on the bottom of the dish, dotting with butter (taken from the larger, main, amount) and sprinkling with salt, pepper and the onion–thyme–bay leaf mixture as you go.

If you can get hold of some lamb stock (I keep a tub or two each of various Joubère stocks in my deep-freeze), pour it over the potatoes. Otherwise you could use any stock you want, I suppose, but I often use just water. Put in the oven and cook for 30 minutes before adding the lamb.

Rub the top of the lamb with the rest of the butter, softened, with the leaves from the remaining sprigs of thyme. Sit the lamb on top of the potatoes and put back in the oven for 1 hour, then raise the heat to gas mark 8/220°C and cook for another 30 minutes. This should give you pink, but not underdone meat. But test after about 1¼ hours to see if it's how you like it.

Let the meat rest in the turned-off oven with the door open for about 15 minutes before serving. Even though it doesn't look as lovely, remove the lamb to a board to carve it. You can always put the slices back on top of the potatoes in the tin before you serve it.

RED SLUMP

To make enough red slump for 6 (though it would stretch to 8 – it's just I hate stretching), you need:

for the fruit

1kg red summer fruits
150g (10 tablespoons) sugar, or to taste
4–5 tablespoons water or suitable liqueur (crème de cassis, crème de mûre or an orange liqueur)

for the dumplings

120g self-raising flour
30g caster sugar
15g ground almonds
75g unsalted butter
milk to bind

Put the fruit in a dish – I use one of those oval old-fashioned cream stoneware bowls, but any pie or baking dish that has a capacity of about 3 litres should do. Sprinkle the fruit with the sugar. How much depends on the sweetness of the fruit itself, obviously enough. Start with about 6–8 tablespoons and taste. Add the water or suitable liqueur and put, covered (with lid or foil) in a preheated oven (gas mark 5/190°C). If you haven't got fresh fruit, use frozen red berries (not strawberries). And don't use framboise or fraise liqueur, either.

Leave in the oven while you get on with the dumplings (though you could have made them earlier and left them in the fridge). Sift the flour into a bowl, add a pinch of salt, the caster sugar and ground almonds (almond dumplings are not usual, but I prefer them here). Stir them together and then throw in the butter, chilled and cut into small dice, and rub into the dry ingredients until the mixture is crumbly. You could do this in a free-standing electric mixer, but I wouldn't try a processor.

Pour in enough milk to bind the dough: it should be soft but not too sticky to form into balls the size of small walnuts (remember they will swell while cooking and then they should grow up into the size of proper walnuts); this quantity of dough should make about

24 little dumplings. Take the dish of fruit out of the oven when it's simmering – about 35 minutes if frozen, 15 if not. Take off the lid, stir the fruit and taste for sweetness, adding more sugar if necessary. Put the dumplings in the dish, cover again and bake for another 15–20 minutes by which time the dumplings should be cooked, beautifully swollen and no longer doughy. I like this with ice-cream – this is, after all, an American pudding, but cream, old-fashioned runny cream rather than those stiff restauranty mounds, can be just right, too.

BLACKBERRIES AND CREAM

If you want something plainer, or rather even less trouble, just get masses of blackberries, cover a vast plate with them and do nothing save sprinkle them with caster sugar. Pour a great deal of thick single cream (or even ordinary single cream) into a jug and put it on the table alongside.

This was never going to be a comprehensive list of suggestions, but I am loath to move on without mentioning one more traditional – and this time British traditional – way with lamb: and that's with caper sauce.

Caper sauce in fact goes, or always went, with boiled leg of mutton. But no one eats mutton any more. It's extravagant to boil lamb. It would be awful, though, if caper sauce disappeared: so just make it to go with plain roast lamb instead.

The best way to get some lamb stock to flavour the caper sauce is to roast the lamb for 15 minutes in a very high oven, and then, when you turn it down to about gas mark 6/200°C, add about 400ml water and an onion, halved, to the dish. I've got one of those roasters which is made of a punctured dish over a deeper pan and I put the lamb on the rack, and the water and onion in the tin below. Don't cover the lamb: you want the top to crisp. (For cooking times, check table on page xii.) Otherwise just buy a tub of lamb stock for the sauce.

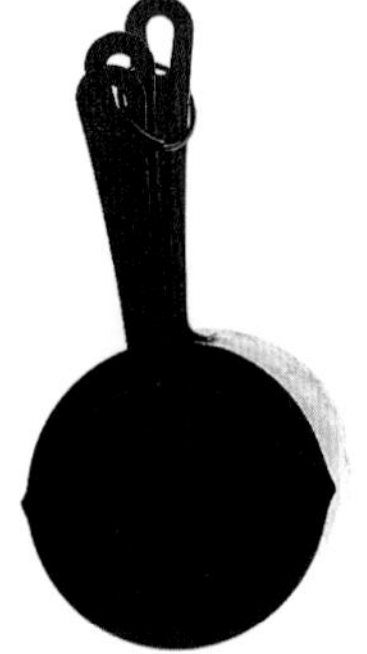

CAPER SAUCE FOR ROAST LAMB

45g butter
45g flour
400ml full-fat milk
200ml lamb stock
3 tablespoons capers plus vinegar from the jar
parsley (optional)

Make this sauce while the lamb is resting prior to carving. If you've braise-roasted the lamb as mooted above, try to remove as much fat as you can from the roasting tin. I am hopeless at it, so what I suggest is that you pour the juices into a measuring jug and mop the top, where the fat is, with some kitchen towel. If you find those gravy dividers effective, use one of them, but I find they make them so big that the top of the liquid – let alone the unfatty part below – never even reaches the spout. Pour 200ml of the juices into the 400ml milk and warm.

Make the roux for the sauce (following recipe for béchamel on page 21), pour in the milk and lamb stock as normal and cook until thick. Stir in the capers (adding more if you want it more capery) and 1 teaspoon vinegar from the caper bottle. Normally I prefer salt-packed capers, but, for this, you want them pickled in vinegar. Taste. I like this fairly sharp and might well add another teaspoon of caper juice, but proceed cautiously. If you like you can also add 1 tablespoon or so of freshly chopped parsley. And do not be reticent with the pepper. For a richer sauce, stir in, at the end, an egg yolk beaten gently with about 5 tablespoons double cream.

To be frank, although it's hardly traditional, I love caper sauce with roast pork, too. Its sour-noted velvetiness goes wonderfully with the densely woven sweetness of the meat. More often, though, I go for onion (or leek) sauce, but habit plays a large part in the Sunday lunch repertoire, I do see.

There's no point in cooking pork at all, if you are going to buy a lean yet flabby supermarket joint. The meat will be tasteless and dry and the fat limp and wet and you won't stand a chance in hell of making any half-way decent crackling. For crackling you need the pigs to roam about, so that their hides get tough and their meat flavoursome.

For regular, ordinary Sunday roast pork I get leg; ask the butcher for knuckle-half. Roast it at gas mark 7/210°C for 1 hour and then turn it down to gas mark 5/190°C. To work out the total cooking time, think along the lines of 25 minutes per 500g plus 25 minutes or 55 minutes per kg plus 25 minutes on top.

If you're going to do just plain roast pork, then follow the instructions for roast potatoes given with the roast beef (see page 281) and work a timetable out for yourself. At least you're not bothering with the Yorkshire pudding so there are fewer major factors to take into consideration. With pork I love sliced green beans and cabbage – huge bowlfuls with butter and black pepper or, as my mother often made it, with caraway seeds. The only time I like red cabbage is with pork, too, so I'll give a recipe for that while I'm about it.

SWEETLY NOSTALGIC LUNCH FOR 6

Roast pork

Roast potatoes

Red cabbage cooked in the Viennese fashion

Stem-ginger gingerbread with sharp cheese, or apple butterscotch tart

ROAST PORK

To make sure the crackling is crackling and not damp chewy rind, make sure you don't cover the pork while it's in the fridge (clingfilm will give it a very sloppy kiss of death). Score it with a sharp knife before roasting. I do it the easy way: I ask the butcher to score it; his knives are better than mine, for a start. Besides, the purpose of going to a good butcher is to make sure the meat is beautifully handled, cut and prepared as well as fresh and well chosen.

If you're stuck with scoring the rind yourself, then take a sharp knife (a Stanley knife for choice) and cut lines on the diagonal at about 2½cm intervals. If you want, you can then do the same the other way, so you have a diamond pattern etched into the rind. But that's not necessary, and it is easier not to.

I like to rub English mustard powder onto the scored, wiped rind (give it a quick go over with some kitchen towel just to make sure it's really dry). Or you can sprinkle salt. Some people dribble vinegar, but I am not convinced.

A tip from my butcher, David Lidgate: to make sure the crackling is properly crunchy all over, when you take the leg out of the oven, quickly peel off the crackling, cut it into 2 or 3 pieces, put it in a hot tray and back into the oven, turning it back up to gas mark 7/210°C as you do so. Start carving and when you're done, take out the crackling, break it into more pieces and put on a plate in the middle of the table for people to take as they like. The pieces of crackling that come from the nether parts of the leg will obviously be damper and take longer to crisp than those from the top part, so don't take all the crackling out of the oven at the same time.

My mother loved red cabbage, so I am fond of this dish. On the whole, I don't like savoury food that's fruity and jammy, but in the right weather and in the right mood, it can be fabulous: aromatic and warming and with just enough edge to stop it from cloying. I prefer it with roast pork to the more usual goose or duck. I think it actually benefits from being eaten with a meat that offers light to its shade. I love it with sausages, too. And it works beautifully with just-fried, still-moussy, calf's liver.

The advantage of fruity stewed red cabbage is that it can be made in advance, and moreover is the better for it. This recipe comes from a lovely book, Arabella Boxer's *Garden Cookbook*, which I picked up at a dusty second-hand bookshop. This book came out in the mid-1970s so it is exactly contemporaneous with my memories of the red cabbage my mother used to cook. I seem to remember, though, my mother always used brown sugar, and a rich treacly one at that. And I had no idea that the culinary style this invoked was Viennese, but I rather love the idea: it certainly adds charm.

RED CABBAGE COOKED IN THE VIENNESE FASHION

1 large red cabbage
1 Spanish onion
75g beef dripping or other fat
2 tablespoons sugar, preferably rich and brown
1 large cooking apple
3 tablespoons red wine or cider vinegar
300ml beef stock
1 tablespoon flour
4 tablespoons cream, sour cream or crème fraîche

Cut the cabbage in quarters, discard the outer leaves and the central core, then shred each quarter finely. Even by hand this doesn't take long. And since this recipe predates the food processor, I tend, nostalgically, to eschew machine cutters here. Illogical of course: I use an electric mixer for pastry happily enough. But then I never saw my mother make pastry.

Chop the onion and melt the fat in a deep, heavy casserole. Cook until it starts to soften and colour. Add the sugar and stir around until all is golden. Put in the cabbage and mix well. Chop the cored but unpeeled apple and add to the cabbage. Add the vinegar and some salt and black pepper. Stir well, cover and cook for 15 minutes over a low flame.

Heat the stock and pour into the casserole. Cook for 2 hours on top of the stove or in a low oven (gas mark 2–3/150–160°C). When the time is up, mix the flour and cream to a paste in a cup and add to the cabbage by degrees, stirring all the time, on top of the stove.

Cook over a low flame for 2 minutes to cook the flour (4 or 5 minutes with ordinary plain flour) and thicken the sauce. Taste and add more sugar or vinegar if necessary – the sweet and sour elements should be nicely balanced, not like the culinary outpourings of a provincial Chinese take-away, so go steady – or more salt and black pepper. Serves 6–8.

If you are making this in advance – which is always a good idea – reheat it, covered, in its casserole for an hour at gas mark 4/180°C, or on the hob for markedly less time.

If you're not making the cabbage, turn to page 364 for a recipe for apple sauce; only I wouldn't strain it here. My grandmother always ate horseradish with her pork; you could think of doing likewise. Similarly, if I weren't bothering with the red cabbage, I'd cook an apple pudding: baked apples, apple crumble, apple pie, or, especially good after the pork, this sour-sweet apple butterscotch tart. Otherwise, dense, wet and aromatic gingerbread (see page 128) and some sharp and crumbly cheese such as Lancashire or Wensleydale would be perfect.

APPLE BUTTERSCOTCH TART

pastry using 120g flour (see page 41)
500g cooking apples (or substitute rhubarb or blackberries)
150g light muscovado sugar
4 level tablespoons flour
2 eggs
4 tablespoons cream

Make a pastry case (to line a 21cm flan case), fill it with the cored, peeled and fairly thinly sliced cooking apples and spread over the top a walnut-coloured butterscotch paste made by mixing the sugar with the flour, a small pinch of salt and the eggs beaten with the cream. Bake at gas mark 7/210°C for 10 minutes and then lower the heat to gas mark 4/180°C and cook for another 20 minutes or so.

If you want a pudding that is altogether lighter (and can be cooked in advance) then try the dusty-rose-coloured rhubarb and muscat jelly (page 345), substituting freshly squeezed orange juice for the muscat if you want something suitably alcohol-free for children (although I wouldn't presume they'd dislike the unctuous grapiness of the wine). There is an established culinary connection, anyway, between rhubarb and pork; the Swedes eat rhubarb purée with pork much as we do apple sauce. I suggest some variation on this theme: just get a stick or two of rhubarb, cook until it turns into a pinky-khaki mush, and when it's cool stir it into a small – cup-sized – bowlful of bought horseradish sauce.

CALMING WINTER LUNCH FOR 6

Roast pork loin with roast leeks

Clapshot with burnt onions

Custard tart

Much as I love proper roast leg of pork with its carapace of amber-glazed crackling, I don't cook it that much: roast boned and rolled loin, without the rind, is my more regular pig-out. I feel at ease with it, even though the flesh can tend to dry stringiness. Ask the butcher for rib-end of loin (hard to carve, but wonderful tasting). And put a little liquid in the roasting pan so the meat grows tender in its own small pool of odoriferous steam. Anything will do: a glass of wine or cider, some stock, water mixed with apple juice, the leftover liquid you've cooked carrots in.

Cooking boned and rolled pork loin bears almost any interpretation or elaboration. By elaboration, I mean not to imply complexity of culinary arrangement but wide-rangingness. If you want, at other times, to add a modern, fusiony note, make a paste of garlic and root ginger and smear that over, rubbing ground ginger into the prepared and removed rind for hot crackling; if you want something altogether less vibrant, then pulverise some dried bay leaves, and press these against the soft covering of white fat. Or rub in ground cloves, cinnamon and cardamom to produce an almost Middle-Eastern waft. Neither of these requires crackling; here you would be after altogether less strenuous eating.

WITH GARLIC AND ROOT GINGER

WITH DRIED BAY LEAVES

GROUND CLOVES, CINNAMON AND CARDAMOM

Get the butcher to remove the bones and give them to you, so you can cook them around the joint, which will make the gravy. And while you're about it, ask him to chop them up small. As for the rind: if you want crackling, ask him to remove the rind, score it and give it back to you; and, even if you don't want crackling, the loin should be left elegantly wrapped in its pearly coating of fat. If there's not enough fat on the joint, it will end up too dry.

ROAST LOIN OF PORK

You will need about 1.8kg boned, derinded weight, which means a joint, before butchering, in the region of 2½kg. If you're a good carver, don't bother with boning. Either way, the crackling should be cooked separately.

Preheat the oven to gas mark 7/210°C. Work out how long the loin needs

– and at roughly 45 minutes per kg, for a 1.8kg joint that's about 70 minutes – and cook the loin in its pan on one shelf, and, putting it in about 45 minutes before you want to eat, the crackling on a rack over a roasting tray on another shelf. About halfway through the pork's cooking time throw a glass of wine (or whatever you're using; cider would be very good here) into the pan.

Some people simply get the rind removed and then drape it over the loin as it cooks. The reason I don't do this is because then you have to do a real number to rid the juices in the meat dish of fat. I am not one of nature's gravy makers, and therefore I do everything to make life easier for myself – and frankly suggest you do too. As for this gravy: all you need to do – having cooked the crackling in a separate pan – is pour the winey juices from the meat dish into a sauceboat or bowl, removing fat if you can and if you need to. Taste it: you may need to add a little bit of water, you may just want to use it as is. I am not on the whole a thick-gravy person: you may be. For a recipe for apple sauce to go with, see page 364, only again I wouldn't sieve it here.

ROAST LEEKS

For 6 people, get about 8 not too fat leeks (although one each would probably be enough, I'd always rather have over). Once you've made sure they're clean, cut them on the diagonal into logs about 8cm long. Pour some olive oil in a roasting tray and turn the leeks in them so they're glossy all over. Sprinkle over some coarse sea salt and roast for about 30 minutes at gas mark 7/210°C, I usually roast them at a higher temperature and for slightly less time, but it would be absurd to complicate matters since you're going to have the oven at mark 7 anyway.

I love these leeks blistered sweet on the outside, suggestively oniony within their slithery centre. I know that there are going to be onions themselves with the clapshot, but the pork can take the double helping of allium. If you feel otherwise, make a large, iron-dark bowl of butter-drenched kale. Kale, indeed, is a feature of traditional clapshot; this recipe makes do without and it is tempting to make up the shortfall. If you wanted to add a slightly more modern touch, then simply get some pak choi or choi sum (which most supermarkets seem to stock now) and steam or stir-fry it with or without lacily grated ginger.

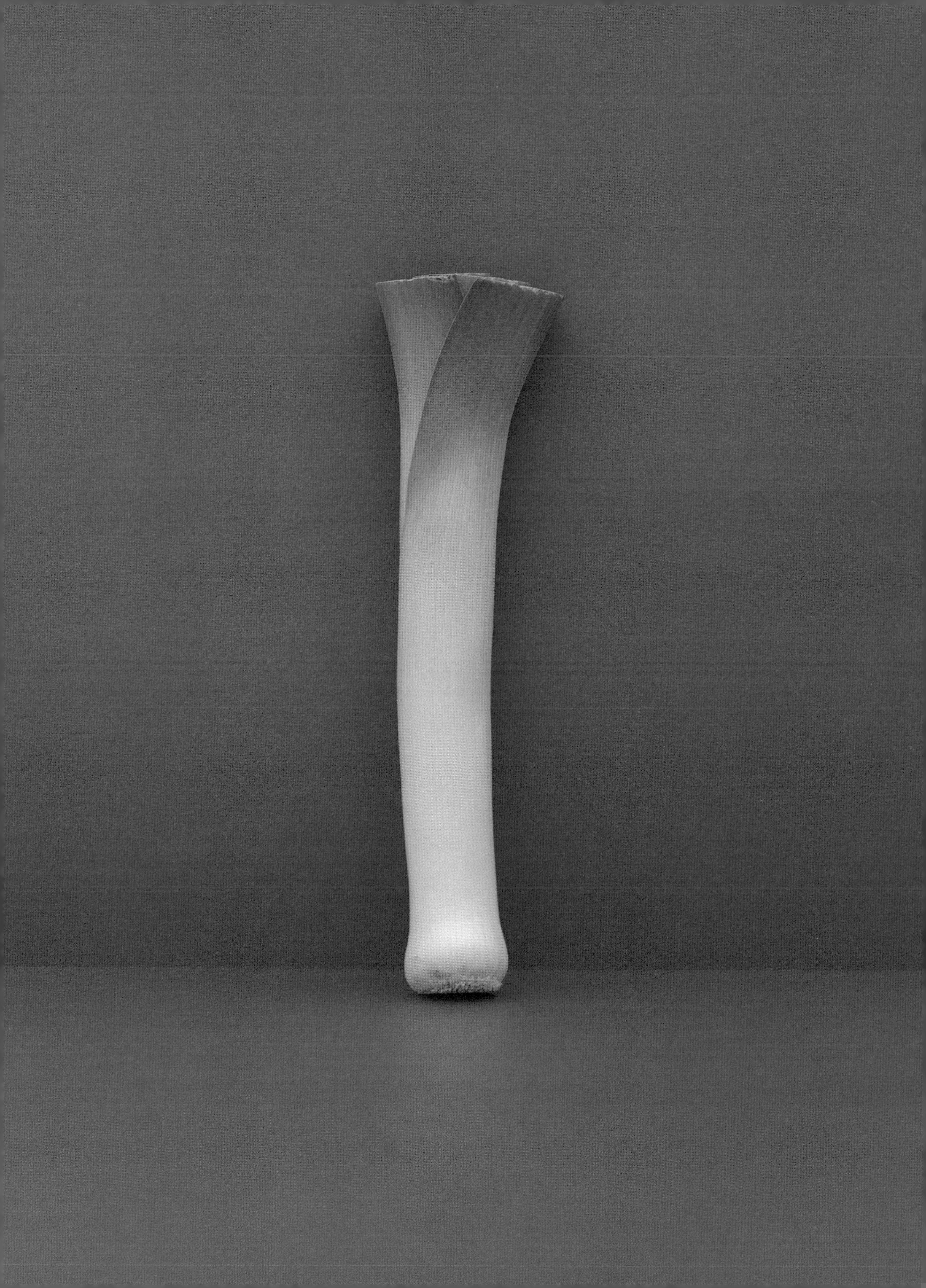

CLAPSHOT WITH BURNT ONIONS

I got the idea for this in the *Tesco Recipe Collection* of October 1996 in an article written by Catherine Brown. It is a modern take on a traditional dish, which was a hodge-podge of various vegetables cooked and mushed together. This is something not so stylish as to be self-conscious, but not so hearty as to be indigestible.

1kg swede, peeled and diced
1kg floury potatoes, such as golden wonder, King Edward or Kerr's Pink, peeled and quartered
100g butter
fresh nutmeg

for the burnt onions
4 tablespoons olive oil
2 large strong onions, very thinly sliced
2 tablespoons caster sugar

First, make the clapshot: put the swede in a pan of boiling, salted water, and simmer for about 5 minutes. Add the potatoes and simmer for about 25–30 more minutes until both are just cooked. Don't overcook or they will disintegrate into potato soup. Drain thoroughly.

Dry the swede and potato slightly by putting them back in the saucepan (which you've wiped dry) and placing it over a low heat. Then mash – with a potato ricer or mouli – with the butter. Season to taste, adding a good grating of fresh nutmeg.

While the potatoes and swede are cooking, get started with the onion-burning. Heat the oil in a heavy-based frying pan over low heat. Slice the onions very finely (I use the processor for this), add to the oil and cook slowly for about 30 minutes until crisp and golden brown, stirring and scraping from time to time. Turn heat to high and sprinkle with sugar and stir continuously for a further 3 minutes or so until the sugar caramelises and the onion darkens.

Put the clapshot in a serving bowl and top with the burnt onions.

CUSTARD TART

I adore custard tart: I love its barely-vanilla-scented, nutmeggy softness, the silky texture of that buttermilk-coloured eggy cream, solidified just enough to be carved into trembling wedges on the plate. It isn't hard to make, but I botch it often out of sheer clumsiness. But now I have learnt my lessons, and pass them on to you. One: pour the custard into the pastry case while the pastry case is in the oven, so that you don't end up leaving a trail from kitchen counter to cooker, soaking the pastry case in the process. And two: don't be so keen to use up every last scrap of that custard, filling the case right to the very brim so that it's bound – as you knew it was – to spill, making it soggy and ruining the contrast between crisp crust and tender filling. If you can manage not to do both those things, then you can make a perfect custard pie. I won't promise it's an easy exercise, though.

If you want to eat it cold, this makes life easier as you can arrange to have free play with the oven the day before. But, at its best, the custard should still have a memory of heat about it. Make it before you put the pork in the oven and let it sit for 1½ hours or thereabouts, gently subsiding into muted warmth in the kitchen.

If you can't be bothered to make the pastry yourself you have a choice: either you can use bought shortcrust or don't bother with a crust at all and make a baked custard. For a baked custard, make double quantities of custard, then pour it into a pie dish (with a capacity of just over 1 litre), stand the pie dish in a roasting tin filled with hot water and bake in a gas mark 2/150°C oven for about 1 hour.

If you don't keep vanilla sugar – although I do recommend it, see page 82 – then just add a few drops of real vanilla extract to the mixture. Of course you can always add an actual vanilla pod to the milk and cream when you warm them, but actually I don't like baked custard with too much vanilla: I like the merest musky suggestion of it.

for the pastry – enough to line a deep flan or quiche case 20cm in diameter

see recipe in Basics Etc, page 43

1 egg white (leftover from yolk for custard) to seal

for the custard

3 eggs

1 egg yolk

2 tablespoons vanilla sugar

300ml single cream

150ml milk

pinch ground mace

freshly grated nutmeg

Preheat the oven to gas mark 6/200°C. Make the pastry, line the flan case and bake blind for about 20 minutes, following the instructions on page 44. Take out of the oven and remove the beans and paper or foil. Beat the egg white lightly, brush the bottom and sides of the cooked pastry case with it (the idea being to seal the pastry so the custard won't make it soggy later on) and put back in the oven for 5 minutes. Turn down the oven to gas mark 3/160°C.

Put the eggs, egg yolks and sugar in a bowl and whisk together. Warm the cream and milk in a saucepan with the mace and pour into the egg and sugar mixture. Stir to mix and then strain into the pastry case, as it sits in the pulled-out rack in the oven. Grate over some nutmeg. Push the shelf back in carefully but confidently (tense hesitation can be disastrous: far too jerky), shut the door and leave the custard pie in the oven to bake for about 45 minutes. Take a look though, after about 35 minutes. The custard, when it's ready, should look more or less solid but still with a tremble at its centre.

Take out of the oven, grate some more nutmeg over and leave until it reaches tepid heaven.

If pork is not cooked often enough, salmon is over-exposed. It can, though, be just right. One proviso: get in early, towards the end of spring. Once summer starts, even as we edge towards it, the torture by poached salmon begins. By mid-June I feel I'll sob if I see another coral-coloured corpse lying flobbily on an enthusiastically displayed plate. But when I eat it unexpectedly, I am surprised at how much I like it. Another proviso: banish the identikit English summer lunch of cold poached salmon with new potatoes followed by summer pudding from your repertoire.

In theory wild salmon should be available from February (until the end of August); in practice you may be lucky to get much until April, which is when I am setting my fictional lunch.

SPRING LUNCH FOR 8

Salmon baked in foil

Tabbouleh and fennel salad, or peas, avocado and mint

Almond sponge with orange syrup

This is the perfect menu for a sprightly April: the salmon makes you feel summer's on the way, and the fragrant and tender sponge offers comfort because it isn't.

SALMON BAKED IN FOIL

My grandmother swears that the way to cook a whole salmon is to cover it with cold water, bring it to the boil, let it simmer for 10 minutes then turn it off. When it's cold, she says, it will, whatever its weight, be perfectly à point.

If you don't own a fish kettle (as I don't) then baking salmon in the oven, wrapped in foil, is the best and simplest way to cook it. Everyone has their own way, and I notice that cooking at high temperatures is gaining fashionable ground, but this is the basic method. Heat the oven to gas mark 2/150°C. Get a piece of foil large enough to wrap the fish loosely, and butter it if you are going to eat the fish hot, oil it if you're going to eat it cold. Lie the fish on top of the greased foil, season with salt and pepper, squeeze over the juice of ½ lemon, then twist the edges of the foil together lightly. The foil envelope should be well sealed but baggy.

Put the parcel into the oven and cook as outlined below. For 8, you should have a salmon of about 2½kg, which is probably as big as you can get in your oven. I always put the foil parcel directly on the shelf, not having a tin big enough. I rely on my Aunt Fel's way, which is to cook the fish at this fairly low heat for 12 minutes per 500g. If you like your salmon fashionably orange in the middle, rather than flakey peachy pink, cut overall cooking time by about 15 minutes. I also pass on a tip from the fishmonger Steve Hatt, who reminds to make the join of the tin foil on the back of the fish so that you can quickly unwrap a bit and poke a knife in to see if the fish is coming away from the bone and is therefore ready.

When the salmon's had its time, remove from oven, unwrap the foil and leave it to cool in the opened parcel if it's to be eaten cold. If you're going to eat it hot, let it stand like that for 15 minutes and finish unwrapping and put it on its plate. Either way, surround the salmon with lemon quarters together with watercress if you're going in for a traditional look, otherwise you could supplement the lemon wedges (which are necessary, though of course don't need to be on the same plate as the fish) with rocket, mizuna or flat-leaf parsley. I am not much of a garnish queen, but there is something about an unadorned fish on its platter that makes it look beached.

If the salmon is to be eaten cold, which I do prefer, I might have it with tabbouleh (see page 260) not just to work against culinary expectations but

TABBOULEH

because they are wonderful together. But old pairings do work and I think of peas as going with salmon as much as I think of them partnering ham. My Great Aunt Myra, who was a wonderful cook, used to make a summer salad of peas, avocado and mint (very seventies) and turn to page 382 if you're interested. To go with the tabbouleh, though, just slice some fennel bulbs very, very thinly, drizzle over oil and squeeze over lemon. Add salt, pepper and the finely chopped aniseedy fronds that you removed before slicing. I love this almost medicinally pure taste against the oily denseness of the fish.

PEAS, AVOCADO, MINT

FENNEL, OIL, LEMON

I normally avoid too much same-colour food. However much I resist emphasis on the look, rather than the taste, of what you're eating, appearances do count for something. But all rules, all generalisations, culinary or otherwise, are to be challenged. Here I evince the culinary proof: the pudding I suggest, the almond sponge drenched in orange syrup, is exactly what you want, despite being a tonal echo of the course before; the recipe for it is on page 129.

I know how to observe the proprieties, mutter damply about the cold, exclaim with joy at the prospect of warmth and sun and dusty summer heat, but the truth is I love winter food, winter cooking best. I welcome it, and in January particularly when I make first sightings of early forced rhubarb, as pink as the sticks of Brighton rock my Granny gave me as a child.

WELCOMING JANUARY LUNCH FOR 6

Braised pheasant with mushroom and bacon

Pig's bum

This is such a wonderful winter lunch: in January the memory of all those slabs and plates of meat from Christmas is near enough to make one weepily grateful for a sweetly steamy bowl of stew. The pudding afterwards – as glorious as its name – is the result of a conversation I once had with Antony Worrall Thompson. I'd been, I think, recounting the gastronomic glories of rhubarb; he'd countered by telling me of a steamed pudding he'd had at prep school they always called pig's bum, because of the peculiar form and coloration of this stodgy rhubarb steamed sponge. I, understandably, was entranced. I have no idea how my version of this pudding measures up to his remembered original, my inspiration, but I have grown as fond of it as I could never become of any of the puddings I remember from the school lunches of my past.

The recipe for the pheasant stew is on page 114, and with it I'd have the burghal mentioned there, too; but since the steamed pudding that follows is actually rather light, you could wallow in a pile of buttery mashed potatoes first if you – quite understandably – wanted.

The pudding needs 2½ hours to cook, but you need do nothing to it while it's cooking, so don't regard this as a major problem. Besides, the pheasant stew can be made in advance, so you're hardly giving yourself a terrible Sunday morning in the kitchen.

PIG'S BUM

100g rhubarb, chopped into 4cm pieces
125g plus 1 tablespoon sugar
125g self-raising flour
125g very soft butter
2 eggs
1 heaped teaspoon baking powder
1 teaspoon pure vanilla extract
approx. 3 tablespoons milk

Butter a pudding basin (preferably one with a lid: you can get properly sealing plastic lidded basins which are perfect here) remembering to butter the inside of the lid too; if it hasn't got a lid, you will just have to wrap it all in foil later.

Put the rhubarb in a saucepan with the tablespoon of sugar and 100ml of water, bring to the boil and simmer, covered, over medium heat till it's cooked to a pulp – about 5 minutes. Drain and let cool. Put a full kettle on to heat up the water for steaming later.

Put all the remaining ingredients except for the milk into the food processor and mix till smoothly combined: you must see no lumps of butter, or indeed anything. Then add the rhubarb purée – you should have 4–5 tablespoons – and pulse quickly so that that, too, is combined in the sponge batter, though it doesn't matter if what you have is a pale yellow mixture shot through with strings of pink. If it's still a little stiff, add the milk, a tablespoonful at a time, until smooth and soft. Now dip a spoon in and lick: not because I think you need to add anything, but because the taste of this is better than almost anything; it reminds me of the boiled sweets I used to buy as a child, two-tone affairs called rhubarb and custard, that left the inside of my cheek rough with sugar-shock.

Anyway, pour the boiling water from the kettle into the bottom half of a steamer or just any big pan (in which case, you need the water to come about halfway up the pudding basin), put it on the heat and pour the mixture into the prepared basin. Put the lid on or cover with foil, then wrap all over with foil again, and really wrap, so no water can come in. When the water's boiling, lower the basin in, or set it above on the steamer. Cook for 2½ hours, making sure the water never runs dry or stops bubbling.

You do really need custard with this. How could you think otherwise? I normally like hot custard, but cold is right here. This makes life easier since you don't even have to think of fiddling about with it at the last minute. Turn to pages 35–7 for recipes.

From pig's bum to ham: it's an obvious step. I love ham, or rather gammon (though it doesn't seem to be called that any more), poached in water or cider and then its rind stripped off, the glutinous fatty wrapping underneath pressed with mustard and sugar, scored with a sharp knife and studded with cloves and then glazed in a hot oven. That was my mother's way. If poaching the ham, give it 30 minutes per 500g (see recipe on page 234) plus 30 minutes. When the ham's cooked, either way, strip it, score it (and I have only just worked out how to do this without burning my fingers – leave it to cool, the obvious and right thing to do) and then smear it with glaze before poking in cloves at the interstices of the criss-crossing diagonal slashes. My mother's glaze was simply a stiff paste made of English mustard powder, muscovado sugar and a drop or two of orange juice. Marguerite Patten suggests (in *Classic British Dishes*) a wonderfully malevolent-sounding glaze of black treacle blended with a little crushed pineapple (from a can, presumably) and sugar, which should keep the Hawaiian pizza brigade – and those who sneer at it – happy.

MUSTARD AND MUSCOVADO GLAZE

BLACK TREACLE AND PINEAPPLE

I am much taken with the American way of cooking a ham in Coca-Cola. In an age which solemnly tells you that cooking can produce food only as good as the ingredients that are provided (that's the whole history of French cuisine dispatched then), there is something robustly cheering about this dish. I'd be tempted to stick to the same idiom with pudding, too. By that I don't necessarily mean some sugary example of kitchen kitsch, but one of those unpretentious pies that Americans do so well.

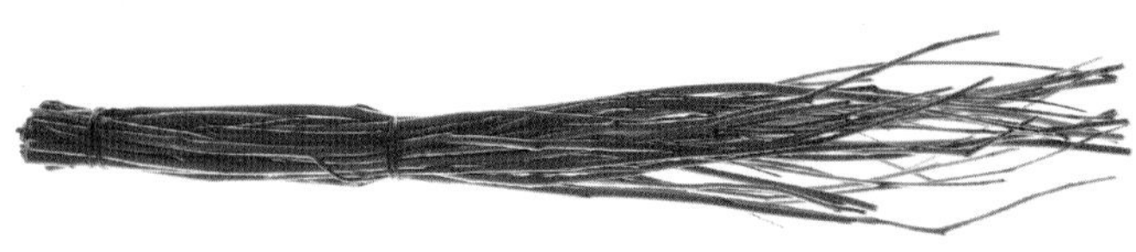

WHITE-TRASH LUNCH FOR 6

Ham in Coca-Cola

Parsley potato, mangetouts and petits pois

Cherry pie

HAM IN COCA-COLA

I cannot urge you to try this strongly enough. The first time I tried it, it was out of amused interest. I'd heard, and read, about this culinary tradition from the deep South, but wasn't expecting it, in all honesty, to be *good*. It is: I'm converted. I have to make myself cook gammon otherwise now; though often I don't bother with the glaze but just leave it for longer in the bubbling Coke instead. But, if you think about it, it's not surprising it should work: the sweet, spiky drink just infuses it with spirit of barbecue. Don't even think of using Diet Coke.

2kg mild-cure gammon
2 litres Coke minus 2 tablespoons (see below)
1 onion, peeled and cut in half
100g freshly made breadcrumbs (made from 4–5 pieces of bread)
100g dark muscovado sugar
1 tablespoon mustard powder
2 tablespoons Dijon mustard
2 tablespoons Coke

I find now, as I've said elsewhere, that mild-cure gammon doesn't need soaking. Follow instructions on page 234 should you need to extract excess salt. Otherwise, put the gammon in a pan, skin side down if it fits like that, add the onion, then pour over the Coke. Bring to the boil, reduce to a good simmer, put the lid on, though not tightly, and cook for just under 2½ hours. (Or, of course, work out timing based on weight of your joint, remembering that it's going to get a quick blast in the oven later. But do take into account that if the gammon's been in the fridge right up to the moment you cook it, you will have to give a good 15 or so minutes' extra cooking time so that the interior is properly cooked.)

Meanwhile preheat oven to gas mark 7/210°C.

When the ham's had its time (and ham it is now it's cooked, though it's true Americans call it ham from its uncooked state) take it out of the pan (do not throw away the cooking liquid) and let it cool a little for ease of handling. (Indeed you can let it cool completely then finish off the cooking at some later stage if you want.) Remove skin, leaving a thin layer of fat. Mix breadcrumbs, sugar and the mustards to a thick, stiff paste with the 2 tablespoons of Coke. Add a drop at a time because the one thing you don't want is a runny mixture. Slap the mustardy crust on the ham, and put it, crust-side up, on a roasting tray and cook in the hot oven for 10–15 minutes until the crust is just set.

Or if you want to do the braising stage in advance and then let the ham cool, give it 30–40 minutes, from room temperature, in a gas mark 4/180°C oven.

With this I'd have a large bowl of floury, large-chunked boiled potatoes, leafily covered with fresh chopped parsley, and I mean covered not sprinkled. But mashed potatoes are wonderful with this, too, truly. Any other vegetable just needs to be green and sprightly and have some crunch to it.

This ham, not surprisingly, is sensational cold, in sandwiches, and the cooking liquid makes a quick, no less fabulous, version of the South Beach black bean soup. I throw 500g of beans in the liquid, adding about 250ml water and the juice and zest of a lime. When cooked and puréed as usual, I eat with some more lime squeezed in, or some drops of balsamic vinegar stirred in, a dollop of smetana or somesuch, and a handful of earthily pungent, eye-searingly green, just-chopped coriander.

CHERRY PIE

My generation is, effectively, American-reared, so I suppose it's not surprising if we have a certain kitchen nostalgia for these foods we've never eaten, only seen in films or read in those exotically demotic stories and novels. And you don't get much more evocatively downhome than a cherry pie. If you were serious about such matters you'd be stoning the fresh cherries yourself, but apart from a brief burst of enthusiasm when I got a friend to bring over a cherry stoner with her when she came to visit, I stick to good bottled ones. Morello cherries in glass jars are just dandy: I'd think twice about using those tins of sweet and squishy black ones, but it could be done.

Serve à la mode – which is American for with ice-cream – or show Euro-cool by dolloping on some good and edgy and far more grown-up crème fraîche instead.

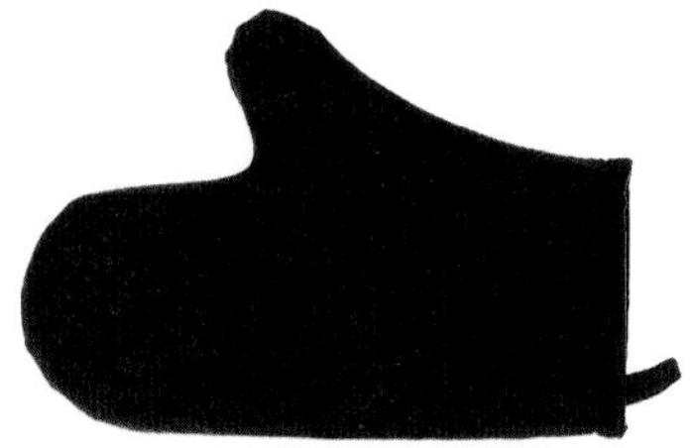

for the pastry
240g self-raising flour
120g butter, cold and diced
2 egg yolks beaten with ¼ teaspoon vanilla extract, pinch of salt and 2 tablespoons of iced water

for the filling
680g jar morello cherries in syrup
30g butter, melted
90g sugar
1 tablespoon flour, preferably Italian 00
1–2 tablespoons juice from drained cherries

Preheat the oven to gas mark 6/200°C. Put in a baking sheet to heat up.

Make the pastry according to instructions on page 42 and then divide into two discs (of about 225g each). Roll out 1 disc to line a 20cm shallowish pie plate. Drain the cherries; you should have about 400g. Make a paste with the melted butter, the sugar, flour and cherry liquid: it will be stiff not runny; the cherries will leak out more as they bake and you don't want soggy pastry.

Roll out the other disc, and then add the cherries and the paste to the pie dish. Moisten edges and top with remaining pastry. Cut off the overhang, crimp the edges and if you're up to it cut out some little cherries to decorate. Make a few slashes in the top with a sharp knife for the steam to escape and then put on the hot baking sheet in the preheated oven.

After 15 minutes, cover loosely with foil and turn down to gas mark 4/180°C and cook for another 18 minutes.

Remove, sprinkle with 1–2 tablespoons caster sugar and let cool for about 40 minutes before eating.

I am aware that the culinary spirit of the age is not ferociously carnivorous and that my blood-oozing joints of well-hung beef and fat-girdled pork risk offending modern quasi-vegetarian sensibilities. But I have wanted to concentrate on this sort of meat cookery simply because it seems to hold such unnecessary terrors for people now. There's enough written on pan-Asian stir-fries and Italo-Thai noodle dishes and you're unlikely to need any more, at least for the time being.

Of course I don't expect anyone to eat this sort of food every Sunday without fail – no one's telling you you can't have pasta, for God's sake – but the particular focus Sunday lunch offers is worth exploiting. For food like this, more than any other sort, is what cooking at home rather than eating in a restaurant is all about.

dinner

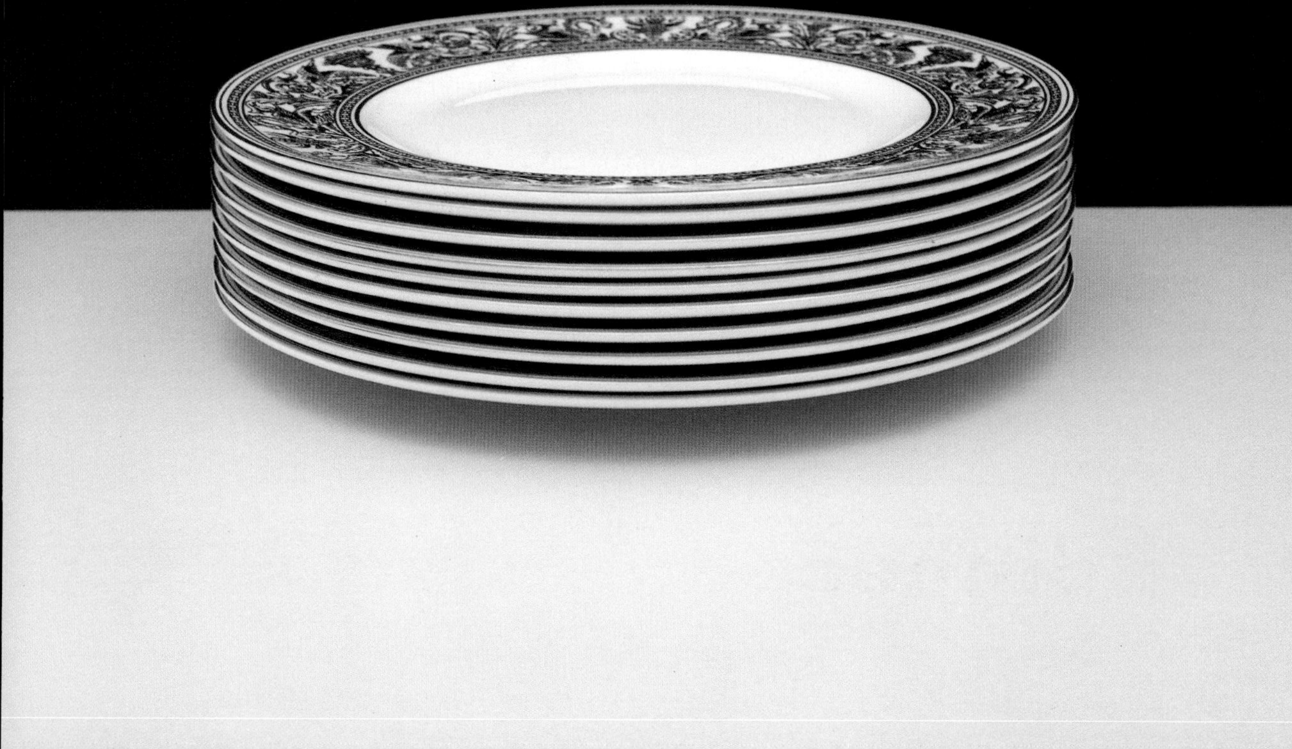

I'm not sure I like the connotations of the term Dinner Party, but I think we're stuck with it. Kitchen Suppers – which is perhaps what this chapter should be called – sounds altogether too twee, even if it evokes more accurately the culinary environment most of us now inhabit. So let's just call it dinner, which is what it is. The modern dinner party was the invention of the post-war, post-Elizabeth David brigade of socially aware operators: this was the age of Entertaining-with-a-capital-E. Not only was the food distinctly not home food, it wasn't even restaurant food: what was evoked was the great ambassadorial dinner. But *autres temps, autres moeurs*: most of us don't even have dining-rooms any more. Yet people still think they should be following the old culinary agenda: they feel it is incumbent on them not so much to cook as to slave, to strive, to sweat, to *perform*. Life doesn't have to be like that. As far as I'm concerned, moreover, it shouldn't be like that. I find formality constraining. I don't like fancy, arranged napkins and I don't like fancy, arranged foods.

That's not to say that I feel everything should be artfully casual: the this-is-just-something-I've-thrown-together school of cookery can be just as pretentious. What I feel passionately is that home food is home food, even when you invite other people to eat it with you. It shouldn't be laboriously executed, daintily arranged, individually portioned. It's relaxed, expansive, authentic: it should reflect your personality not your aspirations. Professional chefs have to innovate, to elaborate, to impress the paying customer. But the home cook is under no such constraints. (Indeed, you don't have to cook much at all if you are prepared to shop well.) I once went to a dinner party a good friend of mine gave, and she was so anxious, she'd been up till three in the morning the night before making stocks. She said scarcely a word to any of us after opening the door, since she was in the middle of the first of about five courses. The food was spectacular: but she spent most of the evening ever-more hysterical in the kitchen. At one point we could, as we stiltedly made conversation between ourselves, hear her crying. The fault wasn't her competence, but her conception: she felt that her dinner party must be a showcase for her culinary talents and

dinner

that we must all be judging her. Some cooks, indeed, seem to resent their guests for interrupting the cooking, rather as doctors and nurses resent patients for interrupting the nice, efficient running of their hospitals.

Restaurants need to be able to produce food in short order. But unless you want to stand in your kitchen handing hot plates out to your friends at the table, you need not and should not. Avoid small portions of tender-fleshed fish that have to be conjured up at the last minute and *à point*, and anything that will wilt, grow soggy or lose character or hope as it sits, sideboard-bound and dished up. Don't make life harder on yourself. I am working on banishing the starter from my dinner-partying life. (Truth to tell, I don't have much of a dinner-partying life: but, in theory, I do invite friends for dinner.) This is not so much because cooking the starter is difficult – in fact it is the easiest course of any of them – but because clearing the table, timetabling the whole meal, keeping the main course warm, can all add to the general tension of the evening.

Besides, our lives are so different now. Because working hours are longer, we eat dinner later. And if dinner doesn't start till nine or nine-thirty, then it is going to be a very late evening if you sit down to three courses. And you don't want to miss out on the general hanging around with a drink beforehand. I am more of an eater than a drinker and tend to get unbearably anxious if the drinking goes on for hours with no sign of the eating to come, so I try to amalgamate the two. I am, in effect, not really banishing the starter, but relocating it, refashioning it. Now, I can't pretend that serving bits with drinks is an original idea, but I suggest that you think of them as the starter. There is no dinner party I would give where I couldn't just make a plate of crostini to eat as a first course.

Normally, I make a couple of different sorts. I don't assemble the crostini in advance, but I often make the mixture with which they're going to be spread days ahead and keep slices for toast, ready-carved from baguette or ficelle, bagged up in the freezer.

CROSTINI

I reckon on getting about 40 usable slices from a ficelle and maybe 50 from a baguette, which seems to be longer as well as thicker. A baguette is commonly used for crostini, but I prefer the ficelle. I like its relative spindliness: the smaller rounds it makes mean you can eat crostini in one bite; and the string loaf seems to have a less tooth-resistant crust. But whichever loaf you're using, cut in straight-knifed rounds rather than diagonally, as usually advised, because it's easier to keep the slices compact and easy to eat that way.

To make the crostini, cut the loaves into slices about ½–¾cm in width. Let your instinct guide you; you probably know yourself just how thick or thin you want them to be. The crostini are no more than slices of bread dabbed with oil and toasted in a hottish oven. Preheat the oven to gas mark 6/200°C and, using a pastry brush or just your fingers, dip in oil and lightly cover each side of each slice of bread. I find 40 slices use up about 8 tablespoons of oil. And, unless specified below, always assume that olive oil (extra virgin, the usual specifications) is indicated. Put the oil-brushed slices on a rack in the oven for about 5–10 minutes. The length of time the bread takes to brown depends in part on how stale it was to start off with (and stale is good here). Turn the bread over as it turns pale gold. Remove when cooked and leave the uncrowned crostini somewhere to get cool. You should toast them no more than 2 hours before you eat them. Don't spread anything on them until wholly cold. And then you can put just about anything on top.

All the quantities below make enough for 20 crostini. I would make at least 5 per person, and probably 2 different kinds.

CHICKEN LIVER

This is your basic crostini, really, the Tuscan version of chopped liver. (Talking of which, if you want to be rakishly cross-cultural, I suppose you could, as the malapropism of a friend's Yiddish-speaking uncle has it, throw *kasha* to the winds and smear this stuff on toasted bagels instead.)

Use whatever grapey alcohol you want: vin santo, Marsala, muscat, white wine, vermouth or sherry. I've specified Marsala because it's what I keep nearest to me by the stove; I suspect a Tuscan would stipulate vin santo. Since you can buy this pretty easily now (depending, of course, on where you live) you could use some in the crostini and keep the rest for dinner: pour into glasses and give people those almond-studded *biscotti* known as *cantuccini* to dunk.

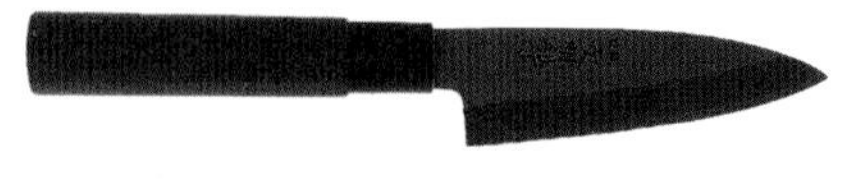

200g chicken livers
milk (enough to cover the livers)
1/3 stick celery
1 clove garlic, peeled
1 shallot, peeled, or 1 spring onion, chopped coarsely
approx. 1 heaped tablespoon chopped fresh flat-leaf parsley
2 tablespoons olive oil
1/2 tablespoon tomato purée
4 tablespoons Marsala (see above)
1 heaped teaspoon capers, rinsed, drained and chopped
2 anchovy fillets, wiped and chopped
1 tablespoon butter

Remove any bits of green or gristle you can see in the chicken livers, then put them in a dish and pour over milk to cover. Leave for about 10 minutes. Put the celery, garlic, shallot (or spring onion) and parsley into the processor and chop finely, or do it by hand. Heat the oil in a thick-bottomed pan (I find a shape somewhere between a frying pan and a saucepan the most useful here) and add the vegetable mix. Cook at low to moderate heat, stirring regularly, for about 5 minutes, perhaps slightly longer, until soft but not coloured. Drain the chicken livers, wipe them dry with kitchen towel and chop them; use a knife or mezzaluna, not the processor. Add them to the pan and cook, prodding, pushing and stirring with your wooden spoon or spatula until that characteristic claret-stained rawness has disappeared; they should still, however, be pink and moussey within. Stir in the tomato purée and cook, stirring, for a minute or so before adding the Marsala. Let this bubble mostly away, then taste and add salt and a good few grindings of pepper as needed. Turn down the heat and let cook gently for another 10 minutes or so.

Then decant the contents of the pan into the bowl of the food processor, add the capers and anchovies and give the merest pulse: you want this chopped but not puréed. (You could always use a knife.) Pour back into the pan with the butter and cook for a few final minutes at gentle heat while you stir. Remove from the heat and let cool before spreading. Sprinkle some more parsley over, once spread.

DUCK LIVERS

Forgo the capers and anchovies, but add instead, at the beginning with the celery mixture, the very finely chopped zest of ½–1 orange. And I use Grand Marnier, either in place of the Marsala, or half-and-half, with a spritz of the orange's juice.

PEA AND GARLIC

I warm to the Day-Glo vibrancy of this concoction; just like the future, so bright you gotta wear shades. But it is seriously good: the sweet pungency of the roasted garlic gives resonance and depth; the parmesan supplies edge and the butter unctuousness. And it's a doddle to make. This amount will give enough for a few extra crostini.

1 head garlic
1 teaspoon olive oil
200g frozen petits pois
1 tablespoon butter
2 tablespoons freshly grated parmesan

Preheat the oven to gas mark 6/200°C. Lop the top off the head of garlic: you want to see the tops of the cloves just revealed in cross section. Cut a square of foil, large enough to make a baggy parcel around the garlic, sit the garlic in the middle of it, drizzle over the oil and then make said parcel, twisting the ends slightly. Put in the oven for 50 minutes to an hour until the garlic is soft.

Cook the peas in boiling salted water as you would normally, only for a fraction longer. Drain and tip into the bowl of the food processor. Squeeze out the soft, cooked cloves of garlic and add them, then the butter and parmesan. Process to a nubbly but creamy purée. Cool before spreading. Sprinkle with mint.

ROAST PEPPER WITH GREEN OLIVE PASTE

If you find the charring and skinning of the peppers too labour-intensive for the effort-sparing strategy of the drinks-accompanying starter, buy them in from a good Italian deli. I buy the Merchant Gourmet green olive paste, spread that on the toast first, and top with a soft tangle of peppers, their skins already burnt off by someone else. If you do want to do your own, you'll need 2 red and 2 yellow peppers; see page 96 for the method. In either case, sprinkle with chopped parsley.

GORGONZOLA WITH MASCARPONE AND MARSALA

Marsala with gorgonzola is a translation of the British tradition of mixing port with stilton. The nutmeg and mascarpone sweeten and blunt the pungency of the gorgonzola; even those who think they don't like blue cheese find this gratifyingly edible. If you're fed up with Marsala, use white port – my mother always kept a decanter of this in the dining-room, and so I have a peculiar nostalgia for it.

This is the easiest crostini topping I can think of. When I make the little toasts, I sometimes anoint them with walnut rather than olive oil.

120g gorgonzola piccante
40g mascarpone
2 tablespoons Marsala
good grating fresh nutmeg
freshly chopped parsley

Put the gorgonzola, chopped, in a bowl with the mascarpone and the Marsala and mash together using a fork. Add a good grating or two of fresh nutmeg and stir again. Cover the bowl with clingfilm and put in the fridge until you need it, but remember to take it out a good ½ hour before you do, to make it easier to spread.

I sprinkle with flat-leaf parsley; a friend of mine tried it with half a slim muscat grape on top: a bit close to the cheesy pineapple of *Abigail's Party*, but good none the less.

LENTIL AND BLACK OLIVE

This looks good on a plate with the paler gorgonzola crostini, above. The idea is adapted from the glorious recipe for black hummus in *Recipes 1-2-3* by Rozanne Gold and is, in effect, just a purée of cooked puy lentils and bought tapenade – I use Merchant Gourmet's black olive paste – with a spoonful of Cognac added. Remember that although it looks suitable for vegetarians it isn't: the tapenade contains anchovies.

60g puy lentils
6 black peppercorns
3 tablespoons tapenade/black olive paste
1 teaspoon Cognac
5 cherry tomatoes
fresh parsley or chives

To make the purée, put the lentils in a saucepan with a generous pinch of sea salt and the peppercorns. Pour over about 500ml cold water and bring to the boil. When boiling, turn down the heat, cover and simmer for 35 minutes, or until the lentils are soft. Drain the lentils, reserving 75ml of the cooking liquid. Let cool for 15 minutes.

Then all you do is put the lentils in the bowl of the food processor with the black olive paste and process until fairly smooth, adding 40–75ml cooking liquid, as needed, to make a spreadable (but still nubbly) paste. Try 2 tablespoons first and then see how you're doing. Remove to a bowl, stir in the Cognac and leave to cool. Cover and stick in the fridge – for days on end, if you like. You might need to add salt, or it might taste very salty, but don't be alarmed: on the toasts and with blanched, peeled and diced tomato and chopped parsley (or chives) dotted on top, it will all mellow and come together.

MUSHROOMS

Get a mixture of wild and cultivated mushrooms from your local greengrocer or buy a supermarket packet of them. If you want to save time, instead of chopping the garlic you can fry the mushrooms in garlic-infused oil.

200g mixed mushrooms
leaves from a couple of sprigs thyme, or pinch dried
1 fat clove garlic
2 tablespoons olive oil
scant tablespoon freshly grated parmesan
flat-leaf parsley

Wipe and then finely chop the mushrooms; I use my mezzaluna here, as I do for finely chopping the thyme and garlic. Pour the olive oil into a pan and when still cold add the minced garlic and thyme. On the heat, cook for about 1 minute, then add the mushrooms, stir and cook until soft and fragrant, and then stir in the parmesan. Salt and pepper robustly to taste. This is best spread while still just warm, sprinkled with flat-leaf parsley. You can put it all in the processor to make a coarsely chopped mixture (easier to spread) but make sure you don't make a purée.

PRAWN AND AUBERGINE

This is not as fiddly as it might sound, since all you do to the aubergine is bake it (if you're making the garlic and pea crostini, you can roast the garlic for that at the same time), and there aren't enough prawns to make peeling them a nightmare. The aubergine tempers the heat of the pepper-spiked prawns, and makes them more spreadable. I get the prawns from the fishmonger or the fish counter of my local supermarket.

1 medium aubergine
1 tablespoon olive oil
1 fat clove garlic, chopped or sliced finely
1 dried red chilli pepper
150g raw tiger prawns, headless but unpeeled
fresh coriander or Thai basil

Preheat the oven to gas mark 6/200°C.

Put the aubergine into the oven, straight on the rack and bake for 1 hour by which time it should be soft-fleshed and cooked. Remove and leave till cool enough to handle, which won't be long. Put a sieve over a bowl and scrape the flesh of the aubergine into the sieve so that it drains. Let it stand there until it's cool, by which time it should be dry and all the excess liquid should be in the bowl.

Put the oil into a heavy-bottomed pan, add the slivered garlic and crumble in the dried red chilli pepper. Turn in the heat for 2 minutes, then throw in the prawns and stir around the hot pan until the livid-grey carapace turns holiday coral: 2 minutes and they should be cooked but still tender. Remove from the heat and, as soon as you possibly can, peel them. Put everything – except the shells – into the bowl of a processor; you really need a mini one for such small amounts. When the prawns are chopped, add the dry aubergine pulp and give another pulse. You need something spreadable but not smooth. Spread onto toasts when you want to eat, and sprinkle with just-chopped coriander. If you were to have any Thai holy basil in the house, that would do fabulously in place of the coriander.

BEANS WRAPPED IN PROSCIUTTO

One doesn't want to wade too deep into canapé land, but I would feel I was doing less than my duty if I didn't faithfully report my other most-relied-upon starter-stand-in: beans wrapped in prosciutto. I saw these little bundles of French beans tied around the middle with Parma ham in the Holland Park Italian delicatessen, Speck, and went straight back home and made my own. Top and tail some French beans and cook them in boiling salted water. Remember that French beans need decent cooking, not mere dunking in hot water. Drain them, wait for them to cool, dip them in balsamic vinegar, then cut the raggedy thin slices of Parma ham in strips and tie them round the bean-bundles.

You may take it for granted that whatever starter I suggest, you can always whip it away and provide the crostini or the fascist beans – I refer to their bundling only: there's no darker connotation here – in their place. I won't say that again. The following menus and recipes are merely suggestions, ideas for you to work on, ignore, play around with as you like. There's no right answer, nor one way only to organise a dinner, compose the food. But at least being shown one path gives you the freedom to study the terrain and choose another.

That choice might often mean not cooking at all, or very little. No one, for example, ever *has* to make a pudding. I am more than happy to get some perfect creation from the pâtissier, to buy ice-cream and good biscuits. But the relatively low effort needed to make any sweet thing will be repaid in gratifying disproportion by the pleasure of your guests. I propose only: you dispose or not, as you wish.

My menus, or sketches-for menus, often give alternatives, an easier route or different seasonal choice. The reasons are simple, but important. Sometimes we've got hours in which to cook, sometimes we haven't, it's as simple as that, and I wanted to show how speediness can be accommodated into a menu without ditching the whole thing. I wanted to show, too, why I thought one starter went with the particular main course, and how those principles or sensory judgements remain true even if their application is somewhat different. Thinking aloud seems to me the best way to offer direction, a sort of enthusiastic culinary companionship, without, I hope, being insufferably bossy. If I were in the kitchen with you, or you with me, these are the things we'd be talking about.

I make a distinction between dinners and kitchen suppers, but it is a slim one. At no time will you find me fiddling about with table decorations or doing clever things with the lighting. But there is a difference between a structured plan to bring people together over food, and just having the usual suspects round after work. I don't get up at five in the morning to buy bucketloads of flowers from the market (and people do, you know) but I do want things to look beautiful. Cheaper than flowers, and more useful because it doesn't interfere with people's line of vision as they're sitting at table trying to talk to each other, is to use food rather in the manner of a still life. A bowl heaped with lemons or limes will always look beautiful. Aubergines, either those skin-stretched vast glossy ones, or the compact, Middle-Eastern purplish babies, look fabulous. As I've said, I don't like bowls of mixed things, but sometimes I have on the table a plate or low bowl of pomegranates mixed with pale, bark-coloured dried figs, their once-red interiors just showing through the split skin, like spiky-toothed gums stained an orange-scarlet with Airfix paint.

Since I am not a vegetarian, I don't ever purposefully arrange a totally meatless and fish-free three-course dinner. And no vegetarian needs tips on meat-free cooking from a committed carnivore like me. But if you want to cater for vegetarians and suchlike, you need to make sure there is food they can eat, without designing the dinner around them. I deal with it by having a vegetable starter (which I do often enough, anyway), soup or salad, say, and then I provide the vegetarian with a plate of wild mushrooms cooked with butter (olive oil for vegans) and garlic and thyme while everyone else eats their main course. The advantage is that a thick dark stew of mushrooms is easy to do while you're getting on with the starter, or before, and can sit in the pan to be reheated when it's needed. And it goes well, without adaptation, with the potatoes and vegetables you'll no doubt be doing anyway. The difficulty with doing vegetarian pasta of some sort is that it sets the eater entirely apart, but with the mushrooms she, or he, has just one different component.

JOHN ARMIT'S WINE RECOMMENDATIONS

There's no need to make a big song and dance about what you drink with what, but I wanted to offer something good in the way of guidance. Following each menu, then, are brief notes by that distinguished but relaxed wine merchant, John Armit. He begins:

In general I have chosen one wine, although you could always choose to have two, say a white with the starter and a red with the main course. Many people would also choose a pudding wine: a muscat or a Sauternes from France, or a sweet German wine.

WINTER DINNER, WITH SUMMER POSSIBILITIES, FOR 6

Caesar salad

Loin of pork with bay leaves, and lentils or cannellini beans

Rhubarb: either in ice-cream, custard, jelly or trifle

This is perfect in January, when the rhubarb is new, trim-limbed and Barbie pink: how you cook it, eat it, is up to you. I have tried to limit my suggestions, but not that hard; I want still to urge you rhubarbwards. This menu works too in summer, when the rhubarb may be nearer khaki-coloured and have slightly more spreading thighs, but will still have that peculiar mixture between delicacy and resonance. In summer I'd cook the pork maybe slightly in advance, and leave it to cool for an hour before slicing it thickly and arranging it on a large, oval plate.

CAESAR SALAD

In my years as a restaurant critic I railed against the messed-about Caesar salad. So many chefs want to do their bit – to shave the cheese rather than grate it, so you lose that fabulous leaf-thickening coating, to throw in whole fresh anchovies, to substitute designer lettuce – and every addition is a loss. Perfection cannot be improved upon. And so what am I doing here, replacing the classic garlic croûtons with small cubes of garlicky roast potatoes? Well, I do this because this is how it happened. Let me explain.

The first time I made the ceviche (see page 348) for dinner one summer, I thought it might be wonderful with some hot and salty croûton-sized, roast, diced potatoes. Reader: I was not wrong. After that, and because anything that's in the oven gives me less grief than anything ever does on the hob, I took to roasting small dice of potatoes and using them in place of croûtons in salads all the time. I get a freezer bag, put in the potatoes unpeeled but diced, about 1cm square, maybe slightly smaller sometimes, throw chopped garlic after them and then add 2 tablespoons olive oil. (When I'm in a hurry, I forget the garlic and use garlic-infused oil instead.) I shake the bag about so that the oil disperses and covers all the cubes of potato, empty them into a tray and then roast them for 45 minutes to 1 hour in a gas mark 6/200°C oven. When they're glistening brown, I take them out of the tin, lay them on some kitchen towel and sprinkle with coarse sea salt. Then I chuck them into some dressed, tossed leaves: and, let me tell you, that's all you need.

As I said, a Caesar salad is perfect in its original incarnation, but if you add potatoes in place of the croûtons for a first-course Caesar salad, you won't need to bother with potatoes for the main course. So that's one less thing to worry about or find hob or oven space for: lentils or cannellini are both vegetable and filler.

This then is what I call, in my notes, *Caesar, mia*.

If you want to add anchovies – which aren't actually a feature of Caesar Cardini's original version, but are so often used they almost count as authentic, and are certainly good in it – just mash one or two up with the olive oil before anointing and tossing the salad.

250g potatoes, diced

2–3 large cloves garlic

6 tablespoons, approx., extra virgin olive oil, or 4 of olive and 2 of garlic-infused oil

2 eggs

4–6 heads baby cos lettuce or 2–3 normal-sized cos
few drops Worcestershire sauce
juice of 1 lemon
30g freshly grated parmesan, probably about 6 tablespoons

Make the croûtons of diced potatoes with garlic and oil as above. You don't want them to go on the salad when searingly hot: so cool on some kitchen towel for about 10 minutes.

Put some water on for the eggs, put a matchstick into the pan (this stops the white flowing out if the shell cracks) and then, when boiling, lower in the eggs and boil for exactly 1 minute. Remove and set aside.

Tear the leaves into eatable sizes and toss with 3–4 tablespoons olive oil to coat well but lightly. Sprinkle over a pinch of salt, several grinds of pepper and toss again. Shake over 6 drops Worcestershire sauce, squeeze on the lemon juice, break in the eggs and toss to blend. Taste for seasoning. Toss with the cheese and then with the potato croûtons at the very last minute, as you bring it to the table – no sooner or it will wilt.

LOIN OF PORK WITH BAY LEAVES

If you've got time, leave the pork in its marinade-rub for 12 or even 24 hours. But otherwise, just do the necessary when you get home in the evening. By roasting the pork at gas mark 6/200°C you can accommodate both croûtons and meat. You want the loin boned and rindless but with a very thin layer of fat still on, and tied at regular intervals. That's why I go to the butcher. And ask him to chop the bones and give them to you to take home while he's about it. The boned, derinded weight of a 2½kg joint should be about 1.8kg.

6 tablespoons extra virgin olive oil
4 cloves garlic, bruised and crushed with the flat side of a knife
6 peppercorns, bruised
6 dried or fresh bay leaves, crumbled, or 2 teaspoons ground
2½kg loin of pork, boned, derinded and rolled (1.8kg oven-ready weight)
1 medium onion
16 more dried or fresh bay leaves, whole
150ml white wine

In a small bowl mix the olive oil, garlic, salt, peppercorns, crumbled or ground bay and a teaspoon of, preferably, rock salt and then put the pork on a large dish or in a large polythene bag, and rub the mixture all over the meat. Cover the dish or tie up the bag and leave in the fridge if you've got steeping time, otherwise – if you're about to start cooking it – just leave it out.

Preheat the oven to gas mark 6/200°C. Finely slice a peeled medium onion and line the roasting tray with it. Strew about 10 bay leaves over the onion. Place the pork, including its marinade, on top and the bones all around, if they fit and if you've got them. Roast in the oven for 1¾ hours, basting regularly.

Remove the pork, scraping burnt bits off, to a plate or carving board and let it sit. On the hob at moderate heat, pour about 150ml wine and 150ml boiling water over the bones, bay, garlic and onion. Let it bubble up and reduce by about a third, and then remove the bones gingerly and strain the liquid contents into a saucepan. Heat, taste, and add liquid as you like to make a good, thin, not-quite gravy.

You can carve, put the slices on a big warmed plate, sprinkle with salt and pour over a little of the juice-gravy, then tent with foil and leave in the turned-off oven while you eat the starter. It is a bit prinky, I know, but it will look fabulous if, when you take it out, you arrange, Napoleonically, some more bay leaves around the edges of the dish with the bay-scented pork.

PUY LENTILS OR CANNELLINI BEANS

Puy lentils or cannellini beans, or indeed any pulses, would do with this. The lentils have the advantage of not needing to be soaked. And I would leave them pretty plain: for 6 people, if it's the only vegetable, just use 500g. Cover with abundant water then bring to the boil, add salt, and simmer for 30–45 minutes. Drain, put the pan back on the heat with some oil (not too much, though, you'll have the meat-juice gravy to pour over later) together with 2 cloves garlic, minced or sliced, and the finely chopped zest of ½ lemon. Turn in the warm oil for a minute or so, then put the lentils back in and toss well, tasting for salt and pepper as usual. Treat soaked pulses similarly, only they'll need longer cooking (you won't get arrested for using canned, but I can't pretend they're as good) and I'd omit the lemon zest and add a little more garlic. Sprinkle over some chopped parsley when they're in their serving dish.

Now for the rhubarb. Even in winter I love this rhubarb ice-cream. It's not just the taste – which is delicate scented perfection – but its very extraordinariness, its almost exotic rarity, which is all the more distinctive for the markedly unexotic nature of its chief ingredient. Now that you can buy so much good ice-cream in the shops, it often seems hardly worth making your own, but this one you couldn't buy. If you haven't got an ice-cream maker (not that ice-cream is impossible without, see page 282) then make the rhubarb custard. To call this an invention would be pushing it, but it is one of my favourite culinary accidents. It came about simply because I was stewing some rhubarb and forgot about it. I felt I really had to do something with the ensuing, practically formless pulp, so I stirred it into some eggs, sugar and milk, poured it into a dish, put that dish in a tin of water and baked it. The result was ambrosial. And typically, because I'd done this as a last-minute damage-limitation exercise I hadn't any precise idea of the ratio of rhubarb to custard. I had to do it three more times before I got it to taste as good as it had the first accidental time. Take it out of the oven about 1 hour before you want to eat it. This really does mean you could do with a double oven if you're eating the pork hot. But you could always bake the custard first: it won't really be warm, but it shouldn't be cool, either.

My rhubarb and muscat jelly is, in a different way, a kitchen accident as well. I'd been making some rhubarb fool, and ended up with half a jugful of excess pink syrup: I decided to make a jelly out of it; muscat seemed like a good idea (and see below). This, in turn, led to the rhubarb, muscat and mascarpone trifle (and refer, you must, to page 121). The last of my suggestions here is the rhubarb meringue pie on page 258; but look up rhubarb in the index if you're up for more.

RHUBARB ICE-CREAM

I can't pretend this is the easy option. If you want to make something simple, cook the rhubarb as below, but just stir it into some whipped double cream and make fool instead.

If you've got vanilla sugar, then use that, otherwise you can add a vanilla pod, halved lengthways, to the rhubarb as you cook it or just stir in a teaspoon or so of best vanilla extract before you freeze the rhubarb–cream–custard mix. And if you're using summer rhubarb, which won't make the perfect blush-pink cream of the early growth, nothing's to stop you adding the merest pin-drop of pink food colouring.

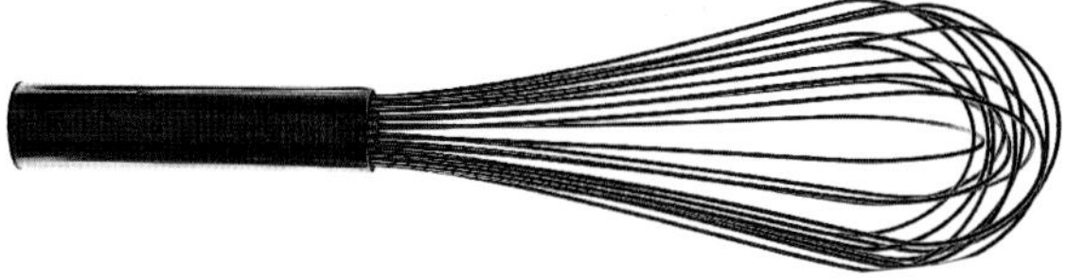

1kg rhubarb (untrimmed weight)
300g vanilla or caster sugar
284ml carton single cream
3 egg yolks
45g caster sugar
284ml carton double cream
approx. 5 tablespoons caster sugar, or more to taste

Preheat the oven to gas mark 5/190°C. Trim the rhubarb and put it in a dish with the 300g sugar. Cover with foil and bake in the oven for 45 minutes to an hour until utterly soft and cooked. If you cook it on the hob, the colour won't stay as bright. Drain, reserving juice, and put the pulp in a bowl to cool. Beat well with a fork so it's smooth.

Put the single cream on to boil, but take off the heat just before it does. Pour it over the egg yolks beaten with the 45g sugar. Half-fill the sink with cold water (this is because you need to stop the custard cooking as soon as it's thickened) and then get on with the custard, by putting the yolk–sugar–cream mixture into a clean pan on lowish heat. Stir with a wooden spoon *constantly*. In about 10 minutes the custard should have thickened (see page 36 if you need more information here). Plunge the pan into the cold water in the sink and carry on stirring energetically for a minute or so. When it's cool, stir in the rhubarb pulp. Then whip the double cream and add to the fruit custard. Taste: you may well need more sugar; add 1 tablespoon at a time, but remember when the mixture's frozen the sweetness will seem reduced. Add vanilla here, too, if you haven't done anything with vanilla earlier.

Freeze in an ice-cream maker, or see page 37.

For some reason this is fabulous with really good bitter chocolate biscuits, or else those plain discs of dark thin chocolate. As for the rhubarb cooking liquid: add a slug or two of muscat (or sugar and water) and boil down till you've got a thick syrup, pour into a small jug and let people dribble it over their ice-cream; or freeze, unreduced, and make jelly with it later.

RHUBARB CUSTARD

100g sugar
1kg rhubarb
100ml water
4 eggs
4 egg yolks
75g vanilla sugar (or caster sugar and vanilla pod or extract)
600ml full-fat milk

Trim the rhubarb, and chop into approx. 3cm slices. Put in a large pan with the water and 100g sugar. Put the lid on and bring to the boil. In about 5 minutes you should have pulp. Pour it into a strainer over a bowl or jug to catch juice, but don't push through the strainer.

Preheat the oven to gas mark 3/160°C. Put the kettle on. Sit an ovenproof dish with a capacity of about 1¼ litres (I use one of those oval cream stoneware dishes, the sort that rhubarb custard was just meant to be in) in a baking tray. In another bowl, beat the eggs, egg yolks and vanilla sugar together with a fork. If you haven't got vanilla sugar, use more caster sugar and add a vanilla pod to the milk and let it steep or just add 1 teaspoon of best and purest vanilla extract to the custard before stirring in the rhubarb. Taste for sweetness.

Put the milk on to boil, but don't actually let it boil. Still beating with a fork, add the milk. When combined, stir in the well-drained rhubarb. Do this gently: you don't want an all-rose affair, but a pale, yellowing parchment cream shot through with that gloweringly intense taffeta pink. Pour into the dish and pour the hot water around the dish, to come around halfway up.

Put in the oven and bake for 45 minutes to 1 hour. When done, remove from pan of water. Check by touching the top: it should be quivering but not liquid. It will continue to set as it stands in the kitchen waiting to be eaten.

RHUBARB AND MUSCAT JELLY

This is spectacular: it's beautiful when the poached rhubarb, fresh out of the oven, sits in its orange-flecked juices; and just so pretty, when it's set and shining and the sweetest dusky rose pink. But because of that colour, don't set it in a ring mould: it makes it look slightly gynaecological. I use an old-fashioned, bulbously curving castle mould. You can get them now made in plastic which is easier to demould than the old copper ones.

When Marks & Spencer sells its beautifully pink prepared rhubarb in 400g packets, I buy a couple of those in place of the 1kg itemised below. When the new season's rhubarb comes in, clementines and satsumas are available, so I often, in place of the orange, just halve one of either, squeeze in the juice by hand and then throw in the consequently crushed and pulpy peel. Blood oranges are, however, best. They intensify the already vivid tints.

If you're nervous about using gelatine (from a practical rather than health or dietary perspective) then the chances are the only gelatine you've ever used is the powdered sort. God knows how anyone can make that work: I always end up with a flabby and collapsing interior margined by a very sandy hard shoulder. Leaf gelatine is the answer (for stockists see page 506). Working on the basis of 4 leaves per scant 600ml (or 1 per 150ml), leave the gelatine leaves to soak in a shallow dish of cold water for 5 minutes, then squeeze them out and beat them in the warm (not boiling) syrup-and-jelly-to-be till it dissolves.

As for the wine: of course use whichever muscat you like; I commonly make this with Frontignan.

1kg rhubarb
340g caster sugar
500ml water
juice and zest of 1 orange
approx. 300ml muscat
8 leaves gelatine

Preheat the oven to gas mark 5/190°C.

Chop the rhubarb into 2–3cm chunks and put into a large ovenproof dish. I find a rectangular one, measuring 30cm x 20cm and 5cm deep, perfect for the job. Sprinkle over the sugar, add the orange juice and zest and the water and cover, either with a lid or with foil. Bake for 1 hour. Take out of the oven, remove lid and let cool.

Strain carefully into a measuring jug: I find this gives about 700ml. Put the pulp aside (you can freeze it for use in the custard or trifle), pour muscat into the juice to make it up to 900ml. Taste: you may want some more sugar or a squeeze more orange or, indeed, more muscat. Remember to add more gelatine if you make more liquid.

Lightly oil a 2-pint jelly mould (I give you it in imperial because they still seem to be made in old measures) by dabbing a kitchen towel in some suitably flavourless oil and then rubbing it over the interior of the mould. Soak 8 gelatine leaves in a dish of cold water until softened. Put 2 ladlefuls of rhubarb and muscat syrup in a saucepan and heat up. Take off the heat, though, before it boils. Squeeze out the gelatine leaves and whisk into the syrup. When they've dissolved pour the contents of the pan back into the jug. If you want to make sure everything's well enough mixed you can pour from jug to pan and back into the jug again. Pour into the jelly mould and place in the fridge to chill and set.

A South African Sauvignon, which is not as austere as the French, and not as obvious as the New Zealand, would be perfect here.

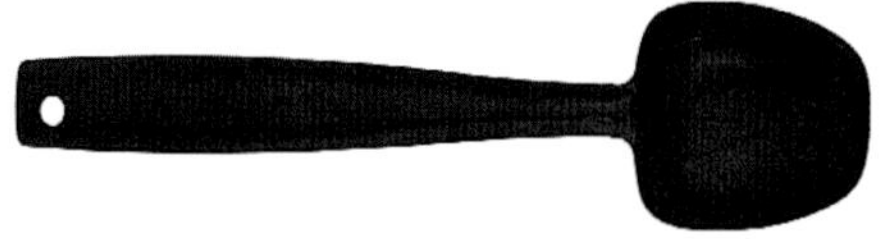

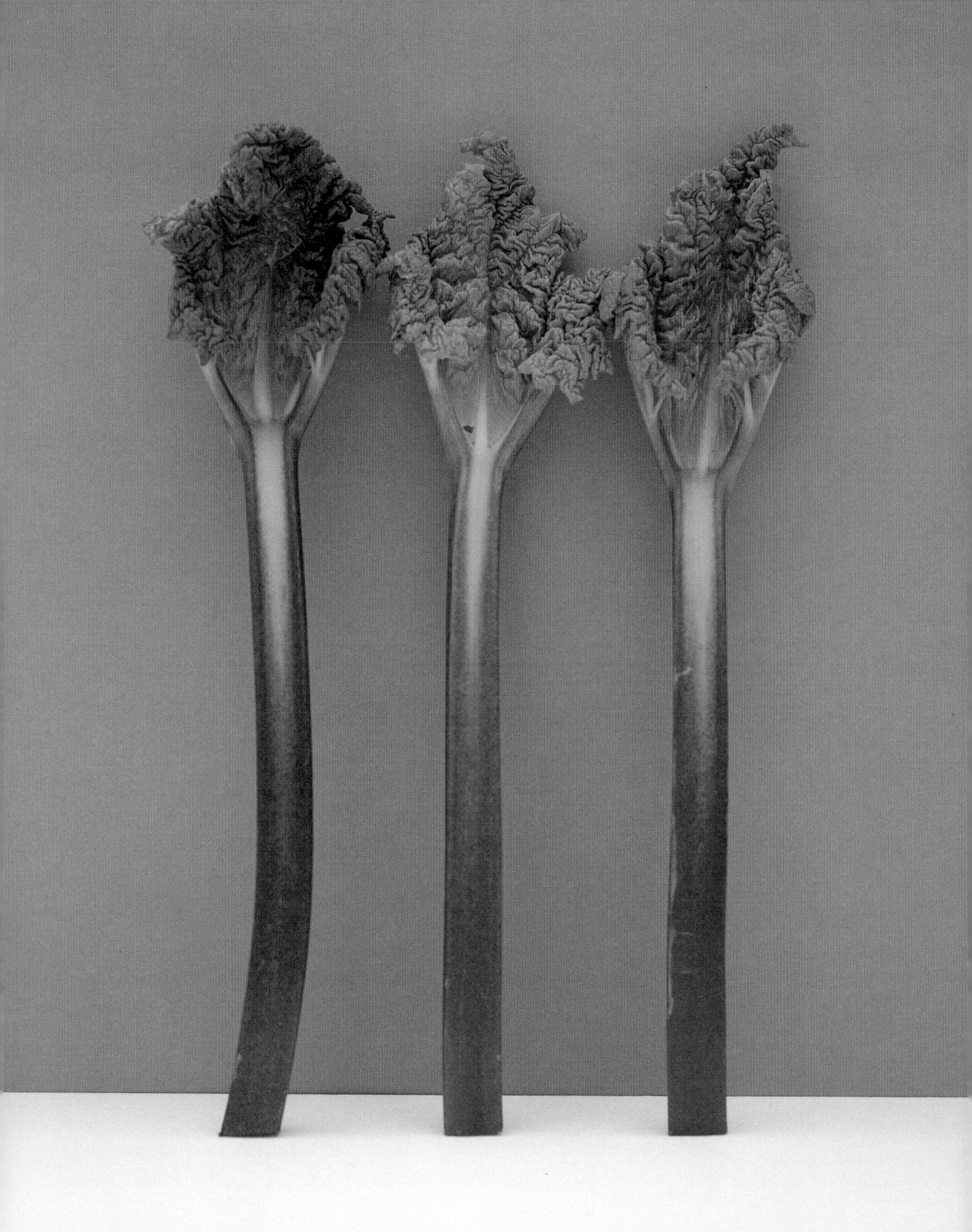

EXTRAVAGANT BUT STILL ELEGANT DINNER FOR 8

Hot sausages with ice-cold oysters, or ceviche with hot garlic potatoes

The tenderest chicken, with green salad and garlic potatoes

Chocolate raspberry pudding cake with raspberries and Greek yoghurt

This is the sort of dinner I dream of: the perfect birthday dinner party for someone who likes oysters and whose birthday (like mine) falls on a suitable date. You can get oysters all the year round now (or some types) but they're still best in winter. Buy an oyster knife at the same time as your oysters: 6 per person. Ask the fishmonger for proper instructions as to cleaning (if necessary) and opening. And you'll need either coarse salt or crushed ice to sit them on. I used to eat oysters and sausages at Alastair Little's first, eponymous, restaurant in Frith Street. He served the most inspired starter in town: cold, cold oysters with hot spicy Chinesey sausages.

My way is to get cocktail sausages (smaller than chipolatas) from my butcher, and then roll them in a roasting tin in chilli oil to spice. If the chilli oil isn't ferociously hot, add some drops of tabasco. Cook them for about 50 minutes in a gas mark 6/200°C oven. Fabulous. But don't forget finger bowls. Cooking them in the oven is the easiest way, but if that creates problems with the chicken, cook the sausages in a pan on the hob.

If you baulk at oysters, replace this course with something that strikes some of the same notes, such as some ceviche, in which the cold, soft flesh of the fish is offset by some searingly hot and salty croûton-sized cubes of garlicky roast potatoes. If you're making this potato-spiked ceviche, you will have to miss out the potatoes with the chicken.

CEVICHE WITH HOT GARLIC POTATOES

Ceviche – fish which is 'cooked' by the acids of a citrus marinade – is about as effortless as you can get. Often, the fish is served with avocado, but I feel that the texture somehow is both too samey and too squashy. I prefer it like this.

The recipe lists turbot, scallops and salmon, but you could use a cheaper combination of fish if you wanted (the salmon, which is farmed, is the cheapest ingredient here). You must, anyway, get the fish from a fishmonger not a supermarket and explain that you will be eating it raw. The fishmonger will tell you which fish are fresh enough and suitable. And don't be put off by the idea of raw fish: it does actually taste – and look – cooked by the marinade.

325g very fresh salmon
275g very fresh turbot
4 very fresh scallops
juice of 3 limes
juice of 2 1/2 lemons
juice of 1 orange
1 tablespoon plus 1 teaspoon balsamic vinegar
325g new potatoes
4 tablespoons olive oil or 2 of olive oil and 2 of garlic-infused oil
3 cloves garlic
1 packet cleaned watercress
fresh coriander for garnish

Slice the fish into strips about 4–5cm by 1–2cm. Cut the scallops into 3 thin discs each and chop the corals or leave whole, or indeed leave out, as you wish. Put in a large dish, cover with the citrus juices and balsamic vinegar and leave in the fridge for at least 6 hours. Before you want to eat, chop the new potatoes up into small chunks much the size of croûtons (in effect you are treating the potatoes as if they *were* croûtons) and then put in a plastic bag with 2 tablespoons of the oil and the cloves of garlic (or garlic-infused oil only), which you have smashed with a pestle and mortar or chopped finely. Put in a roasting tray in a preheated oven, gas mark 6/200°C for about 40 minutes or until brown and crisp.

While the potatoes are cooking, put the watercress on a large plate, take the fish out of its marinade and arrange it on top. Take out 3 tablespoons of the marinade, put in a cup and stir in 1 tablespoon oil and make a dressing (add more oil if you like) to pour over the creviche and watercress. At the last minute, sprinkle some salt on the potatoes and toss them over the watercress and amongst the fish. Chop up some coriander and sprinkle on top.

THE TENDEREST CHICKEN

The title tells no lie. The buttermilk marinade stops the flesh from drying and turning stringy, even after it has been blitzed in a hot oven. Although I would advise getting a proper free-range chicken, this method will work miracles on inferior supermarket birds. Incidentally, despite its name, buttermilk is very low in fat, which makes it useful if you want to keep a skinless portion (for virtuous reasons) as moist as possible. Buttermilk is sold in supermarkets (often next to the yoghurts).

1 litre buttermilk
10 cloves garlic, minced
2 tablespoons Dijon mustard
1 tablespoon soy sauce
2 large chickens, each cut into 8 (or same number of portions)
3 tablespoons butter, melted
3 tablespoons olive oil

Pour the buttermilk into a large bowl and stir in the garlic, mustard and soy. (You may find this easier to do in 2 batches in separate dishes.) Add the chicken pieces, turning to cover, and then pour the entire contents into 2 plastic bags and tie with elastic bands. Leave in a cool larder for about 8 hours – longer if in the fridge as the flavours take longer to steep the colder it is.

Remove the chicken from the marinade and wipe totally dry with kitchen towel. Preheat the oven to gas mark 7/210°C. Melt the butter and stir in the olive oil, sprinkle with salt and pepper. Arrange the chicken, skin side up, on 2 oiled baking trays, brush over with the melted butter and oil, mixed, and put in to cook. It's difficult to say exactly how long it will take: evidently it depends on the size of the chicken. Poke and test. I tend to give the brown meat portions 30–40 minutes, breasts 20–25. Either take the breasts out first and keep them warm, or put the thighs and legs in 10 or so minutes before the breasts.

The chicken can be kept warm, but the potatoes most definitely cannot wait: they must stay in the oven till the very last minute, so put them in the oven 50 minutes before you plan to eat the starter. For 8 people, I'd get 8 decent-sized (175–225g) baking potatoes, and leave them unpeeled but cut them into square chunks of about 1cm. Get 2 heads garlic and throw the cloves, separated but unpeeled (or use garlic-infused oil), with the potatoes into a roasting dish. Slick the potatoes and garlic with oil and cook at gas mark 7/210°C for 60–70 minutes. When you take them out of the oven, sprinkle with coarse sea salt and fresh chopped parsley.

GARLIC POTATOES

GREEN SALAD

As for the green salad, go for one with plenty of crunch and absolutely no garlic in the dressing. And I'm presuming you've had bread on the table since the first course, so we needn't even mention it now.

Now, for pudding. First, the logistics. You want this warm, not hot, so you can cook it before putting the chicken in, taking it out in time to allow the oven to get hotter for the meat. The sausages can go into the oven with the pudding at gas mark 4/180°C, but for 10–15 minutes longer than if they're cooked at gas mark 6/200°C. Reheat them on the hob and they'll brown up in the pan then.

CHOCOLATE RASPBERRY PUDDING CAKE

I call this a pudding cake because its texture is simply a mixture between pudding and cake, though lighter by far than that could ever imply. Think, rather, of a mousse without fluffiness: this is dense but delicate with it. And it's heavenly at blood heat, when the cakiness of the chocolate sits warmly around the sour-sweet juicy raspberries embedded within, like glinting, mud-covered garnets. This should be eaten an hour or so after it comes out of the oven. It gets more solid when cold, and loses some of that spectacular texture. If you have any left, wrap it in foil and heat it up in the oven, or warm it up a slice at a time in the microwave before eating it.

Use fresh raspberries or well-thawed frozen ones, adding more if frozen. But the cake works unfruited, too. Just replace the raspberry liqueur with a tablespoon or so of dark rum and serve with coffee ice-cream.

This is so easy to make (a little light stirring, that's all) that it's almost more work to type out the instructions than to make the cake itself.

185g self-raising flour
30g cocoa powder
250g unsalted butter
2 tablespoons crème de framboise or 1 tablespoon eau de framboise
95g caster sugar
95g muscovado sugar
250g good dark chocolate such as Valrhona
185ml black coffee and 185ml water, or instant coffee made up with 2 teaspoons instant coffee and 370ml water
2 eggs, beaten slightly
250g raspberries plus more to serve

Preheat oven to gas mark 4/180°C.

Butter a 22–23cm spring-sided cake tin and line the base with baking parchment.

Sift the flour and cocoa powder together in a bowl, and set aside.

Put the butter, framboise, sugars, chocolate, coffee and water in a thick-bottomed saucepan and stir over low heat until everything melts and is thickly, glossily smooth.

Stir this mixture into the sifted flour and cocoa. Beat well until all smooth and glossy again, then beat in the eggs. This will be runny: don't panic, and *don't* add more flour; the chocolate itself sets as it cooks and then cools.

Pour into the prepared tin until you have covered the base with about 2cm of the mixture and then cover with raspberries and pour the rest of the mixture on top. You may have to push some of the raspberries back under the cake batter by hand. Put into the preheated oven and bake for 40–45 minutes. Don't try and test by poking in a skewer as you don't want it to come out clean: the gunge is what the cake is about. But when it's cooked, the top will be firm, and probably slightly cracked. Don't worry about that: a little icing sugar will deflect attention. When it's ready, take the cake out of the oven and put on a rack. Leave in the tin for 15 minutes and then turn out.

When you're just about to eat, dust with a little icing sugar pushed through a tea strainer. Serve with lots more fresh raspberries, and Greek yoghurt, whipped double cream or crème fraîche.

Sancerre, the perfect wine with oysters, will not be overawed by the spicy sausages; a good Bordeaux has the harmony and complexity to suit the garlic and buttermilk-marinaded chicken.

TARTED-UP HOMEY DINNER FOR 6

Chicory and mustard salad
Ham with pea orzotto and roast leeks
Poached pistachio-sprinkled apricots stuffed with crème fraîche

One of the reasons I love this menu is for its central side dish, if this is not a contradiction in terms. The pea orzotto is a kind of barley risotto or stew, only this is better, sharper, smarter. Because pearl barley has less gluten than rice it doesn't get sticky if it stands around after it's been cooked. It's true that the actual stirring and whole process of the absorption of the stock to make a risotto takes longer with pearl barley than with rice, but an extra 15 minutes' effort in advance is nothing compared to the hell of having to get everything ready from scratch at the last minute.

But another reason I'm keen on this menu is that it shows how by changing the details you can change the whole: with boiled potatoes and carrots, the ham in cider is a not particularly partyish weekend lunch (which, indeed, is where you'll see the recipe, and turn to page 234, only lose some of the veg); with the orzotto and oven-charred leeks, the chicory salad and the pistachio-sprinkled apricots, it is dinner-party food that knows not the word poncy. The ham takes some time to cook, so you've either got to get home from work early, or do it at the weekend. To make your life easier you could buy a cooked ham from the butcher (explain why you want it) and reheat it, either in the cider or as he suggests.

The chicory salad is just the right starter: the salt-sweetness of the ham, peas and barley need the near-wincing astringency of those sword-sharp leaves; the soft-bellied tenderness of the poached dried fruit and its *Arabian Nights* aromatic muskiness complement and elevate what's gone before.

CHICORY AND MUSTARD SALAD

If you see red chicory, or rather that fabulous auburn-tipped stuff, you could get some as well, but I wouldn't worry about using just the normal, greeny-blond *witloof*.

1 tablespoon sherry or cider vinegar
1 scant tablespoon Dijon mustard
2 tablespoon crème fraîche
6 tablespoons extra virgin olive oil
6 small or 4 large heads chicory

To make the dressing, use a fork to whisk the vinegar, mustard, a fat pinch of salt and crème fraîche together in a little bowl or jug and, whisking still, very slowly pour in the olive oil so that you have a smooth, thick, emulsified dressing. I like this with punch. You may prefer a different balance. As with all cooking, do it a few times until you have exactly what you like best.

PEA ORZOTTO

If you are also making the poached apricots (see below) you may as well use crème fraîche instead of the double cream specified here, since you need it anyway for the pudding, and the salad dressing, above. Though in which case, add a little bit more cheese.

1$^{3}/_{4}$–2 litres stock
90g butter
1 onion, chopped finely
250g pearl barley
100ml white wine or vermouth
300g frozen petits pois, thawed
2 tablespoons freshly grated parmesan
approx. 4 tablespoons double cream

Heat the stock in a saucepan, and keep it just simmering. If you have no home-made stock, use Joubère stock in tubs (the veal, watered down, would be particularly good here) or Marigold vegetable stock powder.

Melt 30g butter, with a drop of oil to stop it burning, in a heavy and large pan. Put in the chopped onion and fry for about 5–7 minutes until it is soft but not brown. Then add the pearl barley and stir well, for about 1 minute, until the grains are coated and glossy with fat. Pour in the wine and let it bubble and reduce, and become absorbed into the onion and barley mixture.

Add a ladleful of hot stock and, stirring the pan, wait for it to be absorbed. Then add another ladleful, and so on-until the stock is all absorbed and the barley cooked al dente. After the first 10 minutes or so you can add a couple of ladlefuls at a time and you needn't be quite as diligent as earlier on about stirring, but don't walk away from the pan. This process will take about 35–45 minutes. You can leave it now and come back and finish the dish off *à la minute*. If you are leaving the orzotto for only an hour or so, then leave it in its pan, adding just a film of stock or hot water so that it doesn't dry out. If you are leaving it for longer (and I have successfully made it a couple of days in advance), you must decant it into a wide-bottomed cold dish, so that it will cool quickly and not carry on cooking. Cover, and put to one side.

Now for the final touch: sauté 120g of the peas in 30g butter for 2 minutes until just cooked, but still sweet, firm and pea-like. If they're not thawed to start off with, they'll take longer. Put aside and sprinkle with a little salt. Sauté the remaining 180g peas in the remaining butter, this time for about 4–5 minutes. Add a ladleful of stock, let it reduce and then liquidize the peas. Just before serving, heat up the orzotto and stir in the whole peas, the puréed peas and 100–150ml (to taste) double cream (or crème fraîche) and the parmesan. If you were eating this without the ham, you should probably triple the amount of cheese. Let stand, loosely covered, for 5–10 minutes (you could eat the starter while it's resting) as this somehow lets the textures and flavours more exuberantly and exquisitely cohere.

If you want to create your own orzotti, you can use the pea orzotto recipe as a guide or follow any risotto recipe, remembering that the barley takes longer to cook, requires more stock and has to have cream for the final stirring or *mantecatura*. (For further use, I particularly recommend making a saffron orzotto, in place of the usual risotto Milanese, to accompany ossobuco).

ROAST LEEKS

As for the leeks: preheat the oven to gas mark 8/220°C and pour some good olive oil into a couple of roasting tins. I reckon on one medium-sized, fairly trim leek per person, based on the supposition that each one gives you 3–4 logs. And

I buy those ready-cleaned, plastic-wrapped ones: getting the mud out myself totally defeats me – and it leaves the leeks too wet to roast satisfactorily. Roll the leeks in the oil, sprinkle with coarse salt and give them about 25 minutes all told, turning them once. Obviously if they're those huge fat ones, add about 10 minutes. When done, they should be bronze and glistening, and burnt in places. Remove to a plate and sprinkle with a little more coarse salt. They'll keep the heat well, so if it makes it easier to take them out of the oven when you eat the salad, do so.

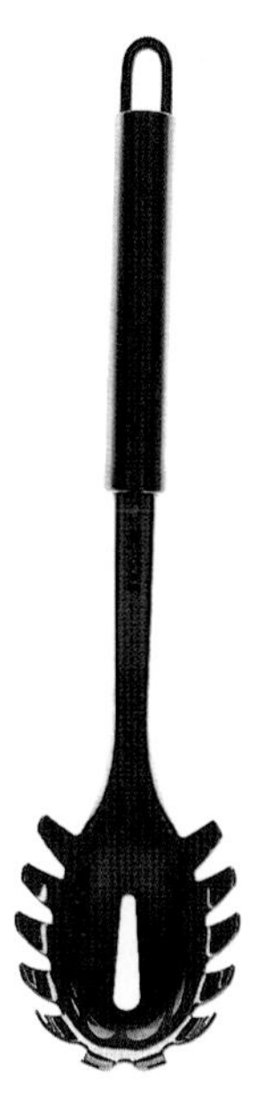

POACHED PISTACHIO-SPRINKLED APRICOTS STUFFED WITH CRÈME FRAÎCHE

This recipe comes via an American book, *The Cooking of the Eastern Mediterranean* by Paula Wolfert (she of the food of south-west France and Morocco). This is another dish you need to start preparing in advance, but since the very fact of a dinner party suggests planning (unless you're ringing round friends at the last minute, in which case we're talking about a slightly different thing), this is an advantage, surely.

Paula Wolfert suggests a mix of mascarpone and double cream as the best imitation of *kaymak*, the thick Turkish buffalo milk cream properly used to stuff the apricots, but I prefer crème fraîche, which is lighter and less cloying. You could also use Greek yoghurt.

300g good dried apricots, preferably Turkish
600ml water
60g sugar
seeds from 6 crushed cardamom pods
2 scant teaspoons lemon juice
200ml crème fraîche
90g pistachios, shelled weight, chopped very finely indeed, to resemble dust almost, or ground in a pestle and mortar

Soak the apricots in the water overnight.

Next day, preheat the oven to gas mark 2/150°C and put in a non-reactive ovenproof container to hold the apricots later. Pour the apricot-soaking liquid into a saucepan and add the sugar, cardamom seeds and lemon juice and bring to the boil. Add the apricots and then pour them and their liquid into the dish that's in the oven. Cover with baking parchment and cook for 1 ½ hours. Remove from the oven and let the apricots cool in the syrup. Chill well.

Before you want to serve them (and I have done this a good half-day before to no deleterious effect) lift out the apricots to drain. Carefully open each one and stuff with 1 teaspoon crème fraîche. Place on flat plate or dish, spoon over some syrup and dust with the very finely chopped pistachios. It is this final touch which makes all the difference, so don't be tempted to leave it out. And don't, either, do what restaurants customarily do and serve straight from the fridge: too-cold food kills the taste and whole pleasure of it.

This is one of those puddings which is so simple that it almost cannot help but become an instantly reassuring part of your kitchen repertoire.

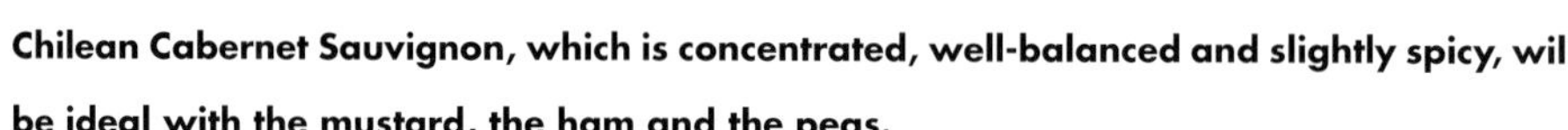

Chilean Cabernet Sauvignon, which is concentrated, well-balanced and slightly spicy, will be ideal with the mustard, the ham and the peas.

EARLY-AUTUMN DINNER FOR 6

Guacamole with paprika-toasted potato skins

Cod wrapped in ham, with sage and onion lentils

Hazelnut cake, with redcurrant and peach salad

This is the sort of food I want to eat when I'm holding on to summer, despite the sad, grey-skied truth of the actual weather on the streets. These are the strong flavours of hotter climates – lime, chillies, coriander, the honeyed saltiness of cured ham – banked down, with mashed potatoes, cod, buttery sage, for northern palates. After this starter, the culinary equivalent of a mariachi band, you need to strike some calmer notes, and the unexotic fish, the sage-and-onion-spiked lentils, do exactly that.

Pudding is another version of cake with berries; here the hazelnut, almost meringuey, sponge and the sharpness of the redcurrants and peaches, provide a foil to the dominant tastes beforehand. When redcurrants aren't around, or the only peaches you can get are stone-hard and green-tasting, substitute whichever fruits you want, but think of something, even if it's just a thawed packet of frozen summer fruits: the cake wouldn't work, here, just on its own.

In most instances I provide a couple of portions extra – 6 pieces of chicken, say, for 4 people – so there's never a cleared serving plate after the food's been doled out. Here, I don't: the guacamole before is more filling than most starters, and there are two carbohydrates to go with. Talking of one of them: I love potato skins with the guacamole (if you're going to go seventies wine bar, you may as well go all the way), and they can scarcely be thought of as hard in what is anyway a very uncomplicated culinary exercise. Baking the skins makes life easier for the second course: you already have your potatoes ready-cooked and more or less mashed, and you've had no peeling to do earlier. But if you are dispensing with the skins and providing tortilla chips instead, don't feel you have to whip up the mashed potato from scratch: just do more lentils and add a lower-effect second vegetable.

But read through all the recipes that make up this menu and you will actually see that this is a very low-effort enterprise. As long as you've got some gadget that whisks the egg whites for the cake, you can handle this dinner after getting home, late and tired, from the office. Just remember, of course, to get started on the cake and put the redcurrants to steep as soon as you get in.

GUACAMOLE WITH PAPRIKA-TOASTED POTATO SKINS

This guacamole doesn't include tomatoes. It makes such a difference: it's fresh and sharp, but instead of the usual burst-boil mush, you end up with a perfect buttery-yellow and jade clay.

The quantities I give are restrained. That's not to say that the portions are mean, but that people will eat as much as you make, and you must leave room for later.

Although it's eaten first, and you can do some chopping in advance, the actual avocado mixture must be made at the last minute.

3 properly ripe avocados
juice of 3–4 limes
4 tablespoons fresh coriander, chopped
½–1 (to taste) fresh green chilli, deseeded and chopped finely
scant teaspoon salt
4 spring onions, sliced finely

Get everything, bar the avocados, prepared when you get home, then just chop them up and mix the whole at the last minute. Even the potato skins (see below) can be done in advance: they aren't eaten hot.

Just before you want to eat, peel and stone the avocados and put the flesh in a bowl. Don't worry about how you do it and how pulpy you make the avocado, as it will be mashed. Dissolve the salt in the lime juice and pour it over. Then add the other ingredients and mash with a fork until you have a rough lumpy mixture. At all costs avoid turning it into a smooth purée: by its nature the avocado will be smooth anyway, but you want as many soft but form-holding clumps as possible.

For the above amount I use 9 baking potatoes, cooked for 1¼–1½ hours at gas mark 7/210°C or until the skins are crisp and the flesh soft. Take them out of the oven, but leave the oven on.

Halve the potatoes lengthways, and with a spoon scoop out the innards into a bowl, leaving a thin layer lining the skins. When all the potatoes have been emptied into the bowl, mash with 300ml warm milk and as much butter, pepper, salt and freshly ground nutmeg as you like. This isn't perhaps as much mash as I'd make under normal conditions, but with the lentils, here, it's fine. Put aside to reheat later (don't put the potatoes in the fridge, just leave the bowl, covered, in a cool place) and get on with the skins.

Halve them lengthways again, so you have 4 long, vaguely scoop-shaped quarters. Mix 1 heaped teaspoon paprika with an equal amount of fine sea salt. Pour about 4 tablespoons olive oil into a bowl. With a pastry brush dab the skins on both sides lightly with oil and then sprinkle the salt–paprika mix over the interior of the long, curving slice. Put in the oven and bake for another 12–15 minutes. Remove to a wire rack and when cool, arrange on a couple of plates. They taste just right with the coriander-heady, mouth-filling creaminess of the guacamole.

COD WRAPPED IN HAM

I use what you could call West Country prosciutto. This is cured ham produced by a small company in Dorset called Denhay, which also makes exceptional bacon (see page 506). Their ham is cut a little bit thicker than Parma ham usually is, so just bear that in mind when you get your prosciutto sliced. Get a few extra slices anyway, for patching up. You can get all your parcelling-up done, and then leave it in the fridge. But you don't want the fish sitting around once it is cooked, so I'd put it in the oven as you sit down to eat the first course.

6 cod fillets, about 175g each
75g unsalted butter, melted
8 slices Parma or other cured ham

Preheat the oven to gas mark 6/200°C. Get out a couple of baking trays, preferably non-stick. Brush the pieces of cod with melted butter, wrap with ham and then brush with butter again. (If you're doing this part in advance, leave the final, ham-coating buttering till just before you bake the fish.) Put in the oven and cook for 15 minutes. Remove and place on top of the lentils.

SAGE AND ONION LENTILS

500g puy lentils
3 whole cloves garlic, peeled, plus 2 cloves garlic, peeled and minced
2 medium onions, peeled but whole
1 large onion, peeled and chopped finely
12 sage leaves
1 stick celery, halved, or 2 sprigs lovage
6 tablespoons extra virgin olive oil
scant ½ teaspoon made English mustard (i.e. not powder)

Put the lentils in a pan, add the whole garlic cloves, the 2 medium onions, 6 of the sage leaves and the celery or lovage. Cover generously with cold water and bring to the boil. When it starts boiling, add a good teaspoon of salt and then lower the heat to a firm simmer and let cook for 35–40 minutes, until the lentils are just cooked. You want some texture to remain, so don't overcook. Drain, and taste the lentils while they're in the colander. If you think they need it, add more salt then and there but remember that the ham is salty.

Put the pan back on the heat, add the olive oil and, when hot, throw in the very finely chopped onion and the remaining sage leaves, shredded or cut any old way into fine strips. Cook for 5–10 minutes (it will depend, among other things, on the diameter of your pan) until the onion has lost its rawness and then some. Stir in the minced garlic and cook for another minute or so and then add the English mustard, before putting the cooked lentils back. Turn the lentils well in the sage and onion mixture. Taste to see if you want to add anything else – lemon juice, more salt, more sage, more oil, some pepper. Leave in the pan until you're ready to eat them, and then turn the lentils onto a large, warmed plate and place the cooked cod on top. This looks wonderful – the pebbly, oil-wet khaki-blackness of the lentils like a cobbled street underneath the cat's-tongue-pink slabs of ham-wrapped fish.

HAZELNUT CAKE

This cake happens to be a brilliant way to use up freezer-stored egg whites. It looks wonderful: a toasty, speckled brown, bulging-sided disc. And it tastes extraordinary: a nutty, tender sponge, with the almost-stickiness of meringue and the aromatic dampness of marzipan. The amount below will probably give you leftovers, but the cake stays all-too-eatable.

I do something that dismays purists and use ready-ground nuts. If you, too, are shocked by the very idea, then you won't need me to tell you to grind the whole, toasted and then rubbed nuts along with the sugar in the processor.

285g ground hazelnuts

300g caster sugar

8 large egg whites

grated zest 1 lemon or ½ an orange

85g plain, preferably Italian 00, flour

Preheat the oven to gas mark 4/180°C. Butter a 23cm springform cake tin, lining the bottom with a disc of parchment.

If you have bought ready-ground hazelnuts, mix them with the sugar; otherwise, see above. Whisk the egg whites with ½ teaspoon salt until you have stiff peaks: I have to say I wouldn't advise doing this without an electric whisk; and if you have a free-standing mixer, so much the better. Fold in the sugar–nut mixture, to which you've added the lemon or orange zest, gradually and gently. Don't get too nervous about this, though: I once tipped about half the bowl in at once and then folded in far too vigorously, and although the cake was a mite flatter than it might have been, it was still fabulous; anyone eating who hadn't seen my characteristic act of clumsiness wouldn't have known anything was other than it should be.

When the sugar, nuts and zest are incorporated into the cloudy mountain of egg whites, sift over the flour. What I do is put the flour into a sieve which I hold over the bowl, giving the sieve a tap every now and again, folding in as I do so.

Pour this mixture into the prepared tin and put it in the preheated oven for 1 hour, or until a fine skewer comes out clean. Take the cake out of the oven and let cool in the tin for about 10 minutes, then release the springlock and remove to a wire rack till cool.

REDCURRANT AND PEACH SALAD

I had the idea of making a redcurrant salad, if that's what we're calling it, to go with the hazelnut cake, out of some vague not-quite-memory of *Ribiselkuchen*, that Austrian pudding cake made of hazelnut-meringue sponge and redcurrants; there seems to be some special affinity between these nuts, this fruit. The peaches or nectarines lend a fleshy mellowness to balance and sweeten, which is needed, since the currants are, even with all this sugar, undeniably sharp. Even though you're going to be pouring mountains of sugar over the redcurrants, you don't actually eat all the syrup it makes. Or not at this sitting. For I can't bring myself to throw this away, but boil it down after and use it to glaze other fruits in open tarts, or to flavour apples in an otherwise plain two-crust pie or, much easier this, to pour over some vanilla ice-cream sprinkled with a fresh lot of hazelnuts, this time roughly chopped.

It's easy to be strict about quantities for baking, but I cannot quite bring myself to sound anything but vague when it comes to what you do to make a fruit salad, especially such a simple, two-fruit arrangement. But let me just say that for 6 people, I'd think along the lines of three 200–250g punnets redcurrants and 3 peaches or nectarines. Remember, this is to be eaten with cake. Put the stemmed currants into a dish and pour 100g caster sugar and the juice of an orange over them; in another hour do the same, and an hour later the same again, so that in total you've used 300g sugar and 3 oranges, though taste as you go along to make sure you need the extra sugar. Turn the currants in the sugary juices every now and again – whenever you think about it. I think these are at their best – sticky, shiny, scarlet jewels, still sharp enough once you bite, but not so sharp that you wince – after 3½–4 hours sitting time, but we're not talking precision timing here. It's fine if you start when you get in; just turn the currants in their syrup more often.

Before you sit down to dinner, put a kettle on to boil and the peaches or nectarines in a bowl, then pour the boiling water over them. Leave for a few minutes, then drain and peel. Or leave them with their skin on. Cut each fruit into about 8 fine slices. Drain the currants and put on a big plate and add the peaches as pleases you. Dribble over the now coral-red sugary orange juices, tasting first to make sure they're as you like them. Leave until the end of dinner when the fruit can join forces on the table with the cake. I serve no cream, of whatever sort; it would taste all wrong with this particular cake. Besides, we're looking for a little uplift here.

A Rhone red or Australian Shiraz – something powerful, ripe and opulent – will suit the ham and lentils. It is important to remember that you don't have to drink white wine with fish or red with meat.

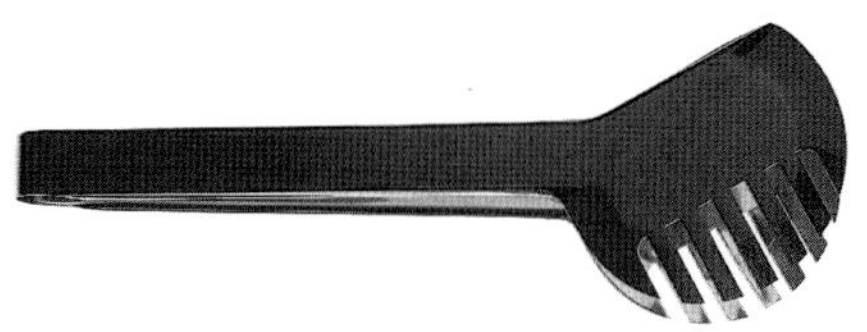

DEEPLY AUTUMNAL DINNER FOR 8

Chestnut and pancetta salad

Roast venison fillet with apple purée and rosemary sauce

Peas and celeriac mash

Quinces poached in muscat with lemon ice-cream, or Marsala muscovado custard with or without muskily spiced prunes

I don't think one needs to be putting on a theme park of the seasons quite, but autumn is a hard one to resist. One can get a little too taken with all those mists and mellow fruitfulness, become a little too parodically bosky, and lost in shades of prune and plum, but this menu seems to me to stop just this side of all that. The chestnuts are coming into the shops (even if I do recommend the vacuum-packed peeled ones), and although venison is available all the year around now, it still feels autumnal, especially when paired with another seasonal – apples. And we have such a short time to take a stab at quinces, we may as well exploit it as we can. For those who don't feel up to tackling this once commonly eaten, now almost exotically unfamiliar fruit, I suggest an eggy and creamy baked custard, buff coloured with Marsala and fudgy muscovado sugar. And if *that's* too much to ask, then all you need to do is provide cheese (gorgonzola, roquefort or stilton and maybe something blander for those who don't know a good thing when they taste one) and a gorgeous plate of those ambrosial fat and sepia-tinged muscat grapes.

CHESTNUT AND PANCETTA SALAD

I got the idea for this from two independently wonderful chestnut and pancetta soups I had, within a few weeks of one another, at Moro and the River Café; these two ingredients seem to do something to one another when put together; they become more themselves – one salty, the other sweet – at the same time as fusing into something greater, transformed. This salad lets them do whatever it is they do even more baldly: there's not just the contrast between salt and sweet, but between crisp and almost fudgily dense. But despite these rich textures and strong flavours, this manages to be a light, unclogging starter. I think the trick is to resist the temptation to boost the quantities of its main ingredients.

Use a slightly bitter leaf, such as escarole, though if that's not to be found frisée will be fine, and make sure you get good, proper Spanish sherry vinegar, otherwise you just get acidity, not intensity.

I'm not stopping you from buying, peeling and preparing your own chestnuts (in which case double the quantities here), but I use those Merchant Gourmet vacuum-packed peeled and cooked chestnuts, which come in 200g boxes from the supermarket. I know it's annoying of me to make you open half a packet, but either throw them all in, or stash them in the deep-freeze, from whose icy wastes they will probably never be retrieved. If you find it difficult to find these chestnuts most of the time, just stock up at Christmas when the shops are awash with them.

1 1/2 escarole lettuces
300g vacuum-packed prepared chestnuts
4 tablespoons and 2 teaspoons best olive oil
225g slab pancetta
1 teaspoon Dijon mustard
1 teaspoon sherry vinegar

Tear the escarole into manageable pieces and cover 2 large plates – mine are 32cm in diameter – with them. Put the 2 teaspoons oil in a pan and place on the heat. Cut the rind off the pancetta and add the rind to the pan to render its fat; give it about 4 minutes. Meanwhile, chop the pancetta into cubes or squat strips and then toss into the pan as well. In about 4 minutes these, too, should have given off a lot of their fat and have become crisp and dark golden in bits. Add the chestnuts and toss them in the hot fat with the pancetta. Don't worry about these breaking, as inevitably they will. I actually prefer it if the chestnuts are slightly rubbly. When they are warmed through, a matter of a minute or so, remove them and the pancetta with a spatula or slotted spoon to the escarole-lined plates. Stir the mustard into the remaining olive oil and, off the heat, stir this into the bacony fat. Mix well and keep stirring and scraping as you add the sherry vinegar. Pour this over the salad, toss deftly and serve.

ROAST VENISON FILLET

This venison has a mixed provenance, as most things do in the kitchen, but its chief inspiration is the recipe for saddle of roedeer from Inverlochy Castle in Fort William, Scotland, to be found in *The Gourmet Tour of Great Britain and Ireland* by Sir Clement Freud.

I know it might look fiddly but you can make the rosemary sauce part-way in advance, and the apple sauce wholly in advance, so all you need to do on the night is cook the venison and reheat the sauces, adding juices from the marinade and the roasting tin to the rosemary sauce.

The weight of venison given is for the prepared, lean meat only: it is expensive if you use fillet, but it will be better. Otherwise you can buy meat labelled simply 'boned venison' in the supermarkets, and you might even get that in one 1½ kg joint; note that you'll need more meat per head if you're not using the stronger-flavoured fillet. You will also need to do two other things: marinate for a couple of days, rather than one, before cooking; and cook at a lower heat and for longer (consult roasting chart on page xii).

1 tablespoon butter
1 teaspoon olive oil
2 x 500g trimmed fillets of venison

for the marinade
1 bottle full-bodied good red wine
1 celery stalk, diced
1 carrot, peeled and roughly chopped
1 onion, peeled and roughly chopped
3 juniper berries, crushed (see pheasant recipe, below)
12 black peppercorns
2 sprigs thyme, or ½ teaspoon dried thyme
2 bay leaves

for the rosemary sauce
750ml beef or game stock
1 carrot, coarsely chopped
1 leek, white part only, coarsely chopped
2 shallots, coarsely chopped
1 stick of celery, coarsely chopped
450ml red wine
bunch of about 8 rosemary sprigs (approx. 25g)
45g butter, cold and cut into cubes

for the apple sauce
50g butter
3 cooking apples, about 1kg, peeled, cored and chunked or sliced
75g sugar
3 cloves
juice of ½ a lemon

Heat the ingredients for the marinade in a saucepan. When it comes to the boil, remove from the heat and let cool. Marinate the venison fillets in this for 24 hours preferably in a cool place, or else in the fridge.

To make the rosemary sauce, put the stock in the pan with the chopped vegetables, bring the stock to the boil, and then cook furiously until reduced by half. Add the wine and rosemary and reduce to about 300ml. If you're doing this in advance you can cook it till this point, reheating and resuming from here on the night. Add 8 tablespoons of the marinade and reduce, again, to 300ml. Strain into a clean pan and, when about to serve, put back on the hob, taste for seasoning and beat in the butter, 1 cube at a time, to make it smooth and glossy.

To make the apple sauce, put all the ingredients in a heavy-bottomed saucepan, with a pinch of salt. Cover, and cook over a medium heat for about 10–15 minutes or until the apples are a soft, collapsed heap. Lift the lid every now and again to prod and stop from sticking. Pass the apple mixture through a fine sieve, tasting to see whether you need more sugar or lemon juice, and reserve till needed. If it's too runny, boil down; if too stiff, add butter and liquid.

To cook the meat, preheat oven to gas mark 8/220°C a good 15 minutes before you want to put the venison in, which is about an hour, more or less, before you want to eat it. In other words, it's coming out of the oven, to rest, when you sit down to eat your first course. On the hob, in a pan that preferably will go in the oven later, melt the butter and oil and sear the fillets on all sides. Transfer to the hot oven and roast for 20–30 minutes. The venison should be browney-puce within (the game equivalent of *à point* pink), but not imperial purple.

Remove the venison fillets to a warmed plate or carving board and wrap or tent loosely with foil to keep warm. If you want, add the juices from the pan to the rosemary sauce. Before you carve the fillets, pour into the gravy, as well, the juices which have run out of them onto the board as they wait.

I would carve the fillets into slices and arrange on 1 or 2 oval plates, so people can take what they like, and hand the sauce round separately, having ladled a little over the soft, sliced meat first. The meat is very intense and 2 to 3 initial slices, even if they're small ones, may be plenty (and you know how I am about portion sizes generally so you know you can trust me here). The same goes for the sauce: only a little is needed; too much would ruin the balance as well as finish the sauce up too soon.

Despite the sweetness of the meat, it seems that it's sweetness, again, you look for in the vegetables. Frozen petits pois come into this category and they rupture the mood of autumnal colour co-ordination, which can't be a bad thing.

And with the peas, I want potatoes, mashed with their own weight of celeriac, lots of butter, plenty of nutmeg. For 8 people, who eat rather than pick at food, you should think along the lines of 1kg of each. Celeriac is no fun to peel, but plenty of fun to eat: suffer in smug silence; your reward comes later.

QUINCES POACHED IN MUSCAT

I'll poach anything in muscat given the chance, but this mixture of honey-sweet wine and fruit from, and perhaps not just metaphorically, the garden of Eden is more than mere culinary opportunism. It is gloriously, impeccably right.

I poach the quinces in the oven rather than on the stove, because it is easier to control the heat this way, and thus to keep the fruit poaching so gently that they keep their form and the liquid its almost ruby clarity. For, as the quinces cook, they become a grainy, glorious burnished terracotta and the wine in which they steep also grows rosier. If you can get hold of some of that Greek red pudding wine, then do: the fruits and their syrup will *glow*.

The only hard bit is the preparation of the quinces, and when I say hard, I mean strenuous rather than labour-intensive. These fruits are rock-hard, and coring and quartering takes strength. But you do nothing to them as they cook, so the trade-off's worth it. They can be done in advance and eaten cold. Four quinces may not seem many for 8 people, but they are so intensely, temple-achingly sweet, that you don't want to eat enormous amounts. A mouthful or two is, however, ambrosial.

4 quinces
700ml muscat
300ml water
500g sugar
1 stick cinnamon
2 bay leaves
3 cloves
3 cardamom pods
6 peppercorns

Preheat the oven to gas mark 3/160°C.

Fill a bowl with cold water and add a squirt of lemon juice to it; this is to put the quinces in to stop them browning. Peel the quinces, quarter them and core them. You might need to do a bit of chiselling with the point of a knife, but don't worry if you can't get every last bit of core out. As you work, submerge the quinces in the acidulated water. Keep the peel and trimmings: they will help the syrup to thicken.

To make the syrup, put the wine, water, sugar and spices in a pan and bring to the boil. Put the peel and cores in the bottom of an ovenproof dish and then put the quartered quinces in on top, pour over the wine, cover – either with a lid or, securely, with foil – and put in the oven for 2½ hours. When you take them out, the quinces will be the colour of old-fashioned Elastoplast. Let them cool in the dish, with the lid on, and when you look at them next, they'll have deepened and darkened further.

When cold, remove with a slotted spoon and put in a glass bowl. Strain the syrup into a saucepan and reduce; taste every now and again (without burning your tongue) to see how far you need to go. Let cool slightly and pour over the quinces waiting in their bowl. A warning, however: the syrup will thicken as it cools anyway; I too often over-reduce it and end up with quince toffee. Any superfluous syrup can be kept, or reduced and kept, to use in place of sugar in apple pies or crumbles. Quinces are traditionally used in these dishes and the syrup gives you that extraordinary mixture between super-homeliness and the exotic without any further peeling.

I suggest lemon ice-cream with this, because in the first instance I love that particular combination and in the second, because there's a no-churn recipe (see page 282) that you can make relatively effortlessly. And I love the ice-cream just with the syrup, too. But no one's going to argue if you just put out a bowl of crème fraîche, or indeed Greek yoghurt, to go with the quinces instead: it's the combination between the grainy, sweet and perfumed fruit and cold near-sour creaminess you're after. It's up to you how you do it.

MARSALA MUSCOVADO CUSTARD WITH MUSKILY SPICED PRUNES

This recipe is really just a variant of the Sauternes custard on page 239: it occurred to me that the particular combination of ingredients in zabaione (and see page 172) worked so well, it might taste equally good translated to the dense fabulousness of a baked custard. (I add muscovado sugar to boost innate tendencies.) It does. I'd consider serving it with some poached prunes, only bear in mind that prunes can never win unanimous support. To cook the prunes, make some tea up with 500ml boiling water and an Earl Grey tea bag (which you discard when the tea's strongish). Pour into a wide, heavy saucepan, adding a cinnamon stick broken in two, a star anise, a clove, the peel of about ⅓ orange, pared from the fruit with a vegetable peeler, 100ml Marsala and 100g light muscovado sugar. Bring to the boil, reduce to a simmer and put 250g (this gives you about 32) pitted prunes into the spicy tea syrup, then poach gently for 20 minutes.

POACHED PRUNES

Leave for at least 24 hours, 36 if possible; these just get better and better. The worse quality they are to start with, the longer you should let them steep. Obviously, this pudding is best with those wonderful, tender-bellied Agen prunes, but I've used tight, wrinkled, hard-skinned ones which look like cheap teddy bears' noses, and they've ended up pretty damn fabulous.

If you want this viscous, conker-shiny syrup even stickier and thicker, strain the poaching liquid (putting the prunes and the beautiful spices into the serving bowl) into a smaller pan, then reduce till you have a tight puddle of almost-liquid molasses. When a little cooler, spoon the quantity you need back over the prunes. And you can eat the rest of the syrup stirred into yoghurt for your breakfast.

450ml whipping cream
150ml Marsala
4 egg yolks
2 whole eggs
4 tablespoons light muscovado sugar
2 tablespoons caster sugar
fresh nutmeg

Preheat the oven to gas mark 2/150°C and put the kettle on. In a couple of saucepans put on the cream and Marsala to boil separately, but take off heat before they do actually come to the boil. Beat the egg yolks and whole eggs in a decent-sized bowl with the sugars. Pour first the hot Marsala and then the heated cream onto the sugar–egg mixture, beating as you do so. Go steady, though: you just want to combine them all, not whip air into them. Put an ovenproof dish – one of those oval bowls with about 1 litre capacity – in a baking tray and pour into the tray from the kettle some just-off-the-boil water to come halfway up the dish. Now pour the custard, through a strainer, into the dish, grate over some nutmeg, cover loosely with some greaseproof paper and bake for about 1 hour, but start checking after 45 minutes. You want the custard just set; it will carry on cooking as it cools. I like this best 1–1½ hours after it's come out of the oven.

Try a relatively young red Burgundy, which has a bit of acidity, but a soft, round, voluptuous, velvety flavour.

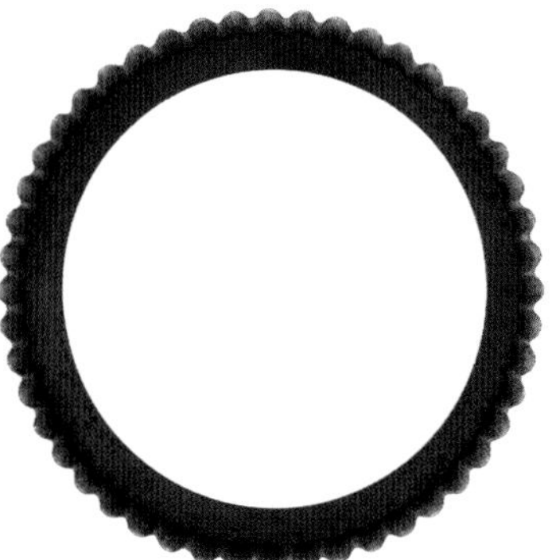

CAMP, BUT ONLY SLIGHTLY, DINNER FOR 6

Little gems with green goddess dressing
Pheasant with Gin and It
Mashed potato, and sweet and sour cabbage
Pavlova

All of these courses may sound like comic turns, a culinary joke made by someone with an overdeveloped sense of kitsch. I admit I am that person, but you don't have to apologise for this menu, or to explain it, or do anything to it other than cook it.

The pheasant is the better for being cooked in advance, and the pavlova can be made the day before. You can store the meringue in a tin before using it, but to be frank I just don't take it out of the oven. I cook it and leave it till I want to anoint it with cream and passion fruit. It is the astringency of the passion fruit which makes this work so well after the sweet herbalness of the gin-and-vermouth-cooked game. You want the soft, sweet, creaminess of the meringue, but you need the sharpness, too.

This is where the starter – a spirit-lifting winter salad – comes in, too. You can get fresh herbs all year round now, so you don't need to turn to the dusty dried stuff, even if the original did.

LITTLE GEMS WITH GREEN GODDESS DRESSING

The original green goddess dressing (created by the Palace Hotel in San Francisco in honour of George Arliss's performance in the play of the same name in the early twenties) was a mayonnaise-heavy affair; I've lightened it slightly, chiefly by using crème fraîche in place of the mayo. But it's much the same otherwise: thick with anchovy, chopped herbs, spring onions and sharp with tarragon vinegar. To the little gems, I've suggested adding some waxy, sliced potatoes (despite the mash that's to come) and cornichons. If you want to keep this sprightlier, lose the potatoes by all means. I love, uncharacteristically, the vinegariness of the cornichons, but if you don't then substitute a handful of raw sugar-snaps.

200g salad potatoes
4 anchovy fillets, drained and chopped fine
2 tablespoons milk
2 tablespoons tarragon vinegar
6 tablespoons crème fraîche
8–10 tablespoons extra virgin olive oil
1 spring onion, finely sliced
3 tablespoons chopped tarragon
4 tablespoons chopped parsley
4–6 little gems
18 whole cornichons, the size of a child's little finger, or fewer gherkins, sliced

Boil or steam the potatoes and when cool, slice into thick coins. I'm happy to leave the skins on, but it's up to you.

Pound the anchovies, preferably using a pestle and mortar, but a fork should do. In a bowl, and definitely using a fork, whisk together the anchovies, milk, vinegar and crème fraîche till smooth. Slowly add the olive oil, still whisking with your fork. Stir in the spring onion, tarragon and 2 tablespoons of the parsley. Check for seasoning. Separate the lettuce leaves and put in a large bowl and add a few tablespoons of the dressing and mix well with your hands to combine, adding the potatoes and more dressing as you need to coat well but not heavily. And this is a thick dressing, so you will have to turn the lettuce leaves in it slowly but for quite a time to make sure it's mixed in smoothly.

Arrange in a large flat plate or a couple, and toss over your little cornichons and sprinkle with the remaining parsley.

PHEASANT WITH GIN AND IT

The method for this stew is based on Anne Willan's recipe on page 114, but the idea is quite other. It came to me one day when I was, as usual, adding white vermouth to something in place of white wine. I wondered when and if ever red vermouth could be used. From there my mind turned to the red vermouth my maternal grandmother used to drink in her Gin and Its, and this thought, in *its* turn, led to this dish.

Juniper berries are conventionally added to game and gin is really just alcoholic juniper. The Martini Rosso adds a quite beautifully rounded herbalness. You end up with a velvety, dark-flavoured gravy. You don't absolutely have to have mashed potatoes to soak it up, but I'd miss them. For 6 people, I'd think 1½kg potato would do, but add plenty of butter, plenty of full-fat milk or cream and a good grating of fresh nutmeg as you mash.

Get hen pheasants if you can, since they're plumper and more tender. Read through the ingredients carefully. I've separated the marinade ingredients from the rest. If you haven't got or can't get hold of any game stock, then use 2 tins Baxter's game soup, strained and made up to 1.2 litres with light chicken stock. All you need to do to crush the juniper berries is lean on them a little with a pestle in a mortar, or put them in a bag and pummel once with a heavy weight, a can of baked beans or something like that.

for the marinade
6 tablespoons gin
450ml Martini Rosso
1 large orange, unpeeled and cut into thick slices
9 peppercorns
9 juniper berries, crushed slightly
1 large onion, peeled and chopped
6 bay leaves
225ml olive oil

for the rest
3 plump pheasants, preferably hen, jointed into 4 pieces each
60g butter
3 tablespoons olive oil (maybe more)
375g portobellini or small chestnut mushrooms, halved or whole depending on size
30 baby onions, peeled (I'm sorry)
300g pancetta, in lardons or diced
4 tablespoons flour, preferably Italian 00
3 tablespoons Martini Rosso
1.2 litres stock (see above)
9 juniper berries, crushed slightly
3 cloves garlic, chopped
shake or two soy sauce

Mix the marinade ingredients together, adding 1/4 teaspoon salt, submerge the pheasant pieces in the mixture and leave for 24 hours. If you can't do it before the morning of the same day, that should just about be OK, but don't cut it any finer. I find it easiest to divide the pheasant and marinade between a couple of polythene bags, well tied.

When you're ready to cook, remove the pheasant pieces and pat them dry with some kitchen towel. Put the butter and oil in a pan that will take the pheasant later – a large Le Creuset, or similar, wide or long rather than deep, would be best – and put it on the hob. When hot, brown the pheasant pieces in it; you may need to do this in batches. Remove to a plate and add the mushrooms to the pan. Soften these and then remove them, too. Next you're going to brown the onions, and you might need to add more fat since the mushrooms may greedily have eaten it all up. The onions should be well browned; devote about 15 minutes to this. Now remove the onions, and add the lardons or diced pancetta and brown in the hot fat. To the crisped lardons, add the flour and cook, stirring, on a low heat for about 5 minutes. Then throw in the Martini Rosso and give a good prod and stir, to scrape up bits and combine. Gradually add the stock and then strain in the marinade. Return the pheasant, onions and mushrooms to the casserole and add the crushed juniper berries, the chopped garlic, a good grinding of pepper and generous shake of soy sauce. Cover, and cook on the hob, at a gentle simmer, for 1½ hours, or in a preheated gas mark 3/160°C oven for 2 hours.

But keep an eye on it. You will probably have to take out the little tender legs after an hour, and let the big, tougher breast pieces (yes, it is that way around) cook for longer. When everything's tender, remove all the pheasant pieces and strain the liquid into another pan, reserving the mushrooms, lardons and onions. If you've got time to let the liquid settle so you can skim off excess fat, so much the better. Reduce the sauce so that it concentrates and thickens; it should be loose and thin, but not watery. Boil it down until it tastes right to you and then put the sauce, pheasant pieces, reserved mushrooms, onions and lardons back in the original pan and reheat gently. And if you want you can keep it in the fridge for up to 3 days until you want to reheat it. Serve sprinkled with chopped flat-leaf parsley.

If you've got any leftovers, bone and chop the meat and reheat with the gravy to make a wonderful sauce for yourself to go with tagliatelle or pappardelle.

SWEET AND SOUR CABBAGE

This has to be cooked at the last minute, but it doesn't take long. You could cook it while someone else is clearing the table after the first course, or as people are helping themselves to the pheasant and mash. If I can bear to get up in the middle of the meal and do this, anyone can.

1½ tablespoons sugar
3 tablespoons white wine vinegar
1 large cabbage, green or white
3 tablespoons light vegetable oil
few drops soy sauce

Mix the sugar and vinegar and add 1½ tablespoons of salt. Slice the cabbage finely, discarding tough bits of stalk. You could use a processor for this if you like the string-thin shreds it makes; the important thing is that it's sliced not chopped. Heat oil in the largest frying pan or similar that you have; if you've got a large wok, then that would do.

Toss the cabbage with a couple of wooden forks or spatulas in the hot oil for 2 minutes until it is all covered in oil and just beginning to wilt. Shake in a few drops of soy and then pour on the vinegar mixture. Toss again in the heat and let it cook for 1 minute or so more and then serve at once, while it's hot and crisp and juicy.

PAVLOVA

This version comes, appropriately enough, from an Australian book, Stephanie Alexander's compendious, addictive *Cook's Companion*. I was taken by her family tip of turning the cooked meringue over before smearing it with cream, so that (in her words) the marshmallow middle melds with cream and the sides and the base stay crisp.

4 egg whites at room temperature
250g caster sugar
2 teaspoons cornflour
1 teaspoon white wine vinegar
few drops pure vanilla extract
300ml double cream, whipped till firm
pulp of 10 passion fruits

Preheat oven to gas mark 4/180°C. Line a baking tray with baking parchment and draw a 20–23cm circle on the paper. I often don't, and just imagine what size the circle should be as I dollop the meringue on. This seems to work fine.

Beat the egg whites with a pinch of salt until satiny peaks form. Beat in the sugar, a third at a time, until the meringue is stiff and shiny. Sprinkle over the cornflour, vinegar and vanilla and fold in lightly. Mound on to the paper on the baking tray within the circle, flatten the top and smooth the sides. Place in the oven. IMMEDIATELY reduce the heat to gas mark 2/150°C and cook for 1¼ hours. Turn off the oven and leave the pavlova in it to cool completely.

Invert the pavlova on to a big, flat-bottomed plate, pile on cream and spoon over passion fruits scooped – pips and all – from their shells. Don't be tempted to add other fruit.

Italian wines from Piedmont – Barolo or Barbera – have wonderful, mineral flavours and will not be overpowered by the Gin and It.

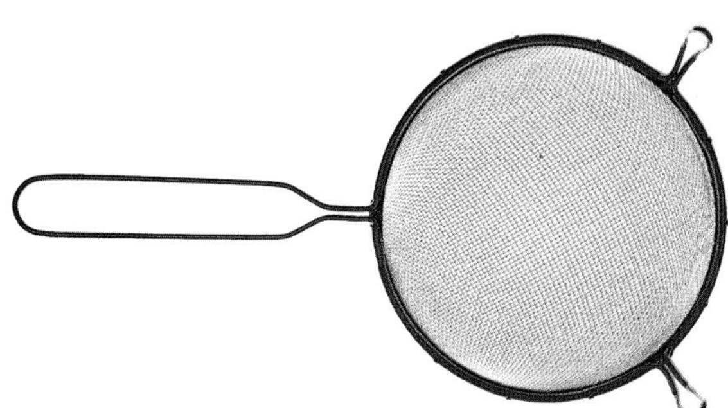

SUMMER DINNER, WITH WINTER POSSIBILITIES, FOR 6

Grilled pepper salad

Marinated, butterflied leg of lamb

Garlic potatoes, watercress and raw mushroom salad

Poached peaches with Sauternes custard or ice-cream, or

Sauternes and lemon balm jelly

In summer, I cook the lamb on the outdoor grill; in winter in a hot oven. You might want to modify the menu otherwise: only you can tell exactly what mood the weather puts you in and how you want, culinarily, to respond. In winter, of course, you won't get the peaches, or if you do they'll be expensive and, worse, probably unsalvageable by poaching. You could, then, just make a baked Sauternes custard (see Weekend Lunch on page 239) and eat it without the fruit to accompany it, or soak and then poach some dried peaches or apricots, or a mixture of each. If you find some peaches you think you could do something with, then follow the recipe for sugar-sprinkled roast peaches in Fast Food (page 189). I couldn't stop myself from adding the recipe for Sauternes and lemon balm jelly, too. The advantage of this – apart from the spectacular but delicate beauty of its taste – is that it is pathetically easy to make. And when it's really hot, it's not just that you don't feel like eating excessive amounts of food, but that you don't want to spend excessive amounts of time in the kitchen.

GRILLED PEPPER SALAD

I never ever, no matter what I'm cooking, use green peppers. If you want to add those expensive Dutch orange ones to this mix of red and yellow pepper, do, but that's as permissive as I'm going to get.

If you like, you can do this the traditional way and arrange the peppers in a dish, make up a plainish oil and vinegar dressing and arrange anchovy fillets in a lattice on top (dotting between the crosses with halved or pitted whole black olives as you wish), but I prefer to make up a salty, khaki-stained anchovy dressing, which may spoil the glazed Chinese lacquer effect of the oil-slicked peppers, but does something extraordinary to blend and transport the flavours – sweet, salty, oily, sharp – so that you have a glorious, explosive fusion.

4 yellow peppers
4 red peppers
5–6 tablespoons best olive oil
2 cloves garlic, peeled and minced
3 anchovy fillets in olive oil, drained and chopped finely
juice of 1/2 lemon
flat-leaf parsley

Char and peel the peppers as directed on page 96. Whatever you do, don't peel them under running water: you will lose all those sweet peppery juices; peel them, rather, over a bowl to catch all those sweet drips. Don't be neurotic about getting every last bit of skin off; most will come off easily enough, the rest you can live with.

Cut the peppers into strips and pile into a shallow bowl. In a thick-bottomed pan, put the olive oil and minced garlic and place on the heat, stirring once you see it's got warm. After about 30 seconds, stir in the chopped anchovies and keep stirring on low heat until they've melted, into the oil. Then pour in the juices you caught from the peppers as you peeled them. Take off the heat. Add 1 teaspoon lemon juice, taste and add more if you like. Pour over the peppers, turn well to coat, then cover tightly with clingfilm and leave to macerate: 3 hours is fine (out of the fridge, though), 24 would be even better. Sometimes I leave this for about half a week in the fridge and it is all the more silkily fabulous for it – as long as you remember to let it come to room temperature before you even think of eating it.

Transfer to a large plate, preferably a white one, to serve, and cover with just-chopped flat-leaf parsley.

There are quite a lot of peppers for 6 people, but that's for two reasons: the first is that I find people want them to stay on the table, within greedy arm's reach, with the lamb; the second is that if you're going to do some peeling, you may as well try for some leftovers later.

MARINATED, BUTTERFLIED LEG OF LAMB WITH GARLIC POTATOES

This is one of my most regular regulars. It is the flattened, boned leg which, opened up, makes a vaguely butterfly shape. In summer I cook it on the grill in the garden. This year I started doing it in winter, as well, in a gas mark 7/210°C oven for about 45 minutes and it was wonderful. Winter lamb may not be as tender as it is in spring and summer, but the taste is deeper and better, really, and the marinade sees off any potential toughness, despite the unforgiving heat of the oven. I don't serve a sauce with this, except for the deglazed meat juices in the pan. In summer there aren't even any meat juices since they've disappeared into the flames, but no one seems to mind.

You must go to a butcher to get the lamb butterflied unless you feel able to do it yourself. I've never tried but I keep meaning to learn. The information below is based on a 2.8kg leg of lamb, which leaves you with a butterflied joint of 2.2kg.

Because it takes so little time to cook, it's a very good way of accommodating a joint of lamb into an after-work dinner-party schedule. And think of it more as a steak: the cooking time is more to do with its thickness than its weight.

1 large leg lamb, butterflied
300ml extra virgin olive oil
zest of 1 unwaxed lemon
4 cloves garlic, squashed with flat of knife
2 x 22cm sprigs rosemary (not that you need to measure), chopped very finely
6 peppercorns
2kg potatoes

Put the lamb with all the rest of the ingredients in a big plastic bag for up to 30 hours, if you can, turning once or twice. Take it out of the fridge when you get back from work (or mid-afternoon if it's at the weekend and if the weather's not too hot) to let the oil in the marinade loosen and warm.

Preheat the oven to gas mark 7/210°C. Take the lamb out of the bag and put in a dish. Pour the marinade into 2 baking trays; these are for the potatoes, which need about 1 hour. The lamb takes 45–50 minutes, but since you need the lamb to rest, put them in at the same time. If you haven't got a double oven it's a squeeze, but not impossible. I cook the lamb in one tray and the potatoes, 1 3/4 kg of them (that's about 6 large baking potatoes) cut into 1cm dice, in a couple of others. And you can always cook the lamb first and eat it lukewarm.

GARLIC POTATOES

Turn the potatoes in the oil marinade in their tins, using your hands to make sure the potatoes are well slicked in the heady oil, and put them in the oven. Transfer the lamb to another tin, reserving the oily juices it leaves behind in the dish, and put that one in the oven, too.

WATERCRESS, RAW MUSHROOM SALAD

I'm lazy and buy ready-washed watercress, a couple of packets, and slice about 175–200g ordinary button mushrooms thinly. For the dressing I just squeeze some lemon juice into the oily marinade the lamb left in the bowl earlier. If this idea appals you, make any other dressing you want.

POACHED PEACHES WITH SAUTERNES CUSTARD

The difficult thing about real custard is the tedium of the stirring and its necessity; the possibility of curdling is never far away. Difficult is perhaps not the right word, but certainly the prospect of making pouring (as opposed to baked) custard can feel too daunting, and I realised I went out of my way to avoid it. Then I hit upon an idea: why not make a runny custard in the oven? I thought I could do it in advance and strain it to make sure no skin got in and then reheat it in a bain-marie on the hob when I wanted it. I doubted it would work because it seemed to me that if it was such a good idea someone would have come up with it before. But it did work; evidently I am either lazier or more fearful than other foodwriters, or both.

SAUTERNES CUSTARD (OR ICE-CREAM)

If you don't want to use Sauternes, substitute any reliably honeyed dessert wine.

500ml single cream
200ml Sauternes
7 egg yolks
60–75g vanilla sugar (or caster sugar, with a vanilla pod steeped in the cream for 20 minutes)

Preheat the oven to gas mark 3/160°C. Boil a kettle, get out a roasting tin and put a wide, shallow bowl or an oval dish with a capacity of about 1¼ litres in it. Put the cream in a pan, the wine in another and bring both to the boil, but watch out that the cream never actually does boil. Remove them both from the heat. With a fork, beat the yolks and sugar together and pour in first the wine, then the cream, beating all the while. Remember, though, you're beating to combine the ingredients, not whisking to get air in. Taste to see if it's sweet enough. Strain the custard into the dish and pour water from the recently boiled kettle into the tin to come up about halfway. Cover the tin with foil; the idea is to make for a steamy atmosphere which will prevent a skin from forming. Put in the oven and cook for 1–1¼ hours (or cook in a pan on the hob as usual).

Take out of the oven and out of the pan of water and let cool for about 20 minutes. Then strain into a bowl which will later fit over a saucepan of simmering water; this is presuming you will want to eat it warm. In fact, you can do three things with this: leave it as it is and let people spoon it over the peaches cold; reheat it till it's warm, not hot, when you're about to serve pudding; or put it when cold into the bowl of an ice-cream maker and follow the manufacturer's instructions. All three options are ambrosial.

POACHED PEACHES

I never think of myself as someone who likes cooked fruit – it's hard to believe that anything could improve on its natural and fresh state – but these peaches are a revelation. I wouldn't poach peaches with flesh as green and hard as young almonds; but ones which are slightly resistant, slightly lacking in that fragrant juiciness that is owing to the peachy estate, take on a plump but well-toned fleshiness and an aromatic roundedness that you couldn't believe could be brought about by just a pan of water and a mound of sugar. It's true that the vanilla you flavour the sugar with, the wine you scent the water with, each do their bit; but even with the plainest syrup, a dull and reticent peach can be transformed.

White peaches are my favourite here. Leave the skins on before immersing them in the softly bubbling syrup, and peel them later: you're left with a plate of perfect, pale mounds splodged pink, like the cheeks of a painted mummer. They look like something out of a children's fairy tale. You feel you should be drinking mead out of a jewel-studded goblet and wearing a wimple with a fetching organza veil.

The procedure is simple.

90ml Sauternes, or the wine you've used in the custard, above
700g vanilla sugar (or use caster sugar and throw a vanilla pod into the pan at the beginning)
8 peaches, or more if you want, preferably white

Put 700ml water, the wine and sugar in a big pan, give a good stir so that the sugar begins to dissolve into the water, put on the hob and bring to the boil. Let boil for 5 minutes. Lower to a firm but not exuberant simmer.

Meanwhile, cut the peaches in half, remove the stones, and lower a few halves at a time – I fit 4 in one go – cut-side down into the simmering syrup. Poach for about 5 minutes or until the peaches feel tender but not flabby. If you know they're in prime condition, then reckon on 3 minutes, but you could need to poach them, gently, for 10. I use a fork to prod into the underside, so the fork marks won't ruin the beauteous display later. With a slotted flat spoon, delicately remove the peaches to a nearby large plate and cook the remaining ones in the same way. Strain the syrup into a jug, remove a ladleful, put it back in the saucepan (freeze the jugful for the next time you make this) and reduce.

You want to end up with a syrup that will cling tightly to the peach cheeks when you pour it over them, but not so much that it sticks. Anyway, let both the syrup and the peaches cool for now, and when they're cool, remove the skins, arrange the peaches on the serving plate and pour the scant amount of syrup over them. They'll be fine for a good few hours like this.

SAUTERNES AND LEMON BALM JELLY

Charlotte Brand, friend and cook, put me on to this recipe from the *Gastrodrome Cookbook*. I've got masses of lemon balm in my garden, but you can substitute an equal amount of lemon grass.

I use a 1¼ litre, or 2-pint, ring mould, and pile pale fruit – golden raspberries and white currants if I can get them – dusted with icing sugar to fill the hole.

Turn to the recipe for rhubarb and muscat jelly (page 345) for comments about gelatine.

340g caster sugar
675ml water
35–40g lemon balm
bottle Sauternes or pudding wine
8 leaves gelatine
juice from 1½ lemons

Bring the sugar and water to the boil and boil for 5 minutes. Remove from the heat and pour off 125ml (or dip in and fill an American half-cup measure). Infuse the lemon balm in the remaining syrup until cold.

Of course you don't have to choose Chateau Yquem, but do select wine good enough to give to friends without making wry-mouthed apologies for it. You don't need a full bottle for the jelly, but since you want some pudding wine to drink with the pudding, there's no point buying a half bottle.

Strain the lemon-balm syrup, measure it and add enough Sauternes, or whatever you're using, to make 900ml. Soak the gelatine leaves in cold water for about 5 minutes, until they're soft. Warm 75ml Sauternes and squeeze out the gelatine leaves, then dissolve them in the hot (not boiling) Sauternes. Mix the lemon-balm syrup, gelatine–wine mix and lemon juice (which should bring the liquid up to 1.2 litres), check the sweetness and add more sugar if needed.

Dab a kitchen towel with vegetable oil (in other words, an oil with as little taste as possible) and smear the inside of the ring mould with it. This will make it easier to unmould later. Pour the jelly mixture in and put it in the fridge and chill for 4–6 hours (or until set, as this depends on the shape of the mould). If it helps, make it the day before.

You might need to place the mould quickly in a sink slightly filled with hot water to turn the jelly out. But make sure it is only quickly. It's better to keep putting it back in if it doesn't come out cleanly and easily rather than leave it in and have it start to melt.

A rich white Burgundy or Californian Chardonnay are rich enough to complement the lamb, the garlic and the mushrooms.

MIDSUMMER DINNER FOR 8

Pea, mint and avocado salad
Fillet of beef with red wine, anchovies, garlic and thyme, or tagliata
Jersey royals, warm spinach and lemon
Strawberries in dark syrup with Proust's madeleines

This, to me, is the perfect dinner: simple, impeccable, beautiful. Of course, it doesn't have to be a June dinner, or even eaten in summer: I cook the beef all through the year and I'm such a fan of the frozen pea that I've got no reason to ration the unfashionable but deeply pleasurable salad, either. But when all the food comes together like this it works at its best. I've given two choices for the beef simply because fillet for 8 is not always going to be a practical suggestion. If you want to make this a more formal dinner, then try the wine and anchovy braised fillet. The tagliata, a fat slab of meat cut all along the rump, marinated, cooked briefly, then carved in squat, juicy slices on the diagonal, is the best thing you can do with your outside grill, *pace*, perhaps, the butterflied lamb of the menu preceding this. But if you're kitchen-bound, a gas mark 7/210°C oven is absolutely fine.

The tagliata needs marinating for a day, and the strawberries need macerating for three hours. If you wanted to strike a more voluptuously grand note, you could end instead with the white tiramisu on page 125.

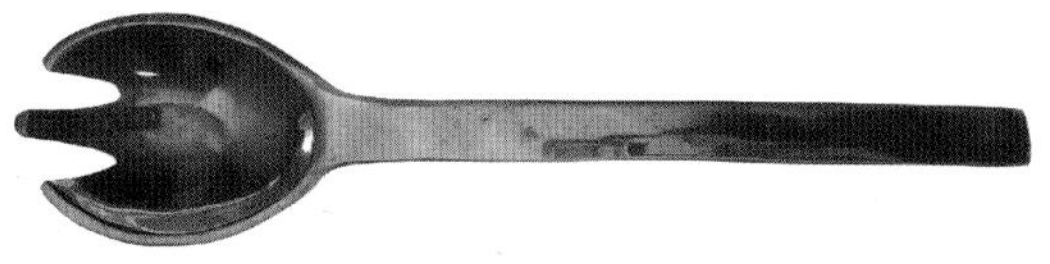

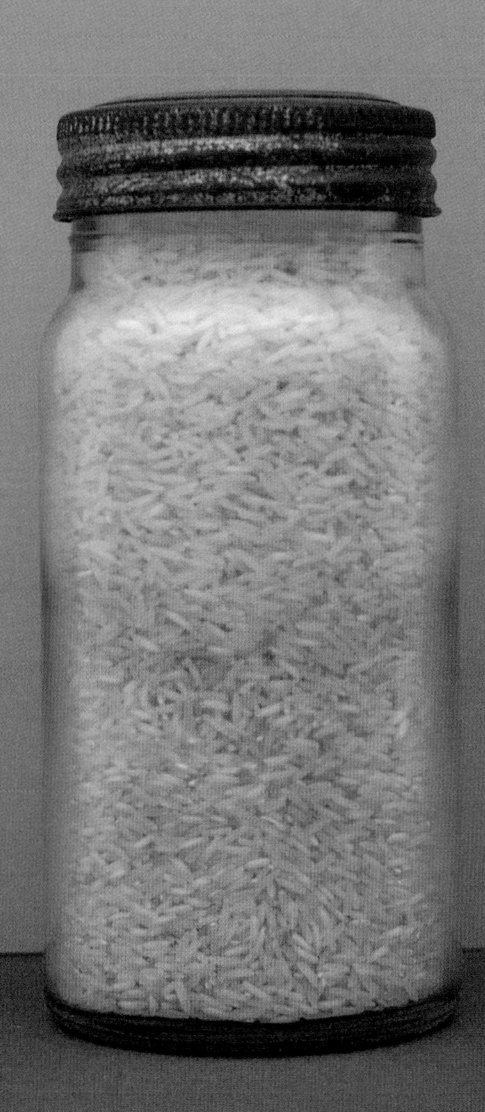

PEA, MINT AND AVOCADO SALAD

This is one of my Great Aunt Myra's recipes. Of course, you can use frozen peas, but it's a pity at midsummer, and feels odd somehow, like having a lightbulb on in brightest daylight. Alternatively – and this is probably the genuine compromise position – you can pod and cook them in advance and leave them steeped in the dressing. Nothing beats freshly podded, just-cooked new season's peas, but we must be prepared to bend a little for our sanity's sake.

9 tablespoons extra virgin olive oil
1 1/2 tablespoon good white wine vinegar
fat pinch caster sugar
bunch of mint
1 1/2 kg peas in pod (approx. 500g podded weight)
assorted salad leaves
2 chicory heads
3 ripe avocados

First make the dressing: put the oil and vinegar and a pinch of sugar into a large bowl and then put in a decent handful of chopped mint. You could use a processor if you've got one with a small insert bowl, but I use either my mezzaluna or a mouli herb mill (hand-held and cheap). Stir well so all is amalgamated. Cook the podded peas for a short amount of time in salted boiling water, just so that they're ready, but not soft. Taste after 2 minutes and then keep tasting. Pour peas in colander and then straight away into the bowl of dressing and let steep for an hour or up to a day.

Just before serving, stir in about a packetful of mixed salad, the chicory, which has been separated into its leaves and the avocado, which should be cut into bite-sized chunky slices. You may need to drizzle a bit more oil in it after tossing. Serve this on a big plate. Sprinkle with some more chopped mint.

FILLET OF BEEF WITH RED WINE, ANCHOVIES, GARLIC AND THYME

I love this particular combination: see, too, the more wintry, homey version in Cooking in Advance, page 112.

1 tablespoon extra virgin olive oil
60g unsalted butter
8 shallots or 4 banana shallots, chopped finely or sliced
good few sprigs thyme to yield 2 teaspoons leaves, or 1 scant teaspoon dried thyme

8 cloves garlic, peeled and squashed with flat of knife
12 anchovy fillets, packed in olive oil, drained and chopped small
2 x 750g pieces fillet of beef, trimmed
2 teaspoons caster sugar
4 tablespoons brandy
300ml good red wine

In a heavy-based pan (I use a cast-iron rectangular casserole; a baking tin, if it's sturdy enough, would do) in which the fillets will fit comfortably (no scrunching at the ends and they mustn't touch each other) heat the olive oil and 30g of the butter. Add the shallots, sprinkle with a little salt, and fry on a lowish heat for about 5 minutes until soft and transparent but in no way colouring. Add the thyme and give 2 more minutes, stirring, then add the garlic and push about the pan too. Now add the anchovies and cook on this low to moderate heat until they've started fusing with the oniony, buttery, oily mess in the pan. Remove this mixture for a minute so you can brown the meat and turn up the heat. Sear the fillets on all sides, sprinkling with the sugar as you do so, till you've got a good crusty exterior. Add the brandy, let it bubble up a bit, then pour in the wine. Return the shallot mixture to the pan. Lower the heat and turn the fillet over. Give the pan a good stir, to make sure the shallots, garlic and so on are not burning or sticking. Cover and leave for 10 minutes: the meat is braising, frying and steaming all at the same time; as it cooks it breathes in flavour. Open the lid, peek in, prod or poke – to see how cooked it is, and how much more time you think it needs – and turn the meat over, cover again and leave for another 5–10 minutes, depending on your findings and taste.

When the meat is almost as you like it, remove it from the pan (it will cook a little more as it rests) and get on with the sauce. And you can do all this before you sit down for the first course. Fish out the garlic by hand. Then turn up the heat and let it bubble up a good bit, and taste to see what, if anything, is needed. You may want to add some water. Take off the heat, but warm up before serving, at which time you should first pour into it the meat juices that have run out of the fillet as it stands and whisk in the remaining 30g butter, cut into small, cold dice. Carve the fillet, arrange on a large, warmed plate and drizzle over some of the sauce, leaving the rest in a jug for people to pour for themselves. If you can find some wild rocket, with those tiny William Morris leaves, use it to edge the borders of the plate. This doesn't just serve a decorative purpose: its pepperiness perfectly offsets the salty pungency of the anchovy–red-wine sauce.

TAGLIATA

If you're going for the tagliata, get two slices, each about 3cm thick and cut along the whole length of the rump, and put each in a large freezer bag to marinate with a clove of garlic squished with the flat of a knife, 100ml extra virgin olive oil, the zest of

½ lemon, a few peppercorns and a heaped teaspoon of fresh thyme leaves or a quarter teaspoon of dried. Tie or knot the bags and put them in the fridge for 12 or so hours. Remove and let get to room temperature before cooking as mentioned above. It's hard to say how long they'll take: it so depends on how you like your meat. I like mine pretty well still quaking and trembling on the plate; 20 minutes or so, depending on how my oven or outdoor grill are behaving. Test by prodding before you start poking knives in: if it's very, very soft and bouncy, it's blue; springy, rare; springy but with resistance, medium-rare to medium depending on that resistance; hard, well, you know the answer to that. Take the steaks out, let them stand for 10 minutes, then carve thickly or thinly as you like, crosswise and on the diagonal. If you've roasted the meat, you'll have some meat juices: deglaze with a little red wine or Marsala, strain, adding a few more chopped thyme leaves to the clear ruby juices, then dribble over the carved meat: there won't be enough for a jug. Put a plate of lemon quarters on the table too, for squeezing over the meat as you eat.

JERSEY ROYALS

Proper Jersey royal potatoes need nothing more than a brisk rubbing before cooking and the lightest anointing with butter after. As to the cooking itself: these are best steamed, but it's pretty well impossible to steam enough for 8 people, so just boil them but make sure you don't overboil them. I'd work on rations of about 200g a head; this sounds a lot on paper, but on the plate it somehow isn't.

WARM SPINACH WITH LEMON

You've got enough going on with everything else, so I'd use packet spinach, or even frozen (providing it's whole leaf, not chopped). Get 4–5 packets of the fresh stuff, 3 of the frozen. And you're not doing much more than wilting the former, thawing the latter. Add butter, olive oil and a bit of lemon juice, or else a good sprinkling of sumac, that sour, citrussy, Middle-Eastern ground-berry spice. Leave some wedges of lemon around the edges of the dish. A little grating of fresh nutmeg does something extraordinary here, too. The spinach should be at room temperature.

STRAWBERRIES IN DARK SYRUP

The darkness of the syrup in question comes from balsamic vinegar. Well, wait: this is not a sprightly, modern, hardly-dressed salad, but one with a syrup of garnet depths and intensity. The balsamic vinegar seems to make the red of the strawberries against it shine with the clarity of stained-glass windows. And it tastes as it looks: deep and light at the same time.

If you have some syrup left over after dinner, you can boil it up so that it reduces and thickens and you'll have the world's best ever, most intensely strawberryish ever, sauce to pour over vanilla ice-cream. There won't be enough this way for more than just you, but do it anyway: it's a heady experience.

Steep 1kg strawberries, hulled and halved, in 2 tablespoons (I find it easier to drizzle this over in 6 teaspoons) balsamic vinegar (the best you can afford) and 10 tablespoons caster sugar. Cover with clingfilm and give the dish a good but gentle shake to make sure all the berries get some sugar and some vinegar on them and leave for 3 hours.

Please: no cream, or similar, with these. But any form of sponge or cake would be fine. Since we are talking ecstatic culinary experience here, it seems entirely appropriate to produce some madeleines. The recipe here comes, naturally enough, from *Dining with Proust,* so we are really talking about:

PROUST'S MADELEINES

Since you need to leave the batter for 1½ hours, you may have to think of baking them as you eat the first two courses. You can eat them – warm and fragrant – as cake-biscuits for pudding. Obviously, you need to buy the special moulds for these shell-shape cakes, but that's not difficult now. I use ones that can take two tablespoons of the mixture below, but are best when you fill them with just one. You may, then, need to bake them in 2 batches.

90g butter, plus more for greasing moulds
1 tablespoon clear honey
2 eggs
75g caster sugar
90g plain flour, preferably Italian 00
icing sugar to serve

Melt the butter over a low heat, then leave to cool. Just before you need to use it, mix the butter with the honey. Beat the eggs, caster sugar and a pinch of salt in a bowl for about 5 minutes with an electric beater, until it's as thick as mayonnaise. Sprinkle in the flour; I hold a sieve above the egg and sugar mixture, put the flour in it and shake. Fold in the flour with a wooden spoon and then add the melted butter and the honey. Mix well, but not too vigorously. Leave to rest in the fridge for 1 hour, then take out and leave at room temperature for 30 minutes. Preheat the oven to gas mark 7/210°C. Melt a tablespoon or so of butter and brush over the madeleine moulds before filling them with cake mixture. About 1 tablespoon should do: don't worry about covering the mould; in the heat of the oven the mixture will spread before it rises.

Bake in the oven for 5–10 minutes. Mine seem cooked after about 7 minutes, but not all ovens are the same, so be alert from 5 minutes. Turn out and let cool on a rack, then arrange on a plate and dust with icing sugar.

A really good Burgundy is always the perfect wine with beef.

INDIAN-SUMMER DINNER FOR 6

Pea and lettuce soup

Lamb with chick peas

Couscous salad

Turkish delight figs with pistachio crescents

This is the sort of food to eat when the days are unexpectedly warm, but the nights are nevertheless beginning to get cooler. You're still in the mood for summer food, but you need ballast too. This food, like that in the previous menu, is as suited for eating on a table in the garden as it is for a windows-shut, curtains-closed dinner inside.

PEA AND LETTUCE SOUP

Shell the fresh peas. Then make a stock with the pods, some parsley stalks, peppercorns, onion, half a carrot and a stick of celery and, of course, water. If I don't feel like tackling fresh peas, or they're not available, I use frozen petits pois and either chicken stock or Marigold vegetable stock powder. I find it easier to start the soup off with thawed peas, but if they're still frozen it couldn't matter less. If you've got any basil-infused oil you can use that for softening the vegetables at the beginning. I know mint is the usual herb here, but basil seems to enhance the fruity sweetness of the peas.

2 tablespoons olive oil

4 spring onions, sliced finely

zest of 1/2 lemon

1 1/2kg fresh peas, podded or 500g packet frozen petits pois

1 English round lettuce, roughly chopped

1 1/4 litres light stock (see above)

1 teaspoon sugar

1 tablespoon dry sherry

3–4 tablespoons double cream

small plant or large handful basil

Put the oil in the pan and when it's warm add the very finely sliced spring onions and lemon zest, stir a bit and then add the peas. Turn well in the oil and then add the lettuce and cook till it wilts and then collapses into the peas. Pour over the stock, sprinkle over the sugar and bring to the boil. Turn down to a simmer and cook gently and uncovered till the peas are soft, about 10 minutes. Purée in batches, in a blender if possible. You don't get that velvety emulsion with a processor, though you can sieve it after processing, which will do it. Or just use the mouli.

Pour back into the saucepan, add the sherry and cook for a minute or so before tasting to see what else the soup needs, bearing in mind you'll be adding some cream and eating it cold. Let it cool a little, then stir in the cream and let it cool properly before putting it in a tureen and into the fridge.

Just as you're about to eat, taste for more salt or pepper, add more cream if wanted, and then shred the basil and add a good bit to each bowlful after ladling it out from the tureen.

LAMB WITH CHICK PEAS

It's up to you whether you use whole noisette rolls, which you roast and then slice, or individual noisette discs, which you grill, griddle or fry; the former taste better, but the latter look better. I can never carve from the entire rolled joint without it unfurling all over the place, but of course you do get the tender, uncharred sides from the middle of the roll. When you cook the individual noisettes, you're sealing each slice in the heat. But the marinade will help to make it tender. Make sure that you're using the best lamb you can afford.

If you're going for the whole-roll option, think along the lines of getting 3 x 400g noisettes (although I might well get 4), and then roast them in a gas mark 7/210°C oven for 20–40 minutes, depending on your oven and the age and thickness of the meat.

As for the individual noisettes, I work on the assumption that you have to give each person 2, and then allow for half of those present to have more.

I think it's easier to cook the chick peas in advance and do the lamb on the evening itself, having put it in its marinade the night before or the morning of your dinner.

THE CHICK PEAS Soak 500g chick peas in abundant water, and with a paste made from 3 tablespoons flour, 3 tablespoons salt and 1 tablespoon bicarbonate of soda (as on page 88). Leave for 24 hours. Drain, running the cold tap over them in the colander as you do so, then put them in a pan with 5 cloves of garlic, peeled and bashed, 2 bay leaves, 2 small onions, peeled but left whole (makes them easier to remove later) and the needles from a large sprig of rosemary. The bitter, boiled shards of rosemary will get in everyone's teeth, and ruin the creamy sweetness of the cooked chick peas, so put them in a bag or tea infuser.

Cover again with abundant water, add 1 tablespoon olive oil, put the lid on and bring to the boil, but do not open the pan; you'll have to listen closely to hear when it's starting to boil. Turn down slightly, and let the chick peas cook at a simmer for about 2 hours. You can check them after 1½ hours, but keep the lid on till then. When tender, drain, reserving a mugful of the cooking liquid. Leave, even up to a couple of days, till you want to eat. It would be better to remove the skins around each butterscotch-coloured pea, and I often start doing this, but have never yet completed the task.

To reheat, put 8 tablespoons olive oil and 6 cloves garlic, peeled and chopped, in a large, wide pan on moderate heat. I like to use a terracotta pot for this. Add to this 1–2 fresh red chillies, seeded and finely chopped, or crumble in a dried chilli pepper. Add the drained chick peas and turn well. Meanwhile, take 3 good-sized tomatoes, blanched, peeled, deseeded, roughly chopped and add to the chick peas. Salt very generously, stir well and taste; you may need to add some of the cooking liquid. You don't want this mushy exactly, but you want a degree of fusion, of fuzziness around the edges. Take off the heat, and cover until you've dealt with the lamb.

THE LAMB For 15 noisettes of lamb, make a marinade out of 10 tablespoons olive oil, 4 cloves garlic, crushed, 1 red onion, peeled and chopped, and 1 small fresh red chilli pepper, seeded and sliced. I find the easiest, most efficient way of doing this is by dividing everything between 2 plastic bags. Leave overnight or for as long as you can.

Just before you're about to sit down for your first course, take the lamb out of its marinade. You can drain the marinade and use that in place of the olive oil for sautéing the chick peas, above; in which case use a smaller amount of chilli. Cook the lamb either by frying in a cast-iron pan on a griddle, or giving it a few minutes each side under a very hot grill, or sear the meat in a pan then give them about 10 minutes in a gas mark 7/210°C oven. To keep the lamb pieces warm, leave them in a low oven on a dish covered with foil while you eat your soup.

When you serve, arrange the chick peas on a big, flattish bowl (again a terracotta one is perfect) or a couple of big plates and place the lamb over them. Chop over some fresh, flat-leaf parsley, or coriander if you feel infused with the mood of late-summer headiness.

COUSCOUS SALAD

Sometimes I provide just a couple of small bowls filled with well-chopped red onion for people to sprinkle over the lamb and chick peas as they like. The alternative is a couscous salad, which in effect is panzanella, only using couscous in place of the bread. I often put basil in it, but this dinner has enough going on as it is without introducing another forceful character, so I suggest parsley.

200g couscous
6 tablespoons olive oil
2–3 tablespoons best red wine vinegar
6 good tomatoes
½–1 small red onion, to taste
1 cucumber
1 bunch parsley, to yield approx. 8 tablespoons chopped

Put the couscous into a bowl with 1 teaspoon salt and pour over 250ml boiling water. Cover and leave for 15 minutes. Fluff up with a fork and add the olive oil, 2 tablespoons of the vinegar and some pepper and put in another bowl (or leave in the same one if you're in no hurry) to cool. Prepare the tomatoes by blanching, peeling, deseeding and dicing, only make sure you don't leave them in the hot water too long. Cut the flesh into neat small dice. Chop the red onion up small. You can leave these, separately, until you want to eat. The rest I'd do at the last minute.

That's to say, when you're about to put the main course on the table, dice the cucumber and stir, along with the tomatoes, onion and 7 tablespoons of parsley, into the couscous with a fork. Add salt and more vinegar if you think it needs it.

Arrange on a plate and sprinkle on the remaining parsley.

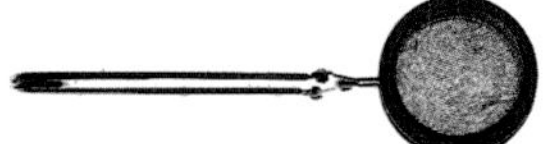

TURKISH DELIGHT FIGS

with thanks to Pat Harrison and Masterchef

How to say this without sounding ungracious? But I would never have expected to find such an easy, straightforward recipe on *Masterchef*. These figs are beautiful but not in an art-directed way: the purple-blue fruits are cut to reveal the gaping red within, so that they sit in their bowl like plump little open-mouthed birds. When they're slicked with the flower-scented syrup, they become imbued with Middle-Eastern sugariness, and the aromatic liquid itself absorbs and takes on a glassy pink from the figs. Perfect symbiosis.

Two figs a head should do it – they are very sweet, very intense – but if you can find only small figs, increase this to 3 per person. They're wonderful, anyway, the next day.

175g sugar
30ml/2 tablespoons rosewater
30ml/2 tablespoons orange-flower water
juice of 1 lemon
12 ripe, black figs

Dissolve the sugar in 175ml water in a small, heavy-based saucepan over a low heat. Increase the heat, bring to the boil and boil rapidly for 5 minutes. Add the rosewater, orange-flower water and lemon juice. Bring back to the boil and simmer for 2 minutes.

Carefully cut the figs vertically into quarters, leaving them intact at the base. Arrange on a flat, heatproof dish and spoon the hot syrup over them. Set aside to cool, basting with the syrup occasionally. Serve at room temperature, with Greek yoghurt and pistachio crescent biscuits (below).

The accompanying biscuits on the show were sesame seed and cinnamon scented. I make instead these pistachio crescents, rich and tender, almost soft and definitely friable. But not hard to do. And the aromatic grittiness and moon-curled shapes give a one-thousand-and-one-nights feel, which is just right with the rosewater scent of the fig-basting syrup.

PISTACHIO CRESCENTS

These are rather like the hazelnut-smoky Middle-European Kipferln sold in expensive late-night supermarkets: densely powdery within, compounded by the blanket of icing sugar with which they are thickly, mufflingly covered. The amount below will make 12 biscuits.

75g pistachios (shelled weight)
60g soft unsalted butter
15g icing sugar, sieved
45g plain flour, preferably Italian 00, sieved
pinch salt

Preheat the oven to gas mark 3/160°C. Grease 2–3 baking sheets or, better still, cover them with Bake-o-Glide (see page 506 for stockists).

Toast the pistachios by frying them in a thick-bottomed frying pan with no fat for a few minutes so that their rich, waxy aroma is released. Pour into the bowl of the food processor and blitz until pulverised. You can buy ground pistachios from Middle-Eastern shops – and I often do – but the varied, both nubbly and dusty, texture of the home-pulverised ones is good here.

With a wooden spoon, beat the butter until creamy – you are getting it ready to absorb the sugar with hardly any additional beating – and then duly add the icing sugar. I just spoon it into a tea strainer suspended over the bowl with the butter and push it through. Beat a while longer, until butter and sugar are light and incorporated, almost liquid-soft, and then add the sieved flour and salt. Keep stirring composedly and then add the ground pistachios, beating until just mixed. The dough will be sticky but firm enough to mould with your hands. If it feels too mushy, put it in the fridge for 10–20 minutes. To make the half-moons, flour your hands lightly and then take out small lumps of the dough – about 1 scant tablespoon at a time if you were measuring it, but I don't suggest you do: this is for guidance only – and roll them between your hands into sausages about 6cm long. Slightly flatten the sausage as you curl it round to form a little bulging snake of a crescent and put on the prepared baking sheet. Carry on until all the dough mixture is used up. And, by the way, don't be alarmed at how green these snakes look: cooked and dredged with icing sugar the intense lichen-coloured glow will fade.

Bake in the preheated oven for about 25 minutes, though start checking after 15. The softness should be just below the surface: take them out when the tops are firm and beginning to go blondly brown. Let the crescents sit on their baking sheets out of the oven for a few minutes and then remove to a wire rack. Go carefully: they are, as I said earlier, intensely friable. Dredge them with icing sugar very thickly indeed (again, I use a teaspoon to push the powder through a tea strainer) and leave to cool. You can do these ahead, and just dust over a little more icing sugar as you serve them.

A Californian Zinfandel has the aromatic spicy quality to be ideal with this meal.

MILDLY WINTRY DINNER FOR 8

Onion tart with bitter leaves

Roast monkfish, pumpkin purée and mixed mushrooms

Almond and orange-blossom cake with red fruit

I think of this as a very calm menu: there's enough food to warm but not so much that everyone will go staggering about afterwards vowing to turn macrobiotic. There aren't potatoes with the monkfish – the pumpkin purée is starchy and filling – so you can comfortably accommodate the cream and the pastry in the tart. The cake for pudding is cooked in advance.

ONION TART

Follow the foolproof pastry recipe on page 41. If you make and roll it out the day before, along with caramelising the onions, all you'll have to do on the night itself is take it in and out of the oven a few times, and beat some eggs and cream together. In other words, it's entirely manageable. Try to arrange things so that the tart comes out of the oven about 40 minutes before you want to eat it. This means that if you're planning to sit down to dinner at 9pm (though you'll be lucky), it should go in, fully assembled, at 7.40. You should get your blind-baking under way, then, as soon as after 7pm as possible.

for the pastry

120g plain, preferably Italian 00, flour
60g cold butter or 30g each lard and butter, diced
1 egg yolk, beaten with a pinch of salt and 1 teaspoon of crème fraîche
iced water as needed

for the filling

30g butter
drop oil
500g onions, sliced very thinly
1–2 teaspoons sugar
4 tablespoons Marsala
2 eggs
1 egg yolk
300ml crème fraîche
fresh nutmeg

Melt the butter with a drop of oil in a heavy-based frying pan, add the onions and sprinkle over with salt, and cook on medium to low heat for 12 minutes, until soft and transparent, then stir in the sugar, reduce the heat further, cover the layers of onions tightly with foil, and cook for another 20 minutes on the lowest heat, until tender (almost mush) and golden brown. Remove foil, turn up the heat and add the Marsala and let cook, on a moderate heat, stirring every now and again to make sure nothing sticks or burns, for another 8 or so minutes. By this time the onions should be a well-stewed, darkish brown tangle. Taste for salt and pepper, and then remove to a bowl to cool a little.

While all this has been going on, roll out the pastry to line a deep, 20cm tart case or 23cm shallower one, and leave in the fridge to rest for 15–20 minutes. Preheat oven, making sure there's a tray in there for the tin to sit on later, to gas mark 6/200°C. Line the pastry case with foil or greaseproof, fill with beans or pulses and bake blind for 15 minutes. Remove the beans and paper, wrap foil over the edges, and give the naked case another 12 minutes. Remove and let it cool a little. Turn the oven down to gas mark 4/180°C.

Make a custard by beating the eggs, egg yolks, crème fraîche and half teaspoon of salt together. Sprinkle in some salt and give a good grinding of black pepper and even more of nutmeg. Line the pastry with the soggy, caramelised onions and then pour over the custard. Leave it rather meanly filled until you've staggered over to the oven and put the tin back on the shelf; then you can spoon or pour in as much of the remaining cream and egg mixture as you dare without it spilling over and down the sides and ruining the pastry. Give another grating of nutmeg on top and bake in the oven for 30–40 minutes. When cooked, it should be set but not firm.

I make a variation on this, replacing the ordinary onions with red onions, the Marsala with red wine, and the crème fraîche with Greek yoghurt.

BITTER LEAVES

To go with the onion tart, make a bitter salad out of reddish chicory, or else chicory and treviso, or, if you're lucky enough to find it, those young greens called *cicorie* by the Italians. Make the anchovy dressing the easy way by adding some drops of anchovy essence to an emulsion of olive oil and lemon juice, adding a pin-prick of honey (very Apicius) if you think the balance needs adjusting. You can dispense with the onion tart altogether and make the salad the focal point, and sole constituent, of the starter. If so, make a dressing by mashing some anchovies to a paste with some thyme, adding a spritz of lemon juice and then as much oil as you need, gradually.

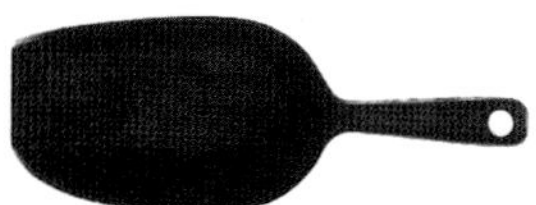

ROAST MONKFISH

Ask your fishmonger for four 500g pieces of monkfish tail; these are going to be easier to get than a couple of great, walloping ones. Trimmed, but with the bone in (it's such a big bone, you can just lift out the fillets as you serve), you should find they weigh about 430g each.

You hardly do anything to them, and what you do you do at the last minute – just before you sit down to the starter.

Preheat the oven to gas mark 5/190°C and, on the hob, sauté the fish a couple of minutes each side in about 3 tablespoons, more if you feel you need it, of butter and a drop or so of olive oil. I use a non-stick frying pan, a Wollpan (see page 506) which has a detachable handle so it will go in the oven later. If you've got any pan that you can use on the hob and in the oven and will fit all the fish, then use it. Otherwise use an ordinary or non-stick pan and transfer to an oven dish, making sure to pour the frying juices over before baking.

When you've fried your fish, sprinkle over some sea salt and a bit of lemon zest, transfer to the oven and bake for 20 minutes. Arrange the cooked monkfish on a large plate, removing each fillet's central bone as you do so. Put the baking tray with its lemony, salty juices on the hob for a moment, stir in some boiling water and grate over some pepper, and then dribble a mere tablespoon or so over the pale firm fish on the plate. But taste and adjust to suit, before doing anything. If you want to strew watercress or big and flat-leafed parsley around the edges of the dish, do.

PUMPKIN PURÉE

If you can, get three small (i.e. 1kg each) pumpkins rather than one huge tough, more watery, less flavoursome one. For each 1kg pumpkin, you need about 60g butter.

Preheat the oven to gas mark 6/200°C. Cut each little pumpkin into four. Remove the seeds (though leave the skin as is) and cut out a square of foil big enough to wrap each chunk in securely. Place each piece of pumpkin in the middle of its foil and dollop one tablespoon unsalted butter, then some salt (this does taste better than just using salted butter, I promise you) and pepper in each quarter's deseeded cavity. Wrap loosely in the foil, but twist the edges tightly to seal it absolutely. Place these packages on one or two baking trays and cook in the oven for 45 minutes.

Remove, but leave in their packages in their tins till cool enough to touch, or – if you're doing this in advance and then reheating as I most often do – leave until completely cool. Then open the parcels over a bowl or pan (or if you want your purée baby-food smooth, over a processor bowl ready and in position) so that all buttery juices are saved, and, using a spoon, scrape out the cooked flesh. Mash with a masher, whip with a wooden spoon or purée any way you like: the pumpkin will be soft enough not to need more than pushing to turn it into purée. There is enough butter in this: you do not need to add anything, except salt to taste, later. Any leftovers make wonderful soup.

MIXED MUSHROOMS

If you can't get such a variety of fresh mushrooms, use about 850g of those mixed mushrooms you can pick up in ready-assembled packages in the supermarket.

- 20g dried porcini
- 100g butter
- 2 tablespoons olive oil
- 2 banana shallots, or about 4 little ones, about 150g, chopped finely
- 2 very fat garlic cloves (use 4 if normal size), very finely chopped
- 200g or 2 large, flat, field mushrooms, chopped into small dice
- 200g button mushrooms, sliced thinly
- 200g chanterelles
- 200g shitake mushrooms, stalks removed, then mushrooms halved
- 30g trompettes de mort
- 2 tablespoonss dry sherry
- 2 tablespoons freshly grated parmesan
- parsley or chives, freshly chopped

Put the dried porcini in a measuring jug and pour on hot but not boiling water from the kettle to come up to the 300ml mark. Put half the butter and the 2 tablespoons olive oil into a pan. Turn on the heat and then add the shallot and garlic and cook on a low to medium heat for about 15 minutes until very soft indeed but not browned. A big, non-stick pan is good for this since the shallot tends to stew rather than fry, which is actually what you want here. After the dried mushrooms have soaked for 20 minutes, strain them, reserving the liquid, and finely chop the reconstituted mushrooms. Add them when the shallot and garlic mixture is soft, and then 2 minutes later add the rest of the butter and all the mushrooms and cook, with the lid on, for about 7–10 minutes, stirring and turning often. You may need longer, but you'll tell at a glance when they've cooked down. Remove the lid, turn up the heat, add the strained mushroom soaking liquid and the sherry and let it all bubble away until the liquid is syrupy. At this point I turn off the hob, and leave the mushrooms to cool and be reheated later.

At which point, warm them up and when hot add the grated cheese. Remove to a serving bowl and sprinkle with the chives or parsley.

The three components of this course not only go well together; the polished-panelling Murillo tones of the mushrooms, the smooth, unsubtle bright orangeness of the pumpkin, the plump, untroubled white of the fish, look wonderful next to one another on the table. And the tastes have the same rightness: the simplicity of the fish, the aromatic earthiness of the mushrooms, the sweetness of the purée; the perfect trio. Don't introduce a salad or anything else – except bread, preferably baguette, to soak up the copiously delicious juices.

PUDDING

Fruit and cake is just what you need here; you don't want to interfere with the simplicity and clarity of what's gone before. The almond and orange-blossom cake needs to be made a day or so in advance (and the recipe for it is on page 129): serve any fruit you want with it; but with a damp cake like this fragrant one, no cream. Raspberries are my favourite, but they may be too expensive or too flavourless, or just non-existent. Some delicatessens stock a German brand of bottled, not-too-sweet red cherries; drained, with some of the syrup reduced and spooned over them, they'd be just right. But never disparage the frozen package of summer fruits: grate some orange zest over before thawing and dust them with icing sugar before serving.

Try a Spanish red, ideally from the Ribeiro del Duero region, which has a fleshy, flinty quality and is harmonious and generous in character.

SIX IDEAS FOR KITCHEN SUPPERS

Since all my meals are eaten in the kitchen, the demarcation between the recipes to follow and those you've just read is meaningless. But, interior design apart, we all know what we mean by a kitchen supper. I take it to be a meal without a procession of courses, just food on the table, and not necessarily much notice in which to plan or cook it (although do look at Cooking in Advance, since most of the recipes there are for just this sort of laid-back thing). As far as I'm concerned, if sausages and mash (with apple rings fried in butter, please, like my grandmother used to make for me) would be appropriate fare, a tub of good, bought ice-cream an acceptable pudding, and it's in the evening, it's a kitchen supper.

All recipes serve 4 abundantly, which is the way I like it.

BLAKEAN FISH PIE

So-called because the intense yellow of the saffron-tinted sauce reminds me of one of those beautiful Blakean sunbursts. The saffron itself adds more than just depth of colour: it headily redeems the bland, cottonwoolly fish you buy in those plastic-wrapped polystyrene trays at the supermarket; useful when you can't get to a fishmonger.

1 carrot
125ml white wine
1 bouquet garni
1kg floury potatoes
125g unsalted butter
225g cod fillets
225g haddock cutlets
225g salmon fillets
approx. 150ml single cream
4 scant tablespoons flour, preferably Italian 00
pinch mace
1 x 0.25g sachet powdered saffron
150g cooked, peeled king prawns
fresh nutmeg

Peel the carrot, halve it lengthways and then cut each half into 3 or 4 and put the pieces in a deep frying pan with 125ml water, the wine, a good pinch of salt and bouquet garni. Bring to the boil and then turn off the heat and let cool. Cook the potatoes in salted water and mash with 80g of the butter. The best instrument for this is a potato ricer: it's cheap and you don't need to peel the potatoes; the skins stay behind as you push the potato through. Set aside until you've cooked the fish and sauce. Alternatively, if it suits better, you can cook the fish and sauce first and set them aside, and do the potatoes after.

Put the white fish in the carroty water and wine, bring to simmering point and poach for about 3 minutes. Remove to a plate and add the salmon and poach for about 3 minutes. Add to this the white fish, strain the liquid (keeping the bouquet garni) into a measuring jug and make up to 450ml with single cream.

Melt 45g butter in a saucepan and stir in the flour and mace. Cook, stirring, for a few minutes then, off the heat, stir in the cream mixture slowly, beating all the time to prevent lumps. When it's all incorporated, put back on the heat and throw in the sodden bouquet garni. Keep cooking and stirring until thickened – about 5 minutes – then add the contents of the sachet of saffron and cook, stirring, for another 5 minutes. Set aside for 10 minutes (or, if you're doing this in advance, let it cool altogether).

Butter a 1¼ litre dish and put in the cooked fish and the prawns. Pour over the saffron sauce (take out bouquet garni) and mix in. Cover with the mashed potato. Make sure the potato completely covers the pie dish so that no sauce can bubble up and spill over. Grate over some nutmeg and cook in an oven preheated to gas mark 5/190°C for 20–40 minutes depending on how cold the pie was when it went in. Eat with peas. You must.

THE IRISH CLUB'S IRISH STEW

When I was a child I remember eating a distinctly nasty Irish stew: watery, greasy and singularly unvoluptuous. I haven't been particularly won round by eating it in Ireland, either. But I recently had a bowlful at the Irish Club in Eaton Square, and it was velvety in its unctuousness, the meat and its gravy both infused with that sweet, tender viscosity. I don't think I have ever been so bowled over by something I've ordered. Actually, I didn't order it, or not initially. I had played safe and asked for the Irish smoked salmon with soda bread. But then I tasted the stew and felt pierced with envy. I am happy to eat from other people's plates; indeed I don't feel there's any point going out if I can't do that. But this was different: I wanted my own, and lots of it. The Irish Club's Irish Stew, with its inclusion of veal stock (and chicken for that matter), may offend purists, but experiences as voluptuous and pleasurable as this are always going to offend them anyway. Don't worry about making your own veal stock – yet again I recommend that made by Joubère – but it's important not to leave it out, as that's what produces, or helps produce, the requisite seductive stickiness.

Give the barley 20 minutes in boiling salted water before draining it and adding it to the otherwise uncooked stew.

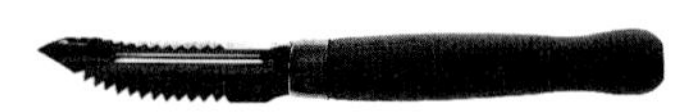

150g pearl barley
1.35kg mutton or lamb chops (gigot or rack chops) not less than 2.5cm thick
5 medium onions or 12 baby ones
5 medium carrots or 12 baby ones
3 large parsnips
needles from a decent sprig rosemary, chopped finely
3 sage leaves, chopped very finely
600ml stock (half veal, half chicken)
8 medium potatoes
1 tablespoon fresh parsley, chopped

Precook the barley as described above, and preheat the oven to gas mark 3/160°C. In a casserole in which you're sure everything's going to fit (and I use my Le Creuset Marmitout, which seems to be exactly the right dimensions for this) brown the lamb, having first cut off all obvious excess fat. You shouldn't need to add any cooking fat to the pan. Remove the meat and start on the onions, carrots and parsnips: if you're using the larger ones, peel and chop them, though don't chop the parsnips that small; if they're baby ones, just peel them. Turn them in the fat in the casserole, cook for about 5 minutes, stirring frequently, then remove to a plate for a moment. Then layer the casserole with the browned lamb, the slightly softened vegetables and the parboiled barley, seasoning well and sprinkling with the chopped parsley, rosemary and sage as you go. Pour over the warmed stock and then peel and slice the potatoes and arrange them, overlapping, like a tiled roof, on top, and season again. Put the lid on the casserole (and the Marmitout is useful as it has a slightly more domed lid than most) so that the potatoes steam inside the casserole. Put in the oven for 1½ hours. If you want the potatoes browned on top, dot with butter and blitz under the grill or in a turned-up oven when cooked.

The whole point of this stew is that it needs no accompaniment – except for bread, and lots of it.

SPANISH STEW

This stew is both plain and yet intensely flavoured: the thickly-sliced, fat-pearled, paprika-bright sausages ooze oily and orange into the sherry-spiked broth; the potatoes cook placidly alongside. It takes a few minutes to assemble, and then you just stick it in the oven. The thing that does make a difference is the chorizo itself: you need the proper, semi-dried (sometimes called fresh) sausages rather than the naturally drier, and stouter-waisted salame. The best chorizo for this seem to come in 200g hoops, so get 2 of those; otherwise 4 100g sausages would do fine, as long as they're the real thing. What you must guard against are those tight-fleshed, too lean and unyielding, so-called 'Spanish-style' chorizo (see gazetteer page 510).

1 tablespoon olive oil
1 small to medium onion, finely chopped
400g semi-dried chorizo sausages
3 cloves garlic, finely chopped
1 bay leaf
100ml dry sherry
1kg waxy potatoes
fresh coriander

Preheat the oven to gas mark 6/200°C. Pour some water into the kettle and switch it on.

Put the oil in a wide rather than deep pan that will go in the oven later – an oblong enamelled casserole or round terracotta dish or such like – and put on the hob on medium to low heat. Add the onion and cook for 5 minutes or so, until beginning to soften. While it's cooking, slice the chorizo into fat coins. Add the garlic and cook, stirring for another couple of minutes. Add the chorizo, the bay leaf and the sherry and stir. Slice the potatoes in half and add to the pot. I just stand by the pot, knife in hand, slicing them in one at a time. When they're all in, stir and pour over water from the just-boiled kettle to cover, but only just; don't worry about the odd potato poking above water-level. Simmer for 10 minutes and taste for seasoning.

Put the dish in the oven, uncovered, and cook for 35–40 minutes. Remove, ladle into bowls, and sprinkle over some fresh chopped coriander as you hand them round. You need lots of (unbuttered) bread with this, but not much else – perhaps a pale, crunchy and astringent salad after.

ONE-PAN CHICKEN

This is very easy, very quick. Don't be too hung up about the quantities below: they're nothing more than a guideline.

olive oil
1½kg chicken, cut into 8 pieces
1kg new potatoes, cut into 1cm dice
3 red onions, peeled and cut into segments
16 cloves garlic
3 red peppers, seeded and quartered
coarse sea salt
bunch flat-leaf parsley

Preheat the oven to gas mark 7/210°C.

Get 2 baking trays and pour in some olive oil to coat. Arrange the pieces of chicken, the potatoes, onions, unpeeled garlic cloves and pepper on them. If you want to use 3 trays and have got the room, do: the less packed everything is, the crisper the potatoes will be. Then drizzle some more oil over, making sure everything's glossy and well slicked (but not dripping), sprinkle with the salt and put in the oven for about 45 minutes.

When done (and taste all component parts) chop over the parsley and – I always do this – serve straight from the baking trays. A green salad's all you need with it, but puy lentils do go well.

ANGLICISED INVOLTINI

I adapted this recipe of Paul Gayler's (in turn his adaptation of a southern Italian recipe) for a *Vogue* column on food for vegetarians. It's anglicised only in so far as the cheese I use for the stuffing is lancashire rather than the more usual, but hard to find, provolone.

Don't serve this piping hot, but warm. The quantities of stuffing make enough for 12 rolls, so I fry only the best 12 slices of aubergines and then stop. If you feel 3 rolls per head will just not do, scale up accordingly. I never salt aubergines: just make sure you buy ones that are bouncily firm and shiny.

olive oil for frying (a lot)
2 large aubergines, cut lengthways into slices 5mm thick
150ml tomato passata
1 ball of buffalo mozzarella

for the stuffing
100g lancashire cheese, cut into very small cubes
75g pine nuts
50g raisins, soaked in water until plump, then drained
4 tablespoons extra virgin olive oil
2 tablespoons fresh white breadcrumbs
1 clove garlic, crushed or minced
2 tablespoons freshly grated parmesan
1 tablespoon chopped fresh basil
1 egg, beaten

Preheat the oven to gas mark 5/190°C.

Heat a generous quantity of olive oil in a frying pan – enough to make a film about 5mm or more thick – and fry the aubergine slices a few at a time until golden on both sides. As they're done, remove them to some pieces of kitchen towel. You will have to add quite a bit more oil as you go, so don't panic about it. Leave the aubergine slices to cool as you make the stuffing. You can always cook the aubergine in advance.

In a bowl mix together the cubes of lancashire cheese, pine nuts, raisins, extra virgin olive oil, breadcrumbs, garlic, parmesan and basil, season to taste and bind with the egg. Lay out the cooked aubergine slices on a table or work surface in front of you and divide the stuffing between them (I find 1–2 tablespoons per slice about right). Roll them up tightly to secure the filling and put them, as you go, into a lightly greased gratin dish into which they'll fit snugly.

Pour over the tomato passata. Cut the mozzarella into about 5mm slices and arrange them down the centre, in a line lengthways like a snowman's buttons. You could always use more lancashire cheese here instead. Drizzle with olive oil, add salt and pepper and bake in the oven for 25–30 minutes. Let stand for a bit before serving.

TAGLIATELLE WITH CHICKEN FROM THE VENETIAN GHETTO

This recipe comes from one of the best food books I've read, Claudia Roden's *Book of Jewish Food*. It is rather far removed from the sort of food I think of as typically Jewish over here, which might be comforting but lacks many of the other culinary virtues.

Of course you can use raisins: I prefer sultanas.

1 chicken (a 1 1/2kg one will feed 4)
2 tablespoons extra virgin olive oil
needles from 2 or 3 sprigs rosemary, chopped very finely
50g sultanas, soaked in warm water for 30 minutes
100g pine nuts, lightly toasted
500g tagliatelle

Preheat the oven to gas mark 4/180°C.

Rub the chicken with oil and sprinkle with salt and pepper, then place it breast down in a baking dish and put in the oven for 1–1/2 hours, until well browned, turning it over towards the end to brown the breast. It's done when the juices run clear, not pink, when you cut into the thigh. When the chicken's nearly ready, put abundant water on for the pasta, salting it when it boils.

Take the chicken out of the oven and take the meat off the bone, leaving all that glorious burnished skin on, and cut it into small pieces. I do much of this by just pulling, without a knife, but if you haven't got asbestos hands, use a knife and fork or wait till it's cooler.

For the sauce, pour *all* the juices from the roasting dish into a saucepan. Add the finely chopped rosemary, the drained sultanas and the pine nuts. Begin to simmer the sauce when you are ready to cook the pasta.

When the pasta's cooked and drained, toss it with the sauce and chicken pieces in a large warmed bowl. I like some flat-leaf parsley chopped over at the last minute. No cheese, please.

The last suggestion in this section is less a recipe than, for me, a way of life: boiled chicken with rice and egg and lemon sauce. This is the food of my childhood, a taste that roots me in my past. When my brother, Dominic, and Rosa got married, this is what he asked me and my sisters to cook him the night before. For us, this is the most significant kitchen supper.

CHICKEN WITH RICE AND EGG AND LEMON SAUCE

Exact quantities would not be in the spirit of things, but all you do is put a chicken, preferably a boiler, or 2 if they're very scraggy, in a pot, throw in chopped carrots, an onion or two, some leeks, a stick of celery, some parsley stalks and peppercorns, cover with water and salt.

Bring to the boil and then simmer for 2–3 hours, often skimming the foam that rises to the surface. About 40 minutes before the end of cooking time, remove as many of the vegetables as you can fish out with a slotted spoon, and add fresh carrots and leeks (and if I'm not in the mood for rice, I might add peeled, halved or quartered maincrop potatoes, too). Sally Soames, the brilliant photographer and old friend, whose chicken soup is one of the many impressive things about her, uses those pencil-thin baby leeks at this stage. But I deviate rarely. Just fat logs of leeks, long chunks of carrots, and the rice to bank them against later. The rice should be plain; and I like basmati.

The egg and lemon sauce, my mother's sauce, is really just a loosened, saffron-streaked hollandaise, without the ceremony. Sit a bowl on top of a saucepan of simmering water, put in it a couple of yolks, a pinch of saffron threads and a grinding of pepper (my mother always used white) and start beating with a whisk. Cube by softened cube, add some butter – until it's thick and pale yellow – then, always beating, add a ladle or so of the chicken stock from the neighbouring pan. Keep whisking, though more gently perhaps now, and when you have a thickened but still runny warm sauce, add a squirt or two of lemon. Remove the bowl from the pan and put it, with a sauce or plate beneath, on the table with its own little ladle.

If you've been able only to get a roasting chicken, you won't need to cook it for so long and the consequent stock will not be much stronger than water. Either boil the chicken in stock, or add a couple of stock cubes in place of the salt.

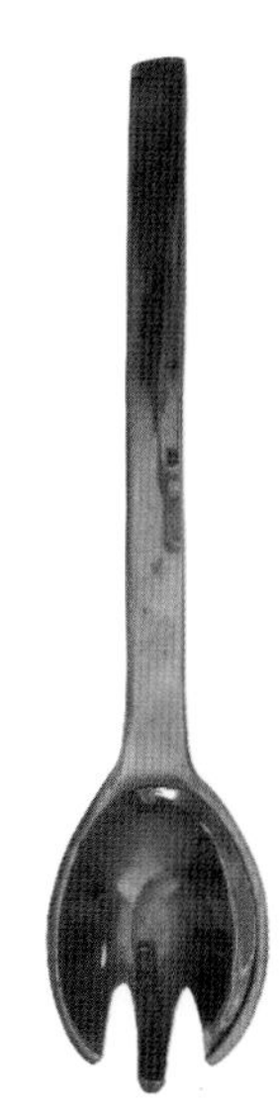

As for puddings: if I'm in the mood to make one, I make what I feel like eating, whether it comes from my dinner-party repertoire or is something I might otherwise think of having after Sunday lunch. By not suggesting any particular puddings here, I'm not depriving you: all the sweet thangs mentioned in any chapter of the book are listed in the Index.

low fat

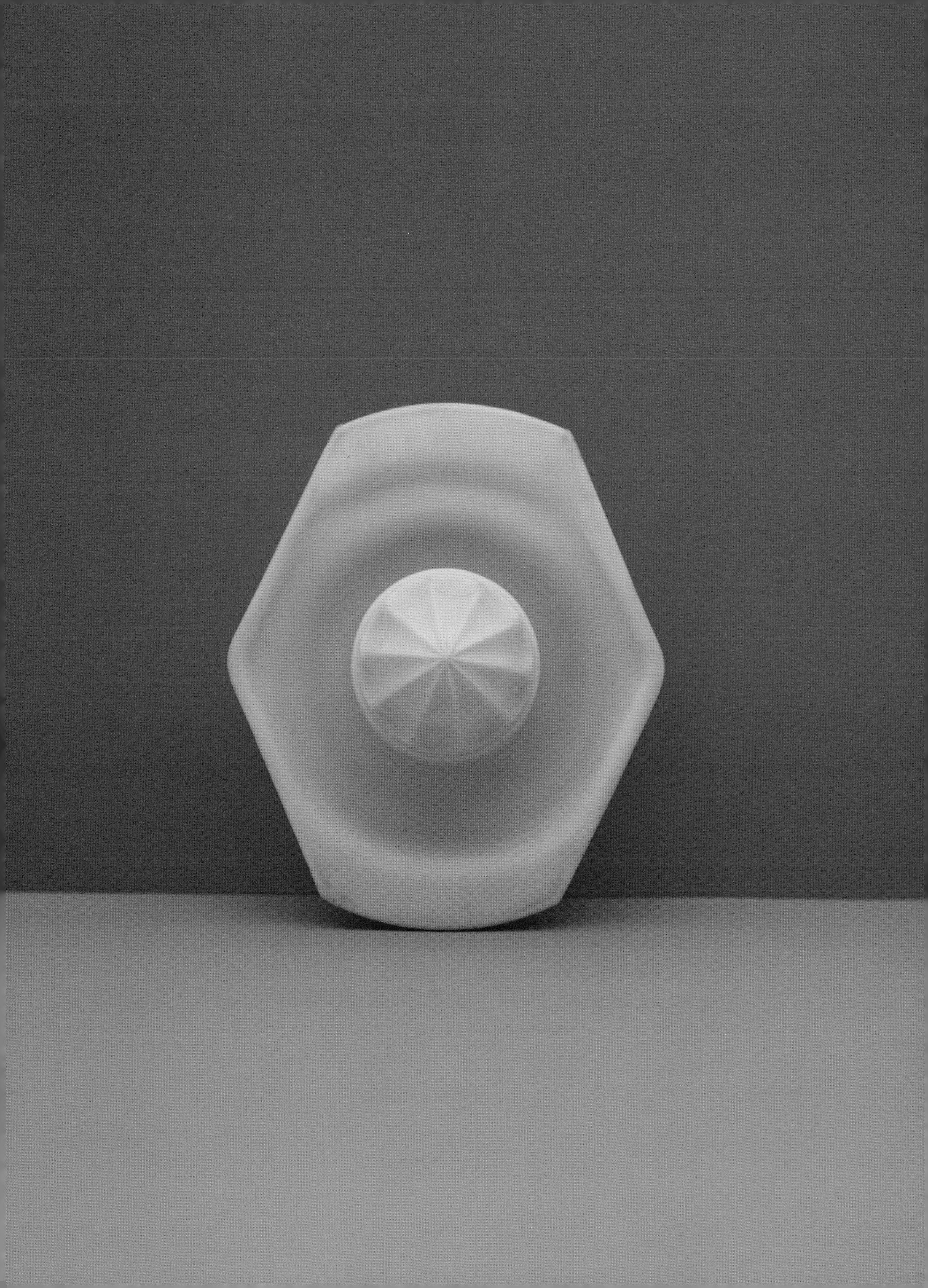

This is not the healthy foods chapter; it's not a healing, nurturing place where bad dietary consciences can come to self-congratulatory rest. You will not read about toxins and chai levels, about chakras and meridians. Nor am I interested in blood-sugar levels or cholesterol. Let's be frank: the issue here is vanity, not health; whether your jeans will do up, not what your oxygen uptake is. No one likes to own up to such a narcissistic preoccupation as mere appearance. Dieting claims almost a moral status when health comes into play. With what piety and smugness do the dietetically pure wave away those wicked, fat-clogged foods and show us, sinners all, the way, the truth and the Lite.

I don't disparage the shallow concerns of the ordinarily vain, which, after all, I share. What I hate is all this new-age voodoo about eating, the notion that foods are either harmful or healing, that a good diet makes a good person and that that person is necessarily lean, limber, toned and fit. Quite apart from anything else, I don't see the muscular morality argument. Why should a concern for your physical health be seen as a sign as virtue? Such a view seems to me in danger of fusing Nazism (with its ideological cult of physical perfection) and Puritanism (with its horror of the flesh and belief in salvation through denial).

So I take it for granted that anyone wanting to read here about low-fat food is doing so because they want to improve their *ligne* not their soul. More, I assume that anyone in need of diminution likes food. It is, after all, those of us who enjoy eating who tend to put on weight in the first place. All too often, though, the sort of people who espouse what I refuse to describe as 'healthy eating' care little for food – and it shows.

Good low-fat food takes time, preparation and thought. This puts a lot of people off, but it's part of the lure for me. I love the whole business of food. One of the things that makes me miserable about diets and dieting (more so than the obvious restraints) is that all too often they reduce food not merely to fuel but to medicine. I like the ceremony of food preparation: the shopping, the chopping, the stirring and attending.

low fat

Calorie intake is crucial. I shouldn't need to say this, it is both so obvious and has been known, and scientifically proven, for so long, but since every contemporary dietary trend is against it, you do need to be reminded and you do need to take note: if your energy intake in the form of calories exceeds your energy expenditure – what it takes to keep you going plus any exercise you want to take to boost it – then you will put on weight; if the latter exceeds the former, you will lose weight. It can't – pending findings, rather than wishful theories, to the contrary – not work. Everyone has their pet excuse, their alternative explanations: it's metabolism, what you eat with what, the intrinsic properties of certain foods, or all down to allergies and intolerances.

Despite, however, a firm belief in the ungainsayable truth of the calorie-intake theory of weight control, I wouldn't begin to suggest that's all there is to it. Put at its plainest, we know that what makes us fat is eating too much: but that says nothing about why we might eat too much, why we get fat, why we might find it difficult to lose those self-destructive, self-sabotaging habits. I'd have found it very difficult to embark on a diet and stick to it unless I'd first tackled *why* I'd put on weight. I don't imagine I'm very different from most women, in that I turn to food when I'm unhappy or under stress. And of course, like most women, too, my eating habits and whole attitude towards food have been influenced by my mother's eating habits and *her* attitudes towards food. I make this point not because I have any particular impulse towards self-revelation, but because I do want to make it clear that I know dieting is not as easy as just eating less. Having said that, you won't lose weight unless you do. And for all my long-held beliefs that fat was a feminist issue, that the modern tyranny of the scales was both ideologically and physically damaging and that intolerance of the un-thin was dangerous, I have to admit that I felt awful when I put on weight after the birth of my first child and better when I lost it.

If you stick to eating foods that are not high in fat most of the time, it is likely your calorie intake will, anyway, be curtailed. I find (when I'm trying to lose rather than just not put on weight) I keep an eye on calories too, as I somehow seem to be able to consume such vast platefuls of food that I can, with relative ease, go calorifically stratospheric while virtuously applying low-fat principles. And if you want to, I refer you to a most indispensible pamphlet brought out biannually by *Slimming Magazine* and called, I'm afraid, 'Your *greatest* guide to calories'. When I draw up my own dietary accounts my sums are not exact or scientifically correct. That's to say, I erroneously zero-rate

Marmite, Bovril, soy sauce, Vietnamese or Thai fish sauce, all herbs, cabbage, carrots, onions, mushrooms, courgettes, mangetouts and sugar-snaps, green or French beans, spinach, chard, pak choi and all that sort of leafy stuff, all lettuces, baby sweetcorn, baby asparagus, turnips, leeks, and pretty well any vegetable that isn't starchy.

But even when I just want to counteract an intensified bout of eating, either as a result of work or in the general run of a greedy life, I would never go below 1,250 calories a day. And on the whole, I don't count the calories, I just concentrate on this (and see the recipes below) type of eating.

Much as I hate the false witnesses of the various new-age health movements, I accept that, in order to make this whole thing work, you need to get in the mood, adopt something of the mindset; you need to shift into the my-body-is-a-temple mode. This way none of it feels like self-denial or deprivation: it feels like giving yourself something, doing something positive for yourself. For all the intellectual muzziness or rapt self-absorption involved, this is crucially important. As the one time Mayor of New York, Fiorello la Guardia, put it: if the ends don't justify the means, I don't know what does.

There is no one easy way to lose weight: different people find different ways; it's a case of what works for you. This is what works for me.

BEFORE YOU START

Since so much of this is about getting your head in gear, what you must do at the beginning is psych yourself up. And since you also need to make it easier for yourself on a practical level by having all the right foods around, you can combine the two by going on a mood- and scene-setting shopping expedition. This does two things: it helps banish any residual feelings of dismay about imminent deprivation (you are, after all, buying things for yourself and moreover things to eat) and it helps propel you into just that arena of obsession that is necessary to the successful outcome of any diet. Yes, yes, yes, to be too obsessed is a bad thing, and no, no, no, I am not for a minute suggesting you totter down the first steps towards anorexia and bulimia and associated eating disorders, but we all know that the less we're trying to eat, the more we think about it, so it makes sense to exploit that. Here, it means getting every little thing right to facilitate the cooking, and later it means thinking at length about what you're going to cook and how. The planning is not only a necessary part of losing weight; it also satisfies the part of the brain which wants, in a normally greedy person – and who else would need to be concerned with all this? – to be occupied with food.

I find just drawing up a shopping list of diet-enhancing ingredients fills me with all the zeal, good vibes and necessary I-can-do-thisness to make me feel positively impatient for it all to start. My stock list would be something like this.

LARDER STUFF

Marigold vegetable stock powder and a small selection of other packet stock including Thai pork and tom yam cubes
about 92,000 types of soy sauce (tamari soy, shoyu, light soy, dark soy, Japanese soy, citrus-flavoured soy, Indonesian Kecup manis, the lot)
teriyaki sauce
sukiyaki sauce (both these are really just soy sauce with other ingredients, itemised below, added for you)
Thai or Vietnamese fish sauce, nam pla or nuoc mam
sake
dry sherry
vermouth
mirin
rice vinegar
miso
instant dashi (sometimes called hon-dashi)
few packs Japanese instant miso soups and ramen noodle soups
Japanese pickled ginger
balsamic vinegar
good red-wine vinegar
various mustards – English, powder and made, Dijon, Meaux, tarragon and other flavours you like
various dry pasta and noodles (Italian short and long and oriental rice, buckwheat and egg noodles)

Tabasco, red and green
chilli sauce or piri-piri
comprehensive collection of spices
dried shitake mushrooms
basmati rice
garlic
onions
shallots (banana shallots for preference)
lemons
limes
dried red chilli peppers
good, bought, low-fat tomato sauce for pasta (check nutrition tables on bottles in the shops and try out till you find one you like; Marks & Spencer's Italian Pasta Sauce is my favourite)
6-pack 25g bags of twiglets
toasted, or fragrant, sesame oil (yes, really)
garlic-infused oil (ditto)

IN THE FRIDGE

There is no way you can make sure of an adequate supply of all the ingredients you might like to use without also having, sporadically, to throw away stuff that's gone off. Even the exotic ingredients can mostly be found at the supermarket. Turn to stockists on page 506 if you have trouble buying any locally.

One each, at least, of each packet of supermarket prepared vegetables
pak choi or similar leafy greens
salad stuff
bunch each of coriander and flat-leaf parsley
lemon grass
Thai basil
fresh rice sticks and somen noodles
shrimp paste

miso (I add it here, too, as it goes in the fridge once opened and I buy squeezy bottles from a Japanese shop, for preference, not burstable plastic bags of it)
fresh chilli peppers
fresh ginger
spring onions
a ready-prepared meal (and see below, in notes to the freezer list)
0-per-cent-fat fromage frais
0-per-cent-fat Greek yoghurt
very-low-fat fruit yoghurts and fromage frais

FOR THE FREEZER

kaffir lime leaves
one or two bagged-up portions cooked rice
some ready-prepared (either by you or the supermarket) meals for one that can be cooked from frozen
24g portions of good cheddar, grated
1 steak, well wrapped
1 boned, skinned chicken breast, well wrapped
sliced bread
frozen whole-leaf spinach
frozen raspberries or summer fruits

Bread, good bread, is one of my weaknesses, and I can eat an entire loaf without difficulty. If I'm having poached egg on toast, or toast and Marmite, as part of my dieting intake, I want to make sure I know I've eaten it. For this I need proper bread. I go to a French bakery and buy a couple of loaves of their *pain du campagne* (sludge-coloured and grainy with a toothsome, tough hide) which I get put through their slicer and bagged-up. I put these bags in the freezer. I can then toast, slice by single slice, as needed, from frozen, and it's not quite so easy to chomp through an entire loaf without thinking.

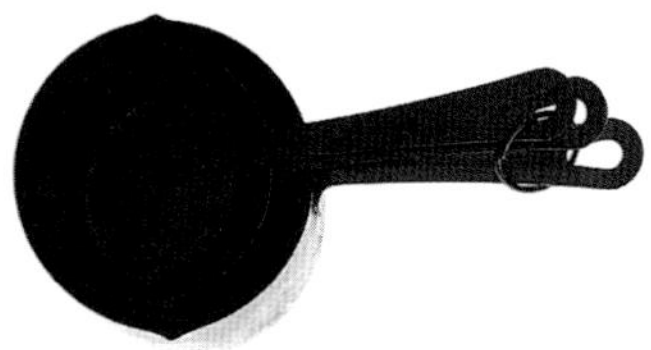

If you're keeping food in the deep-freeze, a microwave is a near-essential piece of equipment. I reckon that most of us who need (and often repeatedly) to lose weight are those for whom instant gratification takes too long. I seek to minimise damage (it's awe-inspiring how many calories you can consume, standing up, just while the dinner's cooking) by having a supply of food I can get from frozen to cooked in a few minutes.

I am not going to suggest that you rush out and buy a great number of gadgets. Many of you will already have a food processor and a microwave. I think there is really only one other essential item and it's a *good* non-stick frying pan. Of all the pans I have tried out, the only ones (thus far) I would recommend are a Finnish make called Panny and a German range called Wollpan. Once I melted some mozzarella in both (not, I admit, suitable to be repeated in a low-fat context) and found that I could clean them out just by wiping with kitchen towel. I think that's a fairly conclusive test. Neither is cheap, but either will save you a great deal of grief (and calories); stockist information is on page 506.

The only other piece of equipment I'd mention isn't essential, but is useful: a griddle. No one needs reminding about plain grilled fish or chicken, but I find too much of this stock-diet food immensely depressing. Most domestic grills are just not hot enough, so that all lean cuts dry out before they are cooked – which is where the griddle comes in. By this I mean one of those heavy cast-iron slabs, ridged on one side for meat and veg, smooth on the other for fish. You do need to oil this to some extent, and I use here an oil and water spray I make myself (pinching the idea from the low-fat culinary evangelist Sue Kreitzman) by buying an atomiser from Boots and filling it with one part best olive oil to seven parts water. By doing this I feel I'm making up for a lifetime of not watching *Blue Peter*. You can, of course, just buy an olive oil spray from the supermarket if it makes life easier. The griddle's good for giving that charcoal-striated edge to otherwise plain foods; and the searing heat that comes over cast iron seems to make food taste more acutely of itself, keep it juicier and make it look better. On the down side, it is very heavy (often I feel just too limp-wristed even to contemplate dragging it out of its drawer beneath the lower oven) and can be nightmarish to wash up; the feel of scourer against cast iron is rather like nails down a blackboard.

Dieting demands exact measurements. You need scales, proper teaspoon and tablespoon measures (the whole set, indeed, comprising ½ and ¼ teaspoon measures, too) and a measuring jug. American cup measures are useful, too.

BASIC PRINCIPLES

Immerse yourself in the desirable ethos before you begin, and settle into good habits once you do. Alcohol is immensely useful in bringing real depth of flavour to food cooked without fat, but if you really want to lose weight, I think you have to give up drinking. I am more of an eater than a drinker so I don't mind, but I know this is difficult for many people. It's not just the calories in the alcohol: even a small drink makes me feel positively insouciant about weight, diet, food, calories, all of it. This is a wonderful feeling while it lasts, but dismal when – several thousand calories later – it stops. Also if I drink enough to give me even a little shadow of a hangover, I have to eat vast amounts of fatty, stodgy food the next day to absorb – or so it feels – all the excess alcohol of the previous evening.

With eating I am less rigid. For just as I find a balance between large portions of low-fat and small portions of relatively high-fat food the best way of maintaining interest in what I'm eating when trying to lose weight, so I find I can stick longer to any diet if I keep a balance between repetition and variety. For example, I find it uncomplicates matters if every day I have the same breakfast and more or less, but not exclusively, the same lunch. Dinner I like to vary, and as much and as thought-consumingly as possible. Those who can't make their own lunch (although most workplaces have rudimentary cooking equipment now) might prefer to swap lunch with dinner, though I must say I'd find it hard to stick to a diet if I ate the same dinner every night. I need to feel dinner is a proper, celebratory meal, when the food I eat is food I can concentrate on, think about, both beforehand and afterwards. Breakfast is about 30g porridge (I use an American ⅓-cup-measure to scoop it out rather than actually weighing it and it must be jumbo oats, preferably organic, or it's just a slimy, too-smooth wallpaper paste) cooked with 2½-3 times its volume of water and eaten with 1 tablespoon golden syrup. If I know I will just stagger into the kitchen in the morning and get that under way, it stops me from deciding on the spur of the moment to put a couple of pieces of toast on, slather them with butter, then heap them with marmalade.

Although a low-fat diet makes things easier in terms of losing weight, for me a low-sugar one doesn't. I found that if I used hardly any sugar (or some ghastly sugar substitute) the food I ate just wasn't as filling. The same's true with hot drinks. I don't take sugar in tea, but I do in coffee. For ages I used one of those powdered ersatz sugars, the sort that fizz up spookily after you add them to the filled-up mug; then I just went back on sugar. What I found was that if I had a mug of coffee with sugar, it filled me up as if I'd eaten food (which of course I had, in the form of the calorie-bestowing sugar). Having said that, I virtually inhale all those fizzy, Nutra-sweetened drinks, the ones we are finger-waggingly told to give up in the name of cellulite-banishment, when I'm trying to lose weight.

BAKED POTATOES

Now, lunch: the most filling and somehow undiet-tasting lunch I found was a baked potato with cheese. Diet books and slimming magazines advocate reduced-fat cheese: I cannot. Despite my love for the well-piled plate, I would prefer to have a small piece of some proper, good cheese than double, quadruple, the amount of some low-fat, depressing variant. (Low-fat yoghurt and 0-per-cent-fat fromage frais, however, somehow taste low-fat even when they're not really, so you may as well go for the low-fat ones.) Food shouldn't be tampered with so that all its rightful, taste-giving properties are taken out of it. Try to find a way of cooking food that's meant to be low fat, rather than strangulated versions of food that was born to be saturated in the stuff. That is one of the reasons why most of my diet-minded suppers (see below) are Thai and Japanese, or otherwise oriental in tone, if not directly; these cuisines quite naturally don't use a lot of fat in many of their dishes, so the food tastes right, is right, cooked like that. Fake diet food, like reduced-fat cheddar, which tastes like bitter rubber, is a waste of your time. In your baked potato, real, strong cheddar in a smaller quantity will taste more, and will melt more seductively into the floury flesh, so that you won't even feel that you're getting less for your calories: 24g of Marks & Spencer's vintage cheddar comes to the same calorie count as 28g of reduced-fat cheese. So we're not even talking about much less in quantity. To be this precise (or obsessive) about calorie-counts, it is easier to buy well-labelled packaged cheese. You also need electronic scales. And the grater and the freezer. Were I to have a chunk of cheddar in the fridge, I'd eat it. So instead I keep a large supply of bagged-up grated cheese, all weighed and uniform, at 100 calories a bag. (And this principle is worth applying to any food that is admissible for your diet in individual portions but not eaten *en bloc.*)

CHEESE

Each lunch-time, I take the little frozen bag out to thaw as I put my potato in the oven to cook. It is a routine, a ritual. If you work in an office which has a microwave, you'll have to make do with that. (I absolutely can't take a packed lunch anywhere with me or I'd eat it by eleven in the morning. I can feel it throbbing away beneath the desk or in my bag, and just can't concentrate until I get rid of it.) This is the advantage of the baked potato option: it becomes routine, which prevents lunch being a significant, decision-provoking issue, but somehow makes it a reassuring fixed point; and it's there, but uncooked till the moment of blitzing, so you can't just wolf it down.

A potato which weighs about 200g raw, which is a goodish-sized potato, plus my 100-calorie package of cheese, makes a lunch of 250 calories. Include my breakfast, of just above 150 calories, and I've still got quite a lot of calories saved for the evening. But I want to offer up one more pearl of dietetic wisdom. Don't allow yourself to get too fiercely and unforgivingly hungry. If you leave eating till you could scrape the wallpaper off and eat that, then two things will happen: the first is that you will be jumpy and depressed; the second is that you'll be so hungry you won't be able to stop eating when you're full up. The more nagging hunger you feel during a diet, the more likely you are to ditch it.

YOGHURT

FROMAGE FRAIS

If you need to eat between meals, don't allow yourself to feel you've failed or that you've given in or whatever it is that makes people inflate with self-reproach and then eat double. Instead, take a low-fat yoghurt or fromage frais from the fridge. They are about 50 calories and, small as they are, they fill you up quite efficiently for a while. Of course it would be better in any number of ways to have an apple or an orange, but sometimes you need the gloop too. Reconcile yourself to this now, count it in and then move on, sister. It's all very well getting hungry when you're at home, because you can be sure to find something suitable to eat. But it's more difficult when you're out. Twiglets, in those small, but not too small, 25g packets, are around 100 calories apiece and low fat with it. And because they're so salty they feel filling (strong tastes do that, see more on this below) plus they're portable. If you had a huge drum of twiglets in front of you, you'd find it difficult to stop eating after your 100-calories' worth; so stick to the little packets. A bar of chocolate with about 250 calories, or a bag of crisps at about 150, are not disasters, either. There are times when chocolate is what's needed and it's better to have just one bar, count it in, and adjust your eating for the rest of the day accordingly, than to brood obsessively on it, have grilled fish for dinner and then go out, buy and eat

TWIGLETS

the entire contents of the all-night garage shop and live, self-flagellatingly, to regret it.

A diet that eliminated *all* fats would be extremely bad for you (and unpalatable). My point is to find balance, not to veer off into extremes. And to vary pace and plate, I often prefer a small portion of something high fat bolstered by forests of green vegetables. One of my regular dinners when trying to lose weight is a Marks & Spencer individual-sized steak and kidney pudding. Now, I am not going to claim that this is a low-fat food, but there is not very much of it, and what there is is very filling. When I'm too hungry or too tired to cook, I have one of those, with a whole packet of ready chopped cabbage and some other green vegetable with strong mustard on the side. Given that this steak and kidney pudding is under 500 calories and I don't count calories in vegetables, this is a trim little dinner all told. Anyway, I can't reiterate too often the need for balance and variation. The thing to remember is to pile, next to almost anything you're eating, a huge amount of soy-dressed or lemon-squeezed leafy or crunchy vegetables.

Much, as Byron wrote in *Don Juan*, depends on dinner. If I eat well at night, and not only eat well but make something of a ritual pleasure out of the meal, I don't feel that edginess, that diet-deprivation thing, that boredom above all else, that can make it all intolerable. Dinner has to feel civilised, or life doesn't feel civilised.

First, stagger the food, so it feels as if you have a wonderful procession of things to eat, not a great mound of stuff on a plate. These quiet rituals – and the low-fat, health-store foods they involve – create a pleasantly virtuous and serene mood. A girlfriend and I refer meaningfully to such meals as templefood. And, as the Japanese know, it makes a difference. If I've decided to have a salmon steak, seared speckly brown and tangerine without, still Tizer-coloured within, and some still-crunchy broccoli with soy and a few pin-prick dots of treacly sesame oil alongside, I might – to prolong my eating evening – make some grilled courgettes to eat before or drink a bowl of miso soup, and, afterwards, peel and finely slice an orange and drizzle over with orange-flower water. This is to make me feel it's something special that I'm eating.

SALMON

COURGETTES

These are a regular supper-enhancer. Get in from work, put the griddle, corrugated side up, on the hob, and then slice a few courgettes, down the length of them, so that you have thin, long, butter-knife-shaped strips. Spritz the griddle with your water and oil spray, then cook the courgette strips briefly on each side till they're tigered brown. Remove, sprinkle with salt, chop over some herbs – parsley, mint, coriander, any one or all three – douse with lemon juice and just eat.

PEPPERS

SEVILLE ORANGES

Another fatless, and in my book calorieless, picking-food is charred, peeled and sliced peppers (see page 96 for method) over which you've sprinkled a drop or two of good balsamic vinegar, squirted a little orange juice, sprinkled a little salt (or use a bit of anchovy essence if you like) and chopped more than a little flat-leaf parsley. And this is transcendental in January when the Seville oranges are around. Their particular biting but fragrant sourness points up the oily sweetness of the skinned and softened peppers. Pomegranate juice (use an electric squeezer) is heavenly, too. (I like to keep this soused tangle of peppers on standby; leave to steep in fridge or larder and add grassy clumps of freshly chopped flat-leaf parsley whenever you eat it. This oil-free peperonata also happens to make a fabulous sandwich filling.)

HERRING

And as long as the Seville oranges are about (which coincides, fortunately, with the clichéd annual post-Christmas clean-up) I like to make as well a dinner of grilled herring, which is put, fiercely hot and sprinkled with salt, on a cold plate covered with paper-thin slices of fennel squeezed over with Seville orange juice.

LEMONS AND NUTMEG

TOMATOES

LEEKS AND ASPARAGUS

But this flavour-intensifying principle works all year round. Just use lemons. It's not only broccoli whose sweetness is made the more vibrant with a squirt of lemon, but all greens. Nutmeg – with all of the above – works in a different, but equally effective, flavour-enhancing way. And any of the soys can be substituted for the lemon. Make a tomato salad, leafy with basil, dressed just with a few drops of good balsamic vinegar. Roasting vegetables also seems to make them taste more emphatically of themselves: leeks (see page 354 and reduce the oil a little), or asparagus, or, indeed, more or less any vegetable can be cooked with a very little oil (if you use none at all you'll just have a wizened limp mess) in a fiercely hot oven. To look at they'll be muted, but the flavours will be kick-started into vibrant life.

FENNEL

The trick is not to become bored, and therefore to use as varied a collection of vegetables as possible. Fennel can be sliced thinly and baked in a small amount of stock in a moderate oven for about 40 minutes, or eaten as a salad with lamb's lettuce and lemon juice. Add an equal amount of white wine to salted water, bring to the boil and add leeks cut into about 10cm lengths and cook until tender. Cauliflower can be broken into florets, dusted with ground cumin and baked in a very hot oven for about 20 minutes until it tastes sweet and charred and spiced; actually, I think this is the best way to eat cauliflower, diet or no diet.

CAULIFLOWER WITH CUMIN

VEGETABLES WITH GINGER AND GARLIC

Chop any vegetable that comes to hand and cook in a method that combines stir-frying with steaming: throw a small amount of stock in a wok and on a high heat add ginger, garlic, spring onions, sugar-snaps, broccoli, fennel, carrots and baby sweetcorn. But all this isn't just to ring the changes with what might otherwise be thought of as standard diet food. The more strongly food tastes, the fuller it makes you. It's the depth of the flavours that helps atone for the lack of fat. In the days when I was the hostage of a sandwich bar at lunch-times, I'd have a low-fat cottage cheese sandwich – no butter – but with anchovies; the saltiness, the aggressive and indelicate invasiveness of those cheap and unsoaked tin-corroded fish made me feel, after it was finished, that something actually had been eaten. Whereas, a plain cottage cheese sandwich, even on brown, hardly has the force of personality to make itself felt. You're not eating, you're giving the mime performance of a woman lunching on a sandwich.

ANCHOVIES

That's where Thai, especially, and other Southeast-Asian cuisines come in: they draw on intense flavours; have a vivid culinary vocabulary; fill you without supplying much in the way of fat. Italian food, it's true, is also strong and direct and robustly flavoured, but it uses more oil, and that oil, green, pungent, evocative, is not an optional extra. It's an essential part of the food. And I know it's supposed to be life-enhancing and healthy but it will still, all oils being equally fattening, make you put on weight. Not that all Italian food uses a lot of it; nor does olive oil have to go completely from your regime. You need only a little. If you add, at the end (rather than at the beginning) of cooking, one teaspoon, a few drops of it even, the glorious taste will come through, virtuous drabness will disappear and flavours will be revitalised. I often, too, stir about a quarter of a teaspoon of garlic-infused oil into some lemon-squeezed spinach; sesame oil makes itself pungently felt in the most minute quantities.

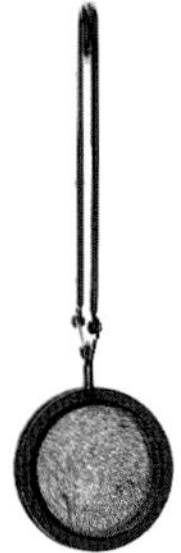

My concern here is how you go about leading the low-fat life in your own kitchen, but there is one important piece of advice to be applied in the world beyond it. Never say diet. By that I don't mean you should banish such a foul four-letter word in favour of the smug-speak term, Healthy Eating Plan, but simply that you should never talk about it. Not out loud. Not in public. In the first instance, talking about dieting is a big bore and in the second, everyone will try, if only out of politeness, to talk you out of it. The third, crucial, element is pure vanity: if you tell people you need to lose weight they will notice that yes, maybe you *do* need to.

The fortunate truth is that no one is really interested in anyone else. If you don't tell them you're on a diet they won't even notice. You can eat as little as you want without drawing attention to it and therefore without inviting comment or sabotage, or allowing yourself to use the excuse of others to sabotage the diet yourself. If you want to diet then you have to take the responsibility yourself, not draft everyone else into the diet police.

When you're invited to dinner, don't warn people of your diet or draw attention to it while you're there. It's so aggressive to do that, so self-centred, and so dispiriting. And you'll just be a party-pooper. Once people know about the diet, they'll feel that you can't really enjoy yourself until you eat and drink to Rabelaisian excess. They'll feel you're being dried up and puritanical and drained of joie de vivre. But if you don't make an issue of it, they won't think of looking at your plate.

I find it very difficult to leave food, but if you really want to and can, then be the one to jump up and clear the plates so no one else sees. You have an easy excuse for not drinking; just say you're driving. But, again, there is no need for anyone really to notice. Just let your glass be filled, but don't drink it.

There may well be nobler spirits out there, but I find the assault on one's vanity the hardest thing about dieting. It's bad enough you need to lose weight, but drawing other people's attention to it is quite intolerable. And it's not just weight gain I don't like people to notice, I can't bear references to weight loss, either. Call me paranoid, but every time someone says, 'You've lost weight!', I hear, 'You were fat!'

There is a vexing circularity about the dieting business: it's easiest to lose weight if you feel self-confident, but it is weight loss that makes you self-confident. But you can work the con trick on yourself. Just as Pascal believed that the act of going to church, of going through the motions of the faithful, led to faith, so if you act thin, you will get thin. Eat like a thin person is the best form of dietary advice. And behave like a thin person, too: which means don't go on about being fat.

Most of the recipes that follow are for one; some are for two. I take the line that that's how we tend to eat when trying to lose weight. Not everyone wants to get into the strict diet account-keeping needed for a calorie-counted diet, but you may follow the recipes below in the knowledge that all the food here is low fat and programmed for diminution.

QUICK STUFF, OR SUGGESTIONS FOR ALMOST-THROWN-TOGETHER SUPPERS

STEAK

Although I subsist mostly on carbohydrates and vegetables when I'm trying to lose weight, I like red meat every now and then when I'm not eating so much; it's filling, it makes me feel better (in France doctors can still prescribe steak and red wine for patients who are run down) and it seems an efficient use of restricted calories. Fillet is the leanest cut, and the easiest one to get in the right, slight, single-portion size (I aim for about 125g to make room for other components, before or after) but if I've got a friend over, or just feel like a meaty blow-out, I buy a 225g 2cm-thick slab of rump, put it on the griddle and cook till crusty without, tender and bloody within. Then I take it off the griddle, sprinkle with salt and leave it to rest on a plate for 5–10 minutes.

Meanwhile I slice some tomatoes and sprinkle with salt and balsamic vinegar or wilt some spinach. I pour off the juices that have collected on the plate with the steak into a bowl, add some soy sauce or bottled (or make your own, and see below) teriyaki sauce. Then I slice the meat in thin slices diagonally across, arrange back on the plate, pour over the blooded soy, and thickly feather with freshly chopped, cave-breath pungent coriander. If you want a more Italianate version, substitute lemon juice for the soy and rocket for the coriander. Either way, I like to eat this with hot English mustard on the side.

FISH

Salmon and tuna are the fish world's equivalent to steak. They are oilier than those pallid, white-fleshed varieties, but they are denser, heavier, too and more robust in flavour. If you can afford the best bass or bream, then just grill and eat. Squirt with lemon, sprinkle with salt and, if you're not being unnecessarily, obsessively strict, dribble over the merest ¼ teaspoon of the most beautiful olive oil (the milder Ligurian for choice) to bring out the sweet, smoky depths of the fish.

Both tuna and salmon can be treated in the same way as steak, either plain grilled or griddled and dressed in soy and herb-sprinkled as above, or coated in crushed pepper and griddled or dry-fried in a non-stick pan to create a juicy piscine take on the bifteck bistro original, poisson au poivre.

POISSON AU POIVRE

Tataki of tuna, in many ways the 1980s equivalent, is well worth reviving in the privacy of your own home. At its most basic, this is just a small, thick, fleshy piece of tuna, cut from the tail, seared on all sides on a smooth griddle and left to cool, dunked in iced water then dried well (see, for interest and comparison, though not for low-fat consumption necessarily, Alastair Little's carpaccio on page 154). Slice some spring onions into 4cm lengths, and cut these in half lengthways, too. Arrange on a plate. Then cut the tuna into very thin slices diagonally across. You will see the outline of the brown-crusted exterior, the ruby fleshiness within. You can dress with ½ a tablespoon lime juice mixed with a pinch of sugar and 1 tablespoonful soy sauce and/or serve a piercingly hot dipping sauce of wasabi powder, made from that green, mustardy, horseradishy root, mixed to a thin paste with soy. And if you want to intensify the contrast between the fish steak's soft, sweet interior and seared, almost bitter, crust, then dredge the tuna in some wasabi powder, too, before griddling it. Sprinkle with coriander and eat with a cucumber salad made by cutting a decent chunk of a cucumber in half, scraping out the seeds and then cutting the two halves finely so that you have a mound of jadelike, glassy half-moons.

TATAKI OF TUNA

From a quirky American book called *Pacifica Blue Plates* by Neil Stuart, I picked up a way of cooking salmon that has contrast and impact. The title – sugar-spiced salmon with Chinese hot mustard – takes almost longer to write than the recipe does to cook. I've adapted the original idea (leaving out the stipulated ¼ teaspoon cocoa), but the result, the almost uncooked Dayglo interior, the crisp, dull bronze but sharp-spiced seared casing around, provides the satisfactions of the original. For a 225g juicy thick salmon fillet (cut from the top end of the fish) mix a ¼ teaspoon each ground ginger, cinnamon, cumin, cayenne, sugar, salt and (Colman's) mustard powder. Heat the griddle (smooth side up) or a non-stick pan and, when hot, thickly dredge the fish in the spice mixture and cook for 2–3 minutes a side. Remove and let stand while you make the purportedly Chinese hot mustard sauce, just by mixing a teaspoon and a half each of sugar and mustard powder with 1 teaspoon of water from the warm tap. I like this with barely-cooked sugar-snaps. And the hot, sweet

SUGAR-SPICED SALMON WITH CHINESE HOT MUSTARD

mustard sauce will jumpstart even the dullest piece of plain grilled farmed salmon. If you can find or afford wild salmon, let nothing interfere, save some lemon or the merest ghost of some freshly chopped tarragon.

RICE

Rice and broccoli, doused in ordinary soy sauce, citrus-seasoned soy or sukiyake sauce, is a quick bowl-to-mouth supper. Basmati rice takes about 10 minutes, though if you keep some frozen in bags you can nuke a portion in the microwave as soon as you walk in through the door in the evening. (I'm not mad about microwaved broccoli, though.) Sometimes a little bowlful of rice eaten immediately can stop you eating everything in the fridge later. In my more temple-food moods, I go in for brown rice, but it takes ages to cook and sometimes feels like a virtuous rather than a pleasurable choice. Where brown rice really works is in a salad: let the rice get cold, keep it in the fridge and then you can make a quick supper by adding soy (by itself or with dashi and mirin added), chopped spring onions, sugar-snaps, mint and coriander.

A LITTLE SOMETHING ON TOAST

Less exotically, you should never forget the filling and comforting properties of baked beans or poached eggs on toast. As long as you get whatever's covering the toast on top of it the minute the toast pops out of the toaster, the lack of butter won't be a lastingly significant loss.

SMALL BIRDS

A 450g poussin is about 400 calories, skin and all, about half that if you can eat it without the skin. I prefer to double my calorific intake by eating it burnished and crisp-skinned; it feels like so much more of a treat. I often cook a couple of these when a girlfriend comes for supper: with it you can make any salad or vegetable you like; I like the lemony, herb-dense, grated beetroot on page 435.

I also love grouse, partridge and quail. Eating the *whole* of something makes you feel less deprived. Roast grouse plain, which is no hardship either in terms of cooking or eating, and almost braise partridge by cooking it in the oven in a little puddle of stock and chopped vegetables. Shred the cooked meat and stir into some carrot, onion and garlic-studded lentils. See also the recipe for lacquered quail, page 434.

Not all the recipes that follow are time-consuming but I feel they come more into the category of thought-about cooking than the let's-just-throw-this-into-the-pan mode of food preparation.

AROMATIC CHILLI BEEF NOODLE SOUP

This satisfies just about every principle of low-fat cookery as far as I'm concerned: it's filling, fragrant, resonant with flavour and beautiful to look at; it feels like a treat. And there's a lot of it. Defatted real stock is best, but you can use good stock cubes, or instant dashi.

60g dried egg noodles

for the stock

400–500ml stock
1 cm piece fresh ginger
1 dried chilli
1/4 teaspoon ground cinnamon
1 clove garlic, smashed but whole

for the beef

120g steak
2 teaspoons soy sauce
1/4 teaspoon ground cinnamon
1 cm fresh ginger peeled and chopped (or put through garlic crusher)
1 clove garlic, finely chopped
1 teaspoon sugar
1 teaspoon piri-piri or chilli sauce

50g sugar-snaps, cut into 2–3 pieces each
75g (small bunch) pak choi, chopped
small clump Thai basil, about 2 tablespoons or so when chopped, or 2 tablespoons coriander, chopped

Cook the noodles as directed on the packet, drain, rinse in cold water and drain again. Reserve till needed.

Heat the stock with its allocated aromatics, bring to the boil, then leave to simmer, covered, while you get on with the beef.

In a bowl mix up all the beef seasonings and then put the beef in, wipe around the bowl to cover one side of the beef with the chilli–cinnamon mixture, then turn over. Leave for 30 minutes. As you put the beef away to marinate, turn the heat off under the stock, but leave the pan with the lid on to let the flavourings infuse the liquid.

Sear the steak on one side in a hot, non-stick pan and then turn over and sear the other side. Cook for 2 minutes more on each side on slightly lower heat, then remove the steak to a board to rest a second while you get on with warming the aromatic soup and noodles.

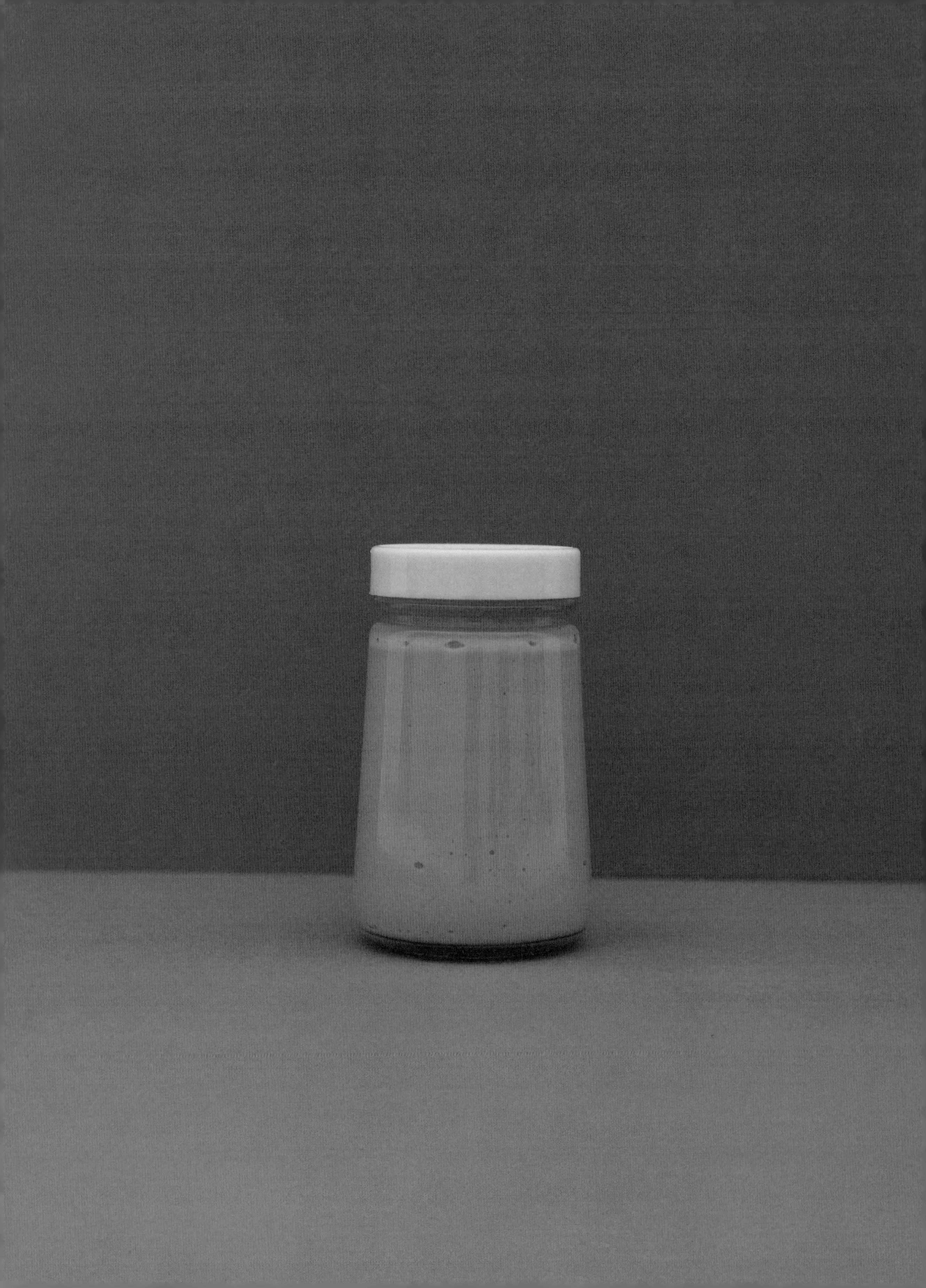

You can either strain the stock into a new saucepan or just fish out the bits as you eat. Do whichever you prefer, but bring the stock back to boiling point, cook the sugar-snaps and pak choi for a minute or so and put in the cold noodles. After another minute, or when the noodles are hot, add the chopped Thai basil (unless you're using coriander, in which case wait to sprinkle it over at the end) and pour into a bowl. Slice the steak into thin slices on the diagonal and lay on top. Eat with a spoon and soy sauce.

Serves 1.

You can do almost whatever you want to this recipe: cut the steak into strips and marinate; use duck breast (fat removed and meat sliced before cooking) or venison (sliced after); use any vegetables; use any sort of noodle. See also the recipe for Sunday Night Chicken Noodle (page 161), only use ½ teaspoon of oil when you stir-fry the chicken shreds.

I often make this for my supper, using thin slices of pork, which have been first dunked, then roasted, in a barbecuey marinade. The recipe for that is included on page 443, but it is probably better to mention here that I use pork stock cubes bought from the Thai shop and use pak choi or choi sum, or other leafy, cabbagey greens.

MUSHROOM UDON SOUP

This is very plain, very calming; the sort of supper I might make myself to get back on track if I've gone out and had pig's trotter – fat, cartilage and all – with mashed potato for lunch.

Dashi is the Japanese stock (what *brodo* is to the Italians) and although you can make it yourself, I advise buying hon-dashi, which is their equivalent to stock cubes. I buy mine in liquid version which you mix in the ratio of 1 teaspoon of hon-dashi to 1 cup water. If you have problems finding the instant dashi liquid, see list of stockists in the Gazetteer, page 506.

5g dried shitake mushrooms, soaked in 300ml hot water
60g fresh udon noodles, or 50g other, dried
1–2 teaspoons instant liquid dashi, or equivalent
few drops soy sauce
few drops sesame oil (optional)
fresh parsley or coriander

Soak the shitake mushrooms in 300ml hot water for 10 minutes. Strain the water into a pan and add a few drops soy sauce and 1 teaspoon of instant dashi. Remove the stalks, then add the mushrooms to the pan. When it all comes to the boil, add the noodles. When cooked, pour into a bowl, and sprinkle over the merest drop or two of sesame oil, more dashi to taste, and some parsley, or coriander if you prefer.

This is enough for 1.

The following recipe has almost the same ingredients, but is very different in character: more bolstering, stronger-flavoured and generally just more solid.

BRAISED DRIED SHITAKE MUSHROOMS WITH SOBA NOODLES

Like the recipe above, once you've got yourself organised, this is a good store-cupboard standby. The braised mushrooms come via the *Japanese Vegetarian Cookbook* by Patricia Richfield; I add them to a capacious plateful of cooked and soy-tossed buckwheat soba noodles. The graininess of the buckwheat is just the right foil to the dense-flavoured and salty shitake.

8 dried shitake mushrooms (or more if you want)
1 teaspoon vegetable oil
1 teaspoon sake
3 tablespoons Japanese soy sauce
4 tablespoons mirin
80g soba noodles
few drops sesame oil
fresh coriander

Soak the mushrooms in hot water for about 30 minutes. Then drain, reserving 100ml of soaking water and straining it if there is grit to get rid of. Remove the stems and discard; squeeze the caps a little to remove excess water.

Heat the oil in a small frying pan, add the mushrooms and stir-fry for 2 minutes. Mix the sake, mirin and 2 tablespoons of the soy sauce with the reserved mushroom-soaking water and pour over the mushrooms in the pan. Bring to the boil and simmer over a low heat, stirring occasionally, until most of the liquid has evaporated – about 15 minutes or so. Meanwhile, cook the noodles according to the packet instructions, drain, rinse with cold water, drain again and toss with the soy sauce and sprinkle with a drop of sesame oil. Toss again, and put on the plate. Pour the mushrooms from the pan on top of the noodles. Sprinkle another drop or two of sesame oil over the noodles; add some just-chopped coriander if desired.

Serves 1.

SEAWEED AND NOODLE SALAD

This is not an authentic dish, in so far as I didn't get it from any Japanese source, just from the happy ransacking of my own larder. Don't worry about which noodles you use. I like the starchy, fresh Japanese ones, but they're not very easy to find: dried Chinese egg noodles will do fine. Neither of these two seaweeds are very hard to get hold of and because all you have to do is soak them briefly, they aren't hard to use. This tastes good, too, just with the fleshy green wakame or without any seaweed at all, just as a plain noodle salad. If you want to forgo the sesame oil, you can: fatless, the dressing is slightly more astringent, but that isn't necessarily a bad thing.

60g fresh Japanese noodles, or 50g soba noodles or Chinese dried egg noodles
8g wakame
8g arame
4 teaspoons Japanese soy sauce
2 teaspoons mirin
1 tablespoon sake
2 teaspoons rice vinegar
½ teaspoon sugar
1 tablespoon dashi (or 1 tablespoon water with a pin-drop of hon-dashi)
1 teaspoon sesame oil (optional)
1 spring onion, chopped finely

Cook the noodles in boiling water for as long as the packet directs, then drain, refresh in cold water and drain again. Set aside. Meanwhile soak the seaweeds in water, again as the packets direct: about 5 minutes for the wakame and 15 for the arame should do it. Drain well.

Make the dressing by putting the soy, sake, mirin, rice vinegar, sugar, dashi and sesame oil, if using, in a small jar and shake, or just mix together in a bowl. Combine the noodles, which should be either at room temperature or cold, and seaweeds and toss with the dressing. Put into a serving dish and sprinkle with the chopped spring onions.

Serves 1.

I like to eat this, perhaps even more in its seaweedless state, with plain mackerel fillets, blistered under a hot grill, then sprinkled with coriander. I love the contrast between hot, crisp-skinned oily fish and cold, slippery noodles.

Salmon teriyaki is more well-known (and by all means substitute a salmon steak or thick chunk of fillet) but I love the preposterously underrated mackerel.

MACKEREL TERIYAKI

2 tablespoons soy sauce

2 tablespoons sake

1 tablespoon mirin

1 teaspoon sugar

1 mackerel, filleted, each fillet cut in half

Put all the ingredients except the mackerel in a saucepan and bring to the boil to dissolve the sugar. Leave to one side for a moment.

Let a non-stick pan get very hot, then put the mackerel fillets in and cook for 2 minutes. Although I like to have the skin still on when I'm just grilling, here the sauce makes it soggy and really the skin is good to eat only when it's crisp, so you might as well remove it before cooking. After 2 minutes turn the mackerel over and add the teriyaki marinade to the pan. Baste the fish and turn once again before removing it with a slotted spatula. Leave the sauce to bubble up in the pan until it's dark and syrupy and thick, but keep an eye on it as you don't want it to burn stickily dry. Pour this reduced teriyaki marinade over the fish. I like this with plain boiled rice or just a huge pile of greens, Chinese or otherwise.

Serves 2.

SALMON MARINATED IN DEN MISO

At Nobu in New York I had *the* most fabulous black cod in miso: the flesh was soft and dense, the crust charred black and sweet with grill-caramelised sake. Black cod – which bears no relation to ordinary cod – seems to be unavailable here, but the recipe works well with any fatty fish, so I suggest using salmon. The miso permeates the fish, but not intrusively. The fact that the preparation needs to be done in advance means you need to plan ahead, but the cooking itself is undemanding.

I've specified quantities for 2. For 1, halve quantities of the marinade only if you've got a dish small enough to fit the one piece of fish snugly, or the amount of marinade won't cover it.

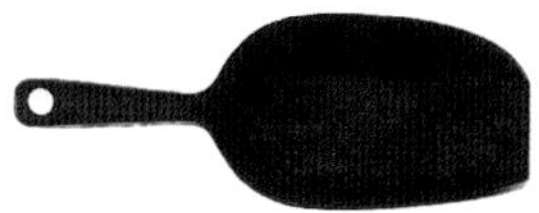

2 chunky pieces of salmon fillet, about 150g each

for den miso

150g white miso

2 tablespoons sugar

2 tablespoons sake

2 tablespoons mirin

Combine all the den miso ingredients, put in a thick-bottomed pan over moderate heat and cook for about 20 minutes, stirring often. You mustn't let the sugar burn and stick at the bottom. Set aside and let cool.

Put the salmon pieces in a shallow dish with the den miso, making sure they are thoroughly covered. Cover with clingfilm and marinate for 2–3 days in the fridge.

When you want to eat, preheat the grill. When it's hot, take the fish out of the marinade and grill on each side until brown and slightly caramelised. This is wonderful served, not entirely Japanese-style, with a bowl of broccoli suffused with lemon or just a huge wigwammed mound of mangetouts.

CAMBODIAN HOT AND SOUR BEEF SALAD

I first ate this at one of Vatchcharin Bhumichitr's restaurants, Southeast W9, and found it spectacular. It's again an example of how the best low-fat food comes from recipes that are not specially adapted to make them so. My version is a slightly anglicised take on the recipe for *plea saj go* as gratefully found in Vatch's wonderful *South-east Asian Cookbook*. I have reduced the number of chillies, used shallot in preference to onion and as Vatch himself suggests, substituted mint for the stipulated chilli leaves. But sometimes, when I can't find mint in the shops and there's none in the garden, I use rocket or a handful of watercress and baby spinach (as found, mixed, in plastic bags in the supermarket) instead. In short, I don't set about doing this as if I were expecting a Cambodian delegation for dinner: I just cook it as I like it.

Although this amount serves 2 if you're eating other things – a dreamy and mild noodle soup to start, a ripe mango for pudding – I often make it just for me: I don't alter quantities; I just don't eat anything else, except perhaps for a sweet, salving banana after.

enough lettuce leaves to cover a serving dish
225g tender steak
2 tablespoons fish sauce
2 tablespoons lime juice (the juice of about 1 lime)
1 teaspoon sugar
1 shallot, sliced finely
1–2 red or green chillies, deseeded and chopped finely, depending on how large they are and how hot you want this
handful mint

Preheat the grill.

Cover a serving dish with lettuce leaves and set aside. Grill the steak; it should be rare, really, but obviously cook it as you prefer. When it's done, remove to a board on which to carve it and pour any juices in the grill pan into a bowl. Cut the steak into very thin slices across and put these with any more juices that run out into the bowl as well. In another bowl, mix the fish sauce, lime juice, sugar, chopped chilli and sliced shallot, stirring well. Then mix the contents of the 2 bowls together, adding the mint leaves (or chilli leaves, or rocket and so on), quickly turn out on the lettuce and serve while still warm.

Serves 2.

THAI-FLAVOURED MUSSELS

I have called these 'Thai-flavoured' rather than 'Thai' because they emanate directly from my kitchen, and I am not Thai and have never even been to Thailand. So this dish is authentic, but in the sense that it is authentically how I cook it. It takes about 2 minutes, and since mussels come cleaned now, there isn't even any debearding or debarnacling to do over the kitchen sink. I use kaffir lime leaves since I keep a stash of them in my freezer, but you can substitute lemon grass. And frankly, it's still worth doing even if you can get neither.

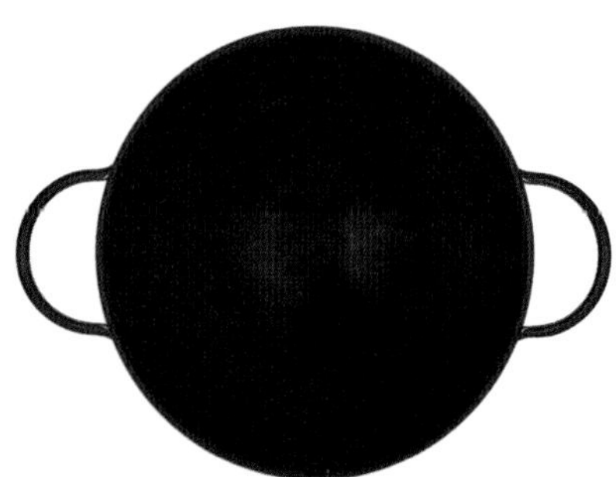

100ml light stock
1 shallot, chopped finely
2 cloves garlic, sliced or chopped finely
3 kaffir lime leaves, chopped or shredded, or one 10cmish stick of lemon grass, chopped finely
1cm piece ginger, chopped finely
20 mussels (approx. 350g)
1 fresh chilli, deseeded and chopped or sliced finely
120ml boiling water
1 tablespoon each lime juice, mirin and fish sauce
good bunch coriander, to yield about 1/2 American cup measure when chopped

Use whatever stock you want here: vegetable, chicken, fish, dashi; from the pot, freezer, tub or packet. Anyway, put it, with the shallot, garlic, lime leaves and ginger in a pan, with the lid on and let it bubble away at a moderate to high heat for 3–5 minutes until you have a thickish, softish mess at the bottom of the pan. Check to make sure it isn't either burning or just getting too dry for comfort and add a bit of water from the kettle if it is. Meanwhile, put the mussels – cleaned if they haven't come from the shop clean – in a sinkful of ice-cold water. Chuck any away that don't sink, and then as you remove them make doubly sure by chucking away any that don't shut when you tap them sharply. I wouldn't expect to have to throw many away, so don't worry unduly.

Add the chopped chilli pepper to the mixture in the pan. Whether you use red or green chilli is immaterial in terms of flavour here; the red one, I think, just looks a little better. After about 30 seconds, or just long enough to get them out of the sink, add the mussels and then throw over the water and then the lime juice, mirin and fish sauce mixed together. Put the lid on, give the pan a shake and leave on a high heat for about 3 minutes, by which time the mussels should have steamed open. Add half the coriander, shake again and pour into a noodle bowl. Sprinkle over the remaining coriander and eat. It's probably just as well this is enough for one, since you will have to spit out the shreds of kaffir lime leaves – or lemon grass if you used that – as you come upon them.

Serves 1.

THAI CLAM POT

This recipe comes by way of an American book that I have to force myself *not* to cook my way through – *Asian Noodles* by Nina Symonds – and, I should own up, is barely scaled down, although its specifications are for 6 people and mine are for 2. I like a lot of liquid: I want an aromatic broth with the noodles and clams submerged in it, and enough of it to drink from the bowl or slurp from a spoon once the noodles and clams have been greedily eaten. But then, I like a lot of noodles, too. And this still works wonderfully with half the amount of noodles, if you're in super-virtuous mode.

Sake you can get in supermarkets now, but Thai basil may be a problem. If you can't find any – I go to a Thai shop near me, indeed I practically live in it – beg and plead with your supermarket to stock it; otherwise settle instead for some fresh coriander. I would make a fuss, nicely of course, since it wasn't that long ago that coriander would have been available only in specialist shops; and Thai basil really is extraordinarily wonderful, as aromatic as liquorice. For that reason, I wouldn't substitute ordinary Mediterranean basil, wonderful as *it* is: they may share the same name, but the celestial pungency, the almost medicinal herbalness of the Thai basil, is not at all the same as the summery and gorgeous scentedness of the Mediterranean plant. Coriander, again, is different, but the quality of pungency is there.

The shells hold up the very gratifying wolfing down, so I remove most of them before ladling the clams into waiting bowls.

800g small clams, preferably palourdes
1 teaspoon bicarbonate of soda, optional (see below)
200g fresh or 125g dried very thin noodles
3 cloves garlic
2 spring onions
1 scant teaspoon safflower or corn oil
1 dried red chilli pepper
300ml water
150ml sake or Chinese rice wine
good handful Thai basil, shredded finely
2 tablespoons fish sauce, or to taste

If you're using venus clams, fill the sink with cold water, add the bicarbonate of soda and leave the clams to soak for an hour. Drain and chuck out any that haven't opened. But if you're using the slightly bigger palourdes, you shouldn't need to soak them.

Heat a large pan of water and when boiling add salt and then the noodles. Cook as instructed on packet or by the shopkeeper (my fresh somen take 1 minute) and then drain, rinse and set aside. Crush the garlic cloves with the side of a knife, then slice finely. Cut the spring onions into 3cm lengths and press down on them with the flat side of a knife, to squash them slightly.

Put a large, heavy pot (big enough to take everything later) on a high flame, add the oil and heat until hot, about 30 seconds. Add the garlic and spring onions, crumble in the chilli and stir-fry for about 10 seconds or until fragrant. Add the water and rice wine, cover and bring to the boil. Add the clams, cover and bring back to the boil. Then reduce the heat to medium (or low, depending on your stove) and cook, shaking the pot from time to time so that the clams cook evenly, for 2–3 minutes, or just until the clams open.

Add the basil (or coriander) to the clams, stir gently, cover and cook for 30 seconds, then stir in the fish sauce to taste. Divide the noodles between a pair of capacious bowls, ladle the clams and broth over and eat immediately. Serves 2.

VEGETABLE MISO BROTH

This is essential to my low-fat eating moments. I cook it more than I cook anything else and every time I do it, I make it differently. Basically, I just boil, in salted water, various vegetables, any that I feel like, putting them in the pan in the order they'll take to cook (thus turnips first, watercress last) and then drain them into a bowl. Over this bowl I pour over a jugful of salty soup made out of some Marigold vegetable powder and 1 tablespoon of miso. Sometimes I add ginger to the broth and stir in some pickled ginger while I'm eating it. But mostly it's just plain vegetables, chunked and still crunchy, with that almost creaturely, emphatically aromatic, miso-thickened broth.

The quantities I give below are to be viewed as sketchy; ignore or add to them as you wish.

2 turnips, peeled and quartered
1 carrot, peeled and cut into large, chunky batons
a few florets broccoli
1 courgette, halved lengthways and then halved across
handful of sugar snaps, each chopped into 2–3 pieces
handful watercress
2 teaspoons Marigold vegetable powder
1 heaped tablespoon miso
fresh parsley or coriander, chopped (optional)

Put a large pan of water on to boil and when boiling add salt. Then add the turnips. After about 5 minutes, add the carrots. After another 7 or so minutes, add the broccoli. Give this 2–3 minutes, then chuck in the courgette, and after another minute the sugar-snaps. Just as you're about to drain the pan, throw in the watercress and then empty the entire contents into a colander in the sink.

Meanwhile make the broth. Pour 500ml boiling water from the kettle into a jug and stir in 2 teaspoons Marigold powder, then 1 heaped tablespoon (or more to taste) miso. Put the drained vegetables into a noodle bowl, then pour over the miso broth. Add chopped parsley or coriander if wished. Eat. Serves 1.

LACQUERED QUAIL

Food that is fiddly, or takes time – artichokes, winkles – is worth considering when you're trying to eat less. It's a variation of the old trick of eating off smaller plates, but piled high, so that you're conned, somehow, into thinking you're eating more.

The lacquer effect is brought about by brushing with pomegranate molasses (which you can get in Middle-Eastern stores and quite a few supermarkets now) mixed with soy sauce, much the same way as the Chinese use maltose to help along that beautiful burnished glow on their roast ducks. You can spatchcock the quails yourself, following instructions on page 149, or just ask your butcher to do it for you.

2 quails, spatchcocked
2 teaspoons soy sauce
2 teaspoons pomegranate molasses

Preheat the oven to gas mark 8/220°C.

Line a small baking tin with foil, shiny side up, and put the quails in skin side up. Put the soy sauce and pomegranate molasses in a pan and bring to the boil on the hob. Let bubble away for ½ minute or so until thick and sticky and pour over the quails, using a pastry brush to dab it all over.

Roast for about 15 minutes, then remove and eat with your fingers as soon as the quails have cooled down just enough for you to bear it.

JAPANESE-FLAVOURED SOUR-SWEET CABBAGE

Sometimes I make myself a bowl of Japanese-flavoured sour-sweet cabbage to eat after this. Shred about 250g cabbage finely, then toss it a hot non-stick pan in which you've already put ¼ teaspoon sesame oil. Keep turning and tossing the cabbage until it wilts impressively, then throw in a mixture made from 1 tablespoon each of soy sauce, mirin and rice vinegar. Give this – still stirring and lifting up the cabbage frantically – another minute, then remove to a bowl and sprinkle over some Japanese seven-spice mixture if you've any to hand. Serves 1–2.

BEET GREENS AND BUCKWHEAT NOODLES

I began this tranche of recipes with noodles and I'll end it with noodles. I love beet greens, but am not mad on beetroot (with some exceptions, and they're listed below, so don't worry about what you're going to do with the rejected roots now). I use Japanese soba noodles for this – also sold at the supermarket – and make a vast plateful; I want nothing else after.

leaves and tender stalks from 1kg bunch beetroot
80g soba noodles
1 tablespoon Japanese soy sauce
1 tablespoon mirin
1 teaspoon rice vinegar
flat-leaf parsley

Put a pan of water on for the noodles, adding salt when it boils. Chop and then put the pink stalks and green leaves in a sink filled with cold water, then remove, drain and cook, in just the water clinging to the leafs and stalks, no more, in a thick-based or non-stick frying pan with the lid on to get the steam rising. Meanwhile cook the noodles, drain them and toss in the soy sauce, mirin and rice vinegar, or use an equal amount of bottled sukiyaki sauce.

Then, when the beet greens are all but ready, sprinkle with salt and throw in the noodles, adding more soy sauce as needed. Stir around in the pan until the buff-coloured noodles take on a deep bronzy pink. Remove to a large plate and cover with freshly chopped parsley.

Serves 1.

The following two recipes are both for beetroot, but since they're for the beetroot you've got left from the recipe above, I make no apology for the purplish onslaught. I had never eaten beetroot raw until I came across Stephanie Alexander's recipe in her *Cook's Companion* for grated beets with lemon juice and chopped herbs, arranged around a central dollop of yoghurt. I cannot tell you what a revelation it is. Something spooky can happen to beetroot when it's cooked (and I don't mean just the vinegar that is often added): it's as if the sweetness has a slightly putrid edge. Raw, the sugariness has a spiky-sharpness about it, which stops it from cloying, even in large quantities.

SHREDDED BEETROOT SALAD WITH YOGHURT

I have adapted the recipe a bit, and also substituted fat-free Greek yoghurt. And since it's what I make to go with roast poussin when a friend comes for a low-key, low-fat supper, I give quantities for 2 naturally big eaters.

good handful coriander
good handful mint
2 large or 4 small beetroots (about 725g)
juice of 1 lemon
150g 0-per-cent-fat Greek yoghurt

Put the coriander and mint leaves in the processor, chop and remove. Take out the double-bladed knife and fix in the grating disc. Peel the beetroot (wearing rubber gloves if you don't want to come over all Lady Macbeth later) and cut them into pieces that will fit into the tube, then push them down until you have a wonderful pile of dark crimson shreds. Toss these in a bowl with the herbs and lemon juice and then arrange them, like a ring, around the edge of a plate. Empty out the tub of yoghurt into the hole in the centre. Change the herbs as you like. With chopped dill and dry-toasted mustard seeds, it's magnificent with salmon, for example. Serves 2 with leftovers.

BEETROOT SOUP

It seems odd not to be convinced about beetroot but to be passionate about this, because in a way this thick, velvety soup is the sweet, smooth essence of beet. It's difficult to say how many it will feed, as I make a big quantity and just keep a jug of it in the fridge for a few days.

2 large or 4 small beetroots (about 725g)
1 teaspoon Dijon mustard
1 tablespoon balsamic vinegar
buttermilk, yoghurt or smetana, optional

Put the beetroot in a large pan, cover with cold water, bring to boil and boil for two hours. Maybe an hour and a quarter if they're small. Beetroot takes much longer to cook than anyone ever tells you (rather like chick peas).

Scoop out the cooked beetroots (retaining the cooking liquid) with a slotted spoon and gingerly pull off skins, before putting in a processor or blender together with the mustard and balsamic vinegar. Purée, adding cooking liquid till the texture is as you like it. Keep some of the cooking liquid, as well, as the soup will thicken as it sits in the fridge and you will need to thin it out later. But if you want just to freeze individual portions you can add water as necessary when you reheat. This soup is wonderful with a slash of buttermilk or yoghurt (or more authentically, smetana) added as you eat it.

RESTRAINED MUSHROOM RISOTTO

A low-fat risotto might sound suspect, but this one works because of its intense, mushroomy depth of flavour. This is the sort of thing I'd make when I have a girlfriend over to dinner, cooking it while we're talking. I have specified garlic-infused oil and Knorr porcini stock just because this makes it easier for a scrabbled-together after-work supper. Boost with 10g of dried porcini, soaked, drained and chopped, plus the soaking water, if you can't get stock.

1 teaspoon butter
2 teaspoons garlic-infused oil
½ onion, chopped finely
200g mixed mushrooms
125g arborio rice
60ml white wine or Noilly Prat
375ml stock, preferably Knorr porcini
2 tablespoons parmesan, freshly grated
parsley

In a small frying pan or medium saucepan, heat the butter and oil. Fry the onion gently until soft but not brown. Add the mushrooms and cook for a few minutes. Stir in the rice and cook for 2 minutes. Pour in the wine or vermouth and let it bubble away until it's absorbed. Add a ladleful of hot stock and cook, stirring, until the stock has been absorbed. Carry on adding ladlefuls and then stirring over a low to medium heat until all the stock has been absorbed and the rice is creamy and just cooked, tender but still firm to the bite. In other words, until it tastes like risotto, which should take 18–20 minutes. Stir in the parmesan and chop some fresh parsley over it. Serves 2.

FINE PASTA WITH CRAB

This is one of the few non-oriental low-fat recipes that you could cook for a dinner party, although I always find pasta panic-inducing in large quantities. Crab meat is so intensely flavoured that fat is not required to add depth. The recipe might seem to be masquerading as an Italian dish, but that is not the intention: really the flavours are borrowed from Thai and Korean crab cakes, but they make a wonderful, resonant pasta sauce. Frozen crab meat, thawed, can be used if you can't get fresh.

1 clove garlic, chopped finely
½ red chilli, sliced finely, with seeds
fresh coriander (¼ bunch or ½ supermarket plastic envelope)
grated zest of most of 1 lime
2–3 spring onions, sliced finely
2 teaspoons olive oil
35g brown crab meat
150 ml white wine
150g egg tagliolini or linguine
60g white crab meat
squirt of lime juice
fresh flat-leaf parsley

Put water on for the pasta. When it's almost boiling, start on the sauce. Sweat the garlic, chilli, half the coriander, half the lime zest and the spring onions in olive oil until softened.

Add the brown crab meat and white wine and simmer for about 10 minutes, stirring occasionally, until it reduces and thickens to an almost sludgy texture.

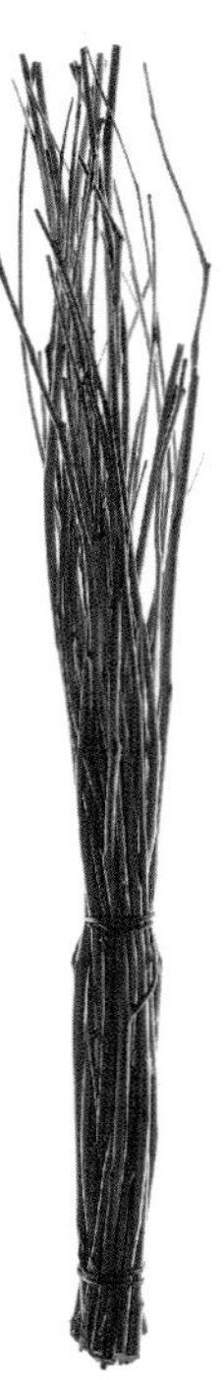

The pasta water should be boiling now, so add salt and then put in the pasta. Fresh egg tagliolini take about 2 minutes, linguine much longer. Whichever you're using, just before the pasta needs draining, stir the white meat with the remaining coriander and lime zest into the brown-meat mixture. Squish briefly with lime so that a drop or two of juice squirts into the sauce. Just before draining the pasta lower a mug into it and fill it up with the pasta cooking water. When the pasta's drained, add to the pan of sauce, or if you prefer, put it into a warmed bowl and stir the sauce into it. Add some more drops of cooking water if the sauce needs help to coat the strands of pasta. Bear in mind, though, that this strong-tasting sauce is meant to cover elegantly and sparsely; in this sense only, perhaps, it is an Italian sauce. Sprinkle with just-chopped flat-leaf parsley, and eat quickly; the thinner the pasta, the faster it clumps as it waits.

Serves 2.

SALAD DRESSINGS

It's one of the fallacies of trying to lose weight that the easiest thing to eat is a salad. There is no such thing as a decent low-fat salad dressing. I have tried everything. So I have come up with dressings which don't exactly duplicate vinaigrette, but will coat leaves without making you wince.

MISO MUSTARD DRESSING

1/2 teaspoon miso
1/2 teaspoon wholegrain mustard
1/4 teaspoon strong clear honey
juice 1/2 orange

Mix everything together well and dress the salad. What else is there to say, except that you could add a splosh of buttermilk as well.

DIJON MUSTARD DRESSING

Having said that low-fat dressing mustn't ape proper dressing, I can see that this one does. But somehow it pulls it off.

1/2 teaspoon Dijon mustard
1/2 teaspoon balsamic vinegar
juice 1/2 orange
drop of soy sauce

Put the mustard in a bowl and slowly stir in the vinegar and orange juice. Taste and add soy as wanted.

THICK MISO DRESSING FOR BEANS

The dressings, above, are runny and good for the robuster leaf salads – radicchio, frisée or something with bite. This, though, is rich and thick and wonderful stirred into warm or cold pulses.

1 heaped tablespoon miso
1 scant teaspoon balsamic vinegar or rice vinegar
drop or two sesame oil

In a little bowl, stir together the miso, balsamic or rice vinegar, and a tiny drop or two of sesame oil and mix to the consistency of a thick paste or dressing by adding a couple of tablespoons of water.

ROAST GARLIC AND LEMON DRESSING

This dressing takes rather longer to make, but you are not required to exert yourself while the garlic's in the oven, so it's still not the biggest deal.

1 head garlic
1 teaspoon vermouth
1 lemon

Preheat the oven to gas mark 6/200°C.

Lop the top off the garlic, just so you see the cloves in cross section. Cut out a square of tin foil, big enough to wrap the garlic in. Place the garlic in the centre of the foil square and bring up the sides, so that when you add the vermouth it doesn't all dribble out. When the vermouth's in, close the parcel by twisting the edges of the foil together and bake for 45 minutes–1 hour. Remove, let cool a bit then squeeze the garlic into a bowl. Squeeze the juice of half the lemon slowly into the roast garlic purée, stirring as you do it. If the dressing is as sharp as you want it to be before it's as runny (though this is meant to be a thick dressing) as you want it to be, beat in a little water. Otherwise, add the remaining half of lemon juice.

THE STATUTORY COOK-AND-FREEZE-AHEAD SECTION

Freezing some low-fat food will get you in the right frame of mind while setting the stage with the necessary props.

VEGETABLE CURRY IN VEGETABLE SAUCE

This is a recipe from Sue Kreitzman's *Low-fat Vegetarian Cookbook* which is so utterly virtuous that I regard it as eating that doesn't count. I don't cook it for other people: it's what I keep for myself to balance out a week of intense going out or overeating at home. This amount makes about enough for 6 huge portions, which I freeze individually and thaw when required. Yes, it can go soggy and fuzzy around the edges, but I don't mind.

If I am being very severe, I eat this with just a raita made with the lowest-fat fromage frais, finely chopped spring onions, grated fresh ginger and chopped mint and coriander. If following a middling path, I add some plain steamed couscous. If I feel I have nothing for which to atone, I buy hot, soft nan bread from my local Indian take-away to mop up the aromatic juices and eat nothing else that night bar some fruit. This recipe is, I admit, time-consuming and labour-intensive, but is the low-fat culinary equivalent of a key text. You should tackle it when you're all fired up to start. Put aside one Sunday evening, and don't think of doing anything else at the same time. It's a worthwhile investment.

- 2 large onions, each cut into 8 pieces
- 2 cloves garlic, crushed
- 1 tablespoon each ground cumin, ground coriander and paprika
- 1/2 teaspoon each ground allspice, ground cardamom and ground ginger
- 1 teaspoon cayenne pepper
- about 600ml stock
- 3 peppers, peeled, deseeded and chopped coarsely
- 3 large carrots, chopped coarsely
- 350g button mushrooms, halved or quartered
- 2 medium white turnips, cut into 1cm pieces
- 1 large cauliflower, separated into florets
- 1 small parsnip, cut into 1cm pieces
- 1 fennel bulb, quartered and cut into 1cm pieces
- 3 celery stalks, cut into 1cm pieces
- juice of 1/2 large lemon
- 3 medium courgettes, cut into 1cm pieces
- 225g runner beans, cut into 1cm pieces

Put the onion pieces, garlic, spices and 300ml stock in a heavy-bottomed saucepan. Cover, bring to the boil, and boil for 5–7 minutes. Uncover and stir in the peppers, carrots and mushrooms. Reduce the heat slightly and simmer, stirring frequently, until the vegetables and spices are 'frying' in their own juices, and the vegetables are tender. Leave to cool slightly.

Purée half the mixture in a blender or food processor, then return the purée to the pan.

Add the turnip, cauliflower, parsnip, fennel and celery. Stir together very well. Add enough stock almost to cover the contents of the pot, season with salt and bring to the boil.

Reduce the heat, cover and simmer for 15 minutes. Uncover, squeeze in the lemon juice, and add the courgettes and beans. Simmer uncovered for 10 minutes more, or until all the vegetables are tender.

Portion this to suit your appetite.

BEEF BRAISED IN BEER

This is pretty much the English version of carbonnade. The beer used should be stout, and I use Sam Smith's Imperial Stout. The prunes – which are authentic, in the sense here of traditional – give a richness and depth, and so very little fat is needed, given it makes up to 6 portions. (In California, incidentally, where they make it their business to know about such things, prunes, puréed, are routinely used to replace their weight of butter in baking.) Like all stews, this is best cooked in advance and then reheated. And since the beef is cooked slowly, you can use very lean stewing steak and it will still be velvety and tender.

175g prunes
150ml water
300ml stout
1 teaspoon English mustard powder
25g plain flour
1kg lean stewing steak, cut into thick strips
2 tablespoons beef dripping or oil, or butter and the merest drop oil
2 onions, sliced finely
300g carrots, cut into batons

Preheat the oven to gas mark 2/150°C.

Pour the water and stout into a bowl and then add the prunes. Ready-to-eat ones need only 2 hours or so soaking, otherwise leave overnight or for at least 6 hours.

Mix the mustard powder into the flour and then coat the beef with it. Heat 1 tablespoon fat and cook the onions for about 5 minutes, stir in the carrots and cook for another 5 minutes. Place the vegetables in a casserole and stir the prunes in with their liquid, with a pinch or two of salt to taste. Add the remaining tablespoon fat to the frying pan and brown the meat, then add meat to the casserole. Cover and cook in the oven for 2½–3 hours.

When it's cool, bag up into 6 equal portions and freeze. Accompany with mounds of green veg. And you could also make a version of the horseradish-chive sauce on page 294 using 0-per-cent-fat fromage frais.

HALF-COQ AU VIN

I don't pretend this is the real thing, in the sense of the Elizabeth David adumbrated original. But it is a good chicken stew, cooked in wine, which borrows from the *cuisine bourgeoise* classic without running too severely into debt. Again, this is something I like to make for myself to reheat and eat alone for dinner when I want something proper and comforting and old-fashioned.

600ml red wine
1 celery stick
1 carrot, peeled and quartered
2 cloves of garlic
1 sprig thyme
few sprigs flat-leaf parsley
3 peppercorns
3 bay leaves
1 tablespoon olive oil
6 skinned chicken thighs
1 medium onion, very finely chopped
75g back bacon, in one piece if possible (otherwise 3 rashers), fat removed, and diced
180g baby button mushrooms
180g tiny onions, peeled
1 heaped tablespoon flour
300ml chicken stock
3 tablespoons brandy

Put the wine, celery, carrot, garlic, sprig of thyme, the stalks from the few sprigs of parsley, the peppercorns and the bay leaves in a pan on the heat. Bring to the boil, reduce the heat slightly and let bubble away until reduced by half.

Then in a casserole, which will take everything later, heat the oil, add the chicken joints and brown a little; you will have to turn often to prevent the chicken from sticking. But persevere: the chicken will colour. Season, turn in the pan, season again, and remove for a while.

The chicken, although it's lean, should have left a few oily juices in the casserole. Add to these the chopped onion and bacon and cook, over medium to medium-low heat, stirring regularly, for about 5 minutes or until soft. Add the mushrooms and baby onions and cook, pushing and prodding, for a further 3 or so minutes. Sprinkle over the flour, stir well to coat and cook out the flouriness, and cook over low heat, for another 3 or so minutes. Gradually stir in the stock and the strained, reduced wine. Replace the chicken thighs. Put on the lid and cook very gently for 45 minutes to an hour.

When the chicken is cooked, heat the brandy in a ladle over a low flame and tilt the ladle until the brandy ignites. Pour this into the casserole and stir well. The sauce–gravy should be just about right now – neither floury nor watery – but should you find it too runny, raise the heat and reduce to thicken a little more. Add the parsley, chopped. You will need, or might want, to add freshly chopped parsley as and when you defrost and eat each individual portion. I get 6 out of this.

CHAR SIU

This, to borrow from Dr Jonathan Miller, is not quite char siu, it's just char siu-ish.

I've given a couple of different marinades for this basically Chinese-influenced barbecued pork. The first is adapted from *Tiger Lily: Flavours of the Orient* by Rani King and Chandra Khan; the second is just something I did with the ingredients I had lying about in the fridge.

In both instances, the pork – a tenderloin weighing just over 300g – is the same, as is the cooking method; it's just the marinade that differs.

4 tablespoons soy sauce
2 tablespoons tomato ketchup
3 tablespoons hoisin sauce
2 tablespoons ginger wine or sweet sherry
2 tablespoons honey
2 scant tablespoons dark muscovado sugar

Mix the marinade ingredients together in a large bowl. Cut the tenderloin in half across. Get plastic freezer bags and put a piece of pork in each; then pour half the marinade in one, and half in the other. Tie both up and squish, seeing that the pork is coated. Lie both bags in a shallow dish and put in fridge for 24 hours.

2 tablespoons soy sauce
2 tablespoons prune juice
2 tablespoons mushroom ketchup
2 tablespoons miso
2 tablespoons mirin
1 tablespoon sesame oil
2 cloves garlic
2 tablespoons light muscovado sugar

Do the same thing with this marinade as you did above.

To cook the pork, preheat the oven to gas mark 8/220°C.

Take the pork out of the marinade (though keep it) and put the meat on a foil-lined baking tin. Roast for 15 minutes, then turn the oven down to gas mark 3/160°C and give it another 20–30 minutes, basting regularly. You want the meat to be tender within. If you think it looks as if it might be drying up, then add a little water to some of the remaining marinade (the second version is more liquid anyway) and spoon it into the pan.

When cooked, remove from oven and let cool. When cool cut into very thin slices, and put 4–5 (about 60g) into freezer bags and freeze (see page 425 above for usage). I keep any marinade that's left over and freeze it for the next batch of pork.

PUDDING

Pudding – in its more solid, substantial and comforting sense – is not the stuff of which low-fat meals are made. That's not to say it is completely out of the dietary question. For one thing, it's important to have something to hand at the end of an anyway abbreviated supper, something to stave off that moment of loneliness and despondency that always threatens to settle when you realise that eating is over for the day.

I have not got a particularly sweet tooth: my weakness will never be biscuits or cakes or puddings; it's bread and cheese that, once I start eating, I can't stop. But somehow when I go on a diet (even if I never even mouth the word to myself, let alone say the word out loud) I suddenly want double-chocolate pecan gâteau or any other revolting concoction so long as it's high fat. It may be psychologically predictable and embarrassing, but there it is. I deal with this in the main by not forbidding myself such stuff: I buy wedges of gooey, icing-encrusted and nut-studded confections, mostly from Marks & Spencer's, since it's all calorie-counted, and reckon it into my overall intake. There are times when it's preferable to eat a vast bowl of steamed greens doused with soy and then a sugar-heavy, fat-saturated pudding for supper rather than a virtuous, balanced and more orthodox combination.

The one thing I don't recommend, though, is trying to concoct low-fat versions of intrinsically high-fat food. Tiramisu made with 0-per-cent-fat fromage frais, cocoa powder and Aspartamame is not the answer (whatever the question is, it's not the answer). It's not just that it will taste horrible, but that you will still feel deprived. Occasional, guilt-free indulgence (to borrow from the slimmer's lexicon) is a much better route. And actually, it's surprising how little you need to eat of something high fat to feel satisfied; in other words, the pudding in its entirety might be vertiginously calorific, but you may not be eating even a couple of bananas' worth of calories of it. Though I do take the point that those of you who truly do manage to eat only a small amount of anything are probably not those for whom this chapter is intended.

And if you can't make smaller portions for yourself, then buy them. If you were to give yourself 100ml of ice-cream, you'd weep: it would hardly cover the bottom of a bowl. But if you buy those little individual 100ml tubs (Loseley Farm make some, and so do Häagen Dazs and their low-fat yoghurt lollies are good, too), you aren't scraping out a meagre portion but eating the entire serving, which feels like more. Again, it's about trying to avoid feeling deprived. Also, you are less likely to speed through the rest of the freezer eating all those unopened little tubs, whereas just lifting off the lid to an already opened large one and digging in, spoon by guilty spoonful, is all too easy. It's like breaking into banknotes.

There's a lot on the market now which comes in pathetically small portions; here, at least, you can work it to your advantage. But beware of distracting yourself, or getting yourself in the wrong frame of mind; so much of all this is in the head, that if you get yourself out of the mood, you can just end up making it harder for, if not actually sabotaging, yourself. This, again, is where the temple-food idea comes in. You want to make a fetish, almost, out of eating the food that's going to make all this easier. So as far as pudding is concerned, this really means fruit. The same principles apply: make it look beautiful, and take longer eating it.

And for this you naturally don't need recipes; the list of ideas that follows is presented just to jolt your memory and help you draw up your shopping lists.

- Peel and de-pith an orange, slice it finely and arrange serenely on a plate. Pour over a drop or two of orange-flower water and sprinkle over a pinch of ground cinnamon.
- Cut a papaya in half, get rid of the seeds, and fill the cavities (avocado-style: v. retro) with raspberries or chopped strawberries.
- Or peel the papaya before scooping out the seeds, then put it cut side down on a plate, slice across thinly and fan out, this time nouvelle-cuisine style, and squeeze the juice of a lime over the fleshy pink slices.
- With a sharp knife, make an incision, skin-deep, all around (lengthwise rather than through its equator) a mango – the best ones are the Indian or Alphonse mangoes, sweet and extraordinarily unstringy – and then peel off

one side's skin. Hold the mango over a plate, and with the knife do some cross hatching, right through to the stone, to form little squares and then take the knife and slice it downwards, scraping the stone and therefore cutting off all the little squares which will then drop into the plate. Do the same to the other half. Or just eat the mango, peeled but otherwise left as is, in the bath.

- Make yourself a kind of Japanese food plate with as much dexterity as you can muster: arrange melon, pineapple, kiwi, orange, artfully chiselled and then, with quiet ceremony, eat them.
- Hull and halve good English strawberries, sprinkle over some balsamic vinegar.
- Cut crosses in figs – as if quartering them without cutting right through them – so that they open like bird-throated flowers. Eat as is if they're perfect; otherwise dust with vanilla sugar, a pinch of icing sugar mixed with ground cinnamon, or honey diluted with rosewater, and blitz them under a searing grill.
- Make a tropical fruit salad by chopping some or all of papaya, melon, mango, pineapple and pour over the seed-crunchy pulp of one or two passion fruits mixed with the juice of half an orange.
- The perfect peach should be eaten alone and unadulterated. But less good, and more prevalent, specimens need both bolstering and camouflage. Tip some blueberries (this, too, symbiotically, is a way of salvaging inferior berries) into a bowl and holding a peach over it, slice into segments, then stir in.
- Never forget watermelon in summer: keep well-wrapped in the fridge and carve off great wedges of it to eat as you want. And make a salad by cutting chunky squares of watermelon, adding pomegranate seeds (and see page 266 for advice as to the best way to release them from their pithy nest) and only a small amount of freshly chopped mint.
- The health farm special: if you can manage to keep pumpkin seeds in the cupboard without raiding it and eating the rest of the opened packet in one go, then keep pumpkin and linseed (the latter less bingeworthy) seeds in store to sprinkle, in teaspoonfuls, over some 0-per-cent-fat Greek or Diet-Bio yoghurt. Add a teaspoon of medium oatmeal and another of runny honey. Dried banana chips are wonderful, but safest to avoid, though a small fresh, sliced banana is worth considering. And try and get Greek mountain honey,

as you get maximum sweetness and flavour for your teaspoonful. Just banana, yoghurt as above and a sprinkling of brown sugar eaten after a couple of minutes' steeping (enough time for the sugar to go caramelly but not enough time for the banana to go black) is wonderful and very – all things being relative – filling.

- Fill a bowl with cold water and ice cubes; to this add, simply, a small bunch of grapes.
- Ditto, but with a couple of handfuls cherries.
- Not quite temple-food, but relatively restrained all the same: fold some raspberries or blackberries into a small bowl of 0-per-cent-fat fromage frais, add a teaspoon of icing sugar and crumble in a meringue.

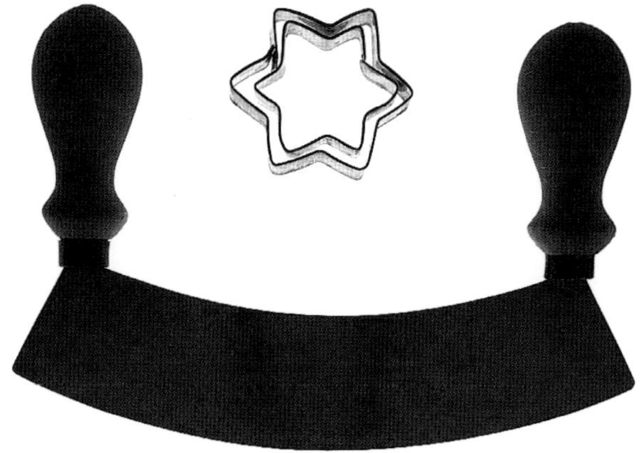

feeding babies and small children

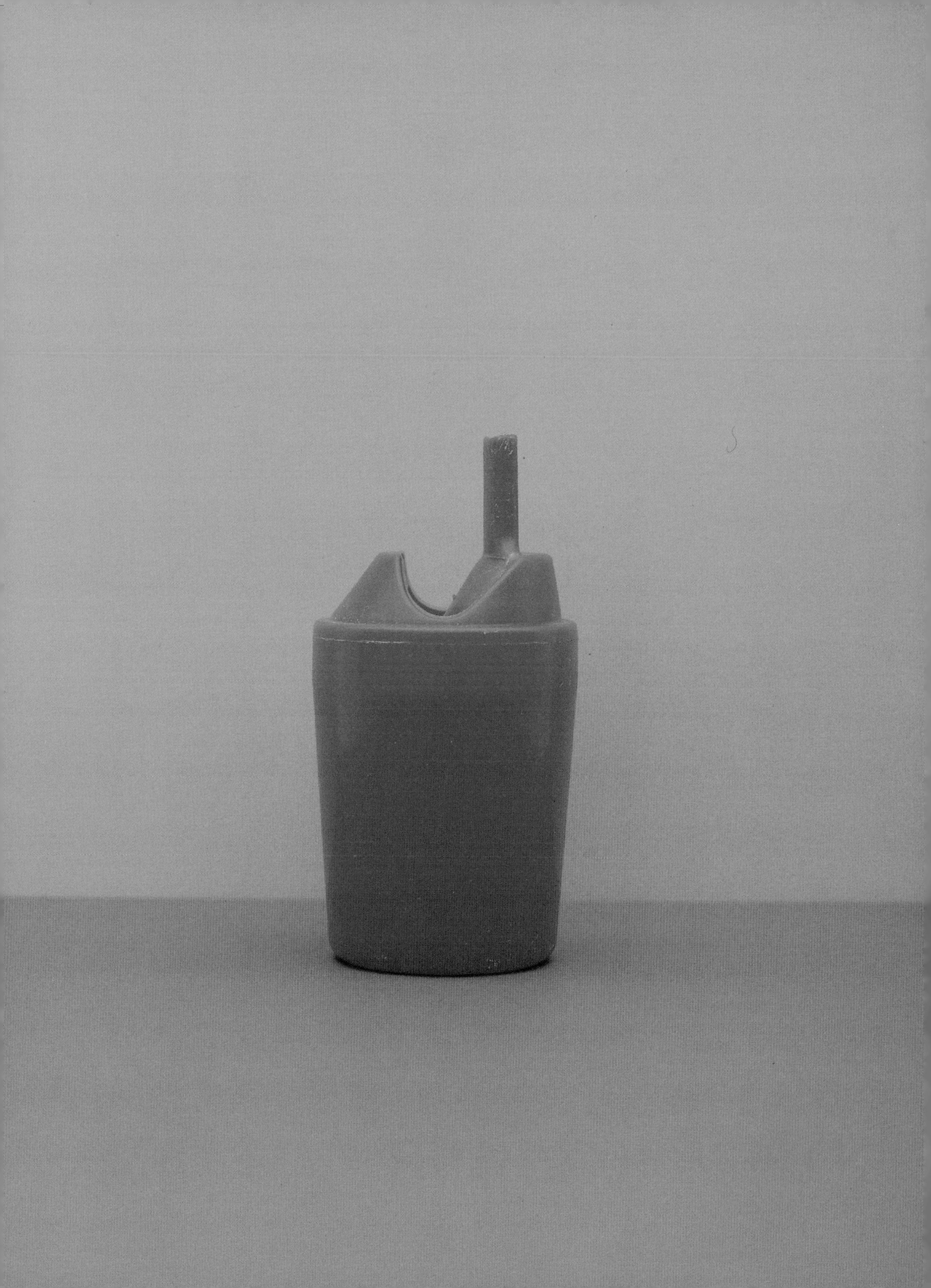

Good eating starts in the cradle. Nutritionists and obstetricians would probably insist that it begins much earlier, but I am talking not so much of the food necessary for good health but the food necessary for a good life. Certainly, they sometimes overlap, and for a child they are inextricably linked. The moment a baby is put to the breast he or she learns that eating is one of the foremost pleasures of life; seeking that pleasure is also how he or she stays alive, and keeps growing.

Latter-day Puritans might think about copying the infant model. In the 1980s there was a comparative study of the eating habits of some workers in the south-west of France and a group of, to use a serviceable but tellingly passé term, health nuts in California. The French ate enormous amounts of red meat and butter and even drank brandy with their breakfasts. But they enjoyed it. The San Franciscans ate few saturated fats, no meat, a lot of alfalfa sprouts, and worried constantly about whether they were eating correctly, whether they had absorbed the right balance of vitamins and nutrients. They were careful to take supplements where they thought necessary. The incidence of heart disease among the Californians was much higher than among the south-western French. It was concluded (I can only believe the scientists in question were French) that a major contributing factor was the anxiety that accompanied the Americans' eating. Since that study some scientists have made other claims about the health-giving properties of red wine. The discrepancy between the sort of diet some Americans feel is a sinful and self-destructive preparation for cardiac arrest, and the low incidence of heart disease in France, has since become known as the French Paradox.

I believe that food should never be thought of as mere fuel. Nor should it be venerated on the one hand, feared on the other. Turning such a life-giving pleasure into a joyless, guilt-ridden and anxiety-provoking but necessary exercise is verging on the criminal. But more – and especially where children are concerned – it is almost bound to be counter-productive.

feeding babies and small children

You can never, alas, ensure good health. But you can learn to enjoy good eating. I'm not sure you can teach it, but you can encourage. If you want children to develop their own taste – and for food other than fish fingers and baked beans – they need to be given good food. I distrust, however, those who have stringent rules about which food is good and which not. The only way to judge whether food is good or not is by tasting it, by eating it. If a child likes baked beans and fish fingers, then it is pointless telling him or her that baked beans and fish fingers are not good to eat. (Anyway, they are.)

There is a lot of fear accompanying judgements about junk and pre-packaged foods. And underneath it all, the fear seems not to be so much about what they will do to the child, but about what they will say about the parent. Too often what passes for love of food is, at best, fashion-consciousness, at worst snobbery. Just as snobbery is in some sense about social insecurity, so food snobbery is really an indication of how frightened and insecure people are about food. They feel that they need to be told what they should like because they have never learnt to trust their own palates. This is why it is crucial to eat well, eat passionately, as a child. Love of food should be something we take in with our mother's milk, not a complicated body of knowledge amassed from the colour supplements in our twenties and thirties. What's good to eat isn't an orthodoxy. But if we don't eat well young, we don't have much to build on. Foundations are everything.

When I was pregnant with my first child, I met the French obstetrician Michel Odent at a party. Of course, during a first pregnancy you are obsessed with it all, and we spoke about babies for as long as I could keep him talking. He told me that one of the reasons breast milk was better than formula was that the taste changed all the time. Whatever a woman's been eating informs the flavour of her milk, and so a breast-fed child has a varied diet from the very beginning. That's to say, the baby learns that unpredictability is in the very nature of food, of life; that change and difference, within a secure context, are not frightening, but desirable and to be savoured. I should admit here that I am a bottle-fed baby who grew up to eat anything. But I certainly ate very little, and that unwillingly, as a child.

M. Odent also told me his research had shown that the children of women who had been instructed to eat fish during pregnancy grew up to adore seafood. I happened to mention this to a friend of mine, who said that when she'd been pregnant she'd had a craving throughout for olives. Her son, from about eighteen months, had shown a marked and otherwise surprising preference for them; they aren't, after all, exactly normal baby-fare. Anecdotal evidence is frowned upon by scientists, but I made a point of eating huge amounts of broccoli while pregnant in the hope of having that rare thing, a child who loved vegetables. I don't mind if it's a coincidence or a result of my intake, but my daughter *does* love broccoli. While pregnant, I also had to have, every day, a bagel with a slice of smoked salmon on it. Maybe that explains my daughter's extravagant, early, and continuing, passion for smoked salmon.

What is the result of genetic predisposition, what of upbringing, I don't know, but they're linked. The way we nurture is part of our nature; the environment we create comes out of what and who we are. It is impossible to convey the pleasures of eating, the real voluptuous joy to be got from food, if we don't feel that joy ourselves. Eating disorders are passed on from mother to daughter (this is not sexist, just – sadly – true) but, even before we get on to such complexities and difficulties, it becomes obvious that our attitude to food colours our children's attitude to food.

From the beginning, you should expect your child to *like* the taste of the food you're offering, rather than nervously expecting it to cause alarm. Nervousness conveys itself to the child. I don't mean that you should force anything. Of course, everyone – child or adult – has their own taste, their own likes and dislikes, and there is no point battling against that. Mostly, though, a child will change, and food given on one day and rejected will be devoured on another day. But that's if you don't push it the first time.

I do think (and given that this is a chapter devoted to the eating practices of the young, I feel justified in rattling this particular cage), that there is a tendency to wean too young in this country. All babies are different and there may well be some who are ready to go on to solid foods at eleven weeks. There is a hopeful theory that babies will sleep for longer once they have solid food and not just milk in their tummies. But giving babies solid food before their digestions can take it is more likely to make them miserable. By the time my daughter was three months, I was being made to feel that I was in some way negligent for failing to offer her solid food (although she was gaining weight well and showed no signs of dissatisfaction with her diet). I then decided to try some baby rice and a little puréed something. She wasn't interested, so I waited until she seemed ready for it. This happened to be at about four-and-three-quarter months. It worked: I offered; she ate. She remains what people call a good eater.

Both my children are growing up in a household where food plays a central part. They see me cooking, see me eating. Food is thus part of the whole fabric of their lives, not just the constituent parts of mealtimes. I accept that when they go to school we will have to enter a less permissive, more picky stage of eating. But I believe that if you give babies and small children the right foundation, if they see you eat with pleasure, and eat pleasurably with you, then, at the end of all the faddiness, they will return to familial normality, if that's not a contradiction in terms. There shouldn't be too much veneration, too much pressure. Let it all just happen. Don't look for trouble.

This brings me to dairy and gluten, and the whole, very contemporary, issue of food intolerances. I don't believe in them. Of course allergies exist, but on the whole allergies manifest themselves radically: you know if you're allergic to some food or other because you are ill, suddenly and as a direct result of having eaten something. The symptoms are incontestably presented. The general malaise that food intolerances are supposed to bring about is much more suspicious. I can't help thinking that adults who are keen to ascribe any number of symptoms – tiredness, lack of energy and enthusiasm – to food intolerance might be better advised to look to their own increasing age for a cause for this insidious drying up of zip, pep and go.

Babies, I admit, don't have the same sort of mechanisms in place (although children certainly can learn very young to use food, or rather the withholding of eating it, as part of the parent–child power struggle: but this is not really a food issue, although you can turn it into one). But we, on behalf of our babies, fuss too much about the wrong things. Our fanatical attention to our children's intake, our obsessive worrying about what terrible things some food can do to them, and our almost primitive belief in the magical properties of other near-voodoo foods, might be doing our children more harm than any of the foodstuffs in question. To live in fear of some food-borne catastrophe is going to be exhausting as well as unhelpful, both day to day and at a more profound psychological level. I should own up here, I suppose, that I did wait until I happened to be in the doctor's surgery with my children before giving them a peanut-butter sandwich for the first time. Although statistically I knew that chances of either of them having some fatal nut allergy were remote, I allowed myself to give in to overprotective maternal neurosis. I am not immune on this score. I worry intermittently about pesticides and shrink from providing adulterated food of indeterminate or covert origin. But I try and resist the notion that children need to be protected from the evils of wheat, milk, sugar and fat.

Because as adults we want – at some time or other – to eat as much as possible for as little calorific spend as possible, many parents think the same virtues hold for their children. This couldn't be further from the truth. No child under the age of five should be given skimmed or semi-skimmed milk. They certainly shouldn't be afraid of big bad fats. They should eat fruit, vegetables, cereals – of course – but don't fill them up with wholewheat pasta and brown rice and don't weight their diet towards the bulky, the hessian weave and stomach-bloating. Children don't have a huge capacity, but they need lots of fuel. In other words, they need food that gramme per gramme is heavily stoked in calories. They eat and run, so you want to make sure that what they eat keeps them going for as long as possible. (Which is why I, nearly every day, thank God for pasta, without which I would be hard-pressed to find food that is maintaining, full of everything that is considered these days dietetically virtuous *and* a useful vehicle for high-fat, calorie-boosting sauces and cheese.) Muesli Malnutrition, the term which doctors apply to the low-fat starvation diet on which many well-meaning, affluent parents keep their children, is a tellingly growing concern.

Of course, it doesn't follow that the higher the fat and the lower the fibre in a child's diet, the better. Even diehard opponents of food faddists and anti-fattists have to accept that huge amounts of saturated fats, day-in day-out, are on the whole unwise. But I believe that animal fats in moderation are good, and in occasional excess unharmful. (And we know that some other fats, such as olive oil, are positively beneficial.) I think it's more important, anyway, to make sure every day that children eat fruit and vegetables, even if they accompany foods that have been fried in dripping or sauced with butter. It's what's missing from a diet that makes the crucial difference.

What you feed your child will go towards forming lifetime habits. It makes sense now not to stoke up trouble for them later. Much as I detest that specious smug and superstitious demarcation between 'healthy' and 'unhealthy' food, I accept that there is such a thing as a healthy diet. Be vigilant, but not obsessive.

For the first months of solid food – which in truth is hardly solid – you are just giving babies slops and purées and beginning the process of giving them food that resembles the food you eat yourself. And you absolutely have to stop yourself minding about the mess: in the first days I wiped my daughter's mouth after each spoonful, but I soon stopped. I had to. You have to learn to live with spilt food and stained clothes or you'll never teach your children to relax around food.

I am not a pediatrician or a nutritionist, and, given the fanatical leanings of most parents, I am almost bound to be a deficient teacher. When we had the builders in, I took out a subscription to *Interiors* and *House and Gardens*; when I was pregnant, I spent sofa-bound evenings reading through parent-and-baby magazines. We are all child hobbyists now, we late-spawning parents of the consumer age; so I take it for granted that somewhere, some if not all of you will have a book on the subject of babies' and children's food, complete with timetables, graphs, nutritional indices and medical advice. If not, trust me, they are widely available. But here, just in case, is a weaning timetable.

BABY-WEANING CHART

Do not add salt to your baby's food until he or she is 1 year or over.

4–5 months	**semi-liquid purées of:** apple, pear, banana, papaya, carrot, cauliflower, potato, courgette, squash, green beans, swede, sweet potato
5–6 months	dried fruit, peach, kiwi fruit, apricot, plum, melon, avocado, peas, tomato, spinach, celery, leek, sweet pepper
6 months	chicken, dairy products, parsnip, foods containing gluten
6–7 months	**minced or mashed foods, which can include:** citrus fruit, berries, mango, sweetcorn
6–12 months	other meats
8–9 months	**chunkier textures, which can now include:** split peas, butter beans, lentils, eggs, fish
over 2 years	shellfish

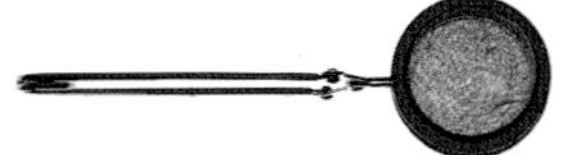

SOLIDS

Many parents start infants off with baby rice. I understand the reasoning – that it is midway between milk and solid food – but in practice it didn't work for my children. One of the fascinating things about how babies and small children eat is that they regulate their intake themselves: they eat as much as they need; if they eat less one day or for several days, they will make up for the deficit in calories later. Whenever I added baby rice to fruit or vegetable purées, my babies would eat as much as they felt they needed, as if what they were eating was just fruit or vegetable. They couldn't, it seemed, detect the rice. For when the grain swelled in their stomachs later, it transpired that they had eaten too much; consequently, and efficiently, they vomited the excess up. This isn't harmful, but I felt it unhelpful to interfere with the fine calibration of their digestive systems.

So for those with small babies who are about to start eating solids, I advise some fresh, cooked, cooled, puréed pear (peeled, obviously) as a first food. I used to cook it by putting chunks of the fruit in a container in the microwave for a few minutes. Bananas, briefly microwaved, then mashed with milk – breast or formula – are also a good first food. The microwave is very good for cooking most fruits. (Vegetables are better steamed, or boiled, I think, as microwaved vegetables have a spooky texture.) Of all fruits, both my children liked papaya best. I'd cut them in half, scoop out the seeds and then blitz them briefly in the microwave. The smell of them, thus nuked, is sickly sweet, almost to the emetic point of putrefaction, or so it seemed to me after pulping too many of these honeyed and puce fruits, but children love the sweet, soft, aromatic flesh.

PEAR

BANANAS

PAPAYA

But ordinary fruit and vegetables are just as good. Variety is important, but a baby's diet doesn't have to include one of every foodstuff known to man. Remember that all foods are new: for a baby, stewed apple is just as exotic as steamed papaya.

For my first child I went into food processing overdrive, filling the freezer with as many different purées and pulped meals as possible. If you're going to peel, cook and purée some carrots you may as well do it once and have enough in the freezer for the month's meals ahead. Apart from anything else, the amount a baby eats is really tiny: even one carrot makes enough for quite a few meals. The only reason I relaxed (rather than abandoned) my bulk preparations of food with my second child was that I was cooking anyway for one child, so fiddling about with an extra bit of fruit or veg or handful of baby pasta at each mealtime didn't seem much trouble.

You do need, however, to be able to feed small babies promptly. If you can prepare baby food in advance, freeze it, and then microwave when needed, you reduce the time you are subjected to outraged, hunger-crazed screaming. But the practical advantage is the least of it. If you slave away cooking from scratch, trying to create some perfect morsel for your baby's edification, you will inevitably take it much harder when she spits it out in disgust or wipes it all over the walls. It isn't wise to put so much emotional pressure on either yourself or your children at mealtimes. If you slave and then freeze the product of your stove-bound slavery, the memory of the effort will inevitably recede and you won't take rejection so badly. This goes for feeding older children, too.

Once a baby has got used to solid food, knows what it's for and enjoys eating it, baby pasta (*pastina*, imported from Italy) is a useful way of making meals. It takes a few seconds to cook (I tended to cook it in milk, defrosted packages of expressed breast milk when they were very little and full-fat cow's milk once they were past six months) and all you need to do is toss it in some butter and grated parmesan. If the baby in question is pre-six months, then you might feel happier adding nothing more, but otherwise use it in vegetable purées, too. It's very fine (or the smallest size is) but the grains retain their separateness: it doesn't become a gluey mass. I rather love it as well, and I think, as far as possible, you should try to give your babies food that you could bear to eat too. This is one of the reasons I cannot bring myself to serve up much bottled baby food. I just feel it must constitute the worst sort of culinary education. I am not neurotically and intolerantly bound to the preciously home-made, however: I always kept a supply of Beechnut baby foods (imported from the United States and increasingly available here) on hand, and often give myself up to the cool but welcoming embrace of the supermarket or Marks & Spencer chill-cook cabinet.

PASTINA

Indeed, Beechnut packages a fine-ground barley meal that I find preferable to baby rice. I gave it to my children for breakfast for ages, before they moved on to Weetabix and then to proper porridge (funnily enough, the baby oats that Beechnut also do weren't as popular). I mixed the barley meal with milk (first breast, then cow's) or sometimes fresh orange juice diluted with water, especially if either of them had a cold.

BARLEY MEAL

PORRIDGE

I used to freeze baby purée in ice-cube trays. Just empty the thickly coloured frozen cubes into plastic bags, label, tie up and throw back in the freezer. I can't advise labelling too strongly. Every time I thought I couldn't possibly forget what this luridly coloured food was, I ended up being mystified at some later date and would defrost apricots when I was after carrots. The brain does go in the aftermath of childbirth: better accept that now.

I quite like pottering about kitchens, so made up quite a few different foods, but you soon realise that more than five or six can be superfluous; babies inevitably favour certain ones over others, and you, as inevitably, choose to defrost the favoured. After the first month or so of plain fruits and vegetables, I got into the habit of creating certain mixtures, and they're useful ones. The compound I was most pleased with was a mush of spinach and sweetcorn – the spinach, with its metallic almost bitter hit, is sweetened, and somewhat de-slimed by the corn. Another – broccoli and carrot – also works well. Though broccoli has a definite sweetness of its own, it also has a cabbagy mustiness which babies, and adults, can warm to less. Carrots intensify the sweetness and seem to neutralise the otherwise enduring Brassica-family brackishness. You will create a sludge of particularly unattractive khaki, but your baby will be able to live with that. When my babies were beyond purées, they ate the broccoli florets whole, a small green tree clasped in each fat pink fist.

SPINACH AND SWEETCORN

BROCCOLI AND CARROT

I started off in fear of salt; indeed, medical advice is that you shouldn't add it to food for a child under 1 year (now I let my children pour rivers of soy over their noodles, but there's nothing like having more than one child for easing one's principles, dietary or otherwise). I did succumb, however, to salted frozen spinach, but drained it and processed it with drained unsalted tinned corn, in about equal measures, before freezing it in cubes. You can, of course, use fresh vegetables, not frozen; or buy organic canned stuff from the health store, which won't have salt added.

I didn't add sugar to any food I gave my daughter, and didn't get into the habit of giving her puddings or biscuits either, and she isn't interested in eating them much now. My son, who has the advantage in this respect of being the second child, loves cake and anything sugary. But maybe (she said a trifle defensively) this isn't entirely because I have relaxed, giving him foods that normally I might not have fed to a baby, but because they have very different palates to start off with.

And that can't be underestimated. Neither I nor my children like baby rice. Your child might adore it. Babies have their own tastes, and to try to change them by force is as idiotic as the once-accepted practice of making left-handed children write with their right hands. Respond to your child but, at the same time, encourage him or her to experiment, to recognise, to enjoy.

SPINACH

One way to encourage your child is to give him or her a small taste of certain foods gradually. I wanted my children to enjoy eating spinach, so I tried to find ways of insinuating spinach into their diet without actually giving them, until they were older, a whole iron-resonant plate of the stuff. Get for your freezer those packs of puréed spinach frozen in lots of tiny spheres. Then all you need to do is defrost one sphere to stir into some other purée or foodstuff. This way, your child will get used to the taste of spinach and will therefore like it. Children respond to the familiar, the known. Just don't make a big thing about it: don't let children know you expect them not to like something before they actually eat it, or show your surprise if they happen to love it.

Pasta sauce, most often pesto; mincemeat, and thus shepherd's or cottage pie; cheesy mashed potato; omelette or frittata; puréed peas; cheese sauce: you don't need me to list all the baby foods into which you can stir a disc of thawed and warmed spinach, but, trust me, it is invaluable later when your child is eating meals rather than slops. But do it before he has reached the stage of looking out suspiciously for green bits.

LIVER

Liver is another food that everyone presumes children will have to be forced to eat against their will. I never found this, but it may be that I am irredeemably extravagant because I fed my children calves' liver and chicken livers, rather than the vile, fibrous, bitter livers I was given at school. People who would never think of asking how much something costs before they eat it themselves, get twitchy about expensive tastes in their young. Whenever I gave my children smoked salmon I was mocked by friends, as if I was making them wear tutus and speak French to one another in the manner of that rich-kid stunt in *High Society*. But children love smoked salmon, which is a very useful meal to bear in mind for hungry, fractious children kept waiting for an inevitably late lunch by an equally fractious parent after a Saturday morning spent shopping in Sainsbury's. After all, it's bad enough having to take the food out of the car into

SMOKED SALMON

the house and then out of the bags into the cupboards. To have to cook any of it would be the final straw. Cut open instead a plastic-wrapped packet of smoked salmon (or smoked trout: it costs less), butter some bread if you must and grate a few carrots if you can. (It's worth knowing, in this regard, that most children seem to like frozen peas, as they are, unthawed, to eat from their own little bowls set out in front of them. It's not wise to let very small children eat these chokingly unyielding vegetable beads, but vigilance is a better route than dietary censorship.)

FROZEN PEAS

Giving children real food, the sort of food we'd eat ourselves, is important. It's why the French eat well, and the Italians: their children are not fobbed off with lesser ingredients and different meals in the erroneous belief that good food or expensive items are wasted on them. I'm not saying that you must bankrupt yourself to provide your angels with luxuries and *bonnes bouches*, but simply that they should not eat worse than you do. If I grate fresh parmesan on to my pasta, why should I insist that theirs comes ready-grated, bitterly musty, smelling of old trainers and trapped in a plastic-lidded drum?

This does not mean that everything your child eats, you will want to eat. One of my infant son's favourite meals was liver puréed with soaked dried apricots. I should not choose to lunch on that. But I added the dried apricots to counter the potentially constipating effects of the liver. Deep within me I must have a fixation with digestive habits: I always feel that the balance between what nannies always used to refer to as the 'binding' and 'loosening' effects of foods has to be maintained. For example, poached egg for tea comes on top of a bowl of sweetcorn.

CHICKEN LIVER

I threw together the apricots and liver in the first place to use up a liver from a chicken I was roasting; real cooking, I can't help feeling, always starts from leftovers. You could use calves' liver, but in which case, because it is less bitter, you should add just a single apricot to the recipe below. I say recipe, but it isn't really anything as precise. For a start, quantities are hard to gauge at any time, but for children, whose ages and appetites vary, it's even harder. But when my son was seven months old, I'd make up a batch of this and reckon it would make 2–3 portions for him. You need a chicken's liver (about 50g) which you fry gently in butter, and 2 cubes of purée made from dried apricot. I reckon that 1 apricot equals 1 cube (or tablespoon), so if you haven't got any ready-made in the freezer, just soak some dried apricots in hot water from a just-boiled

DRIED APRICOT

kettle for an hour or so, and then boil on the hob till soft, drain and purée. Most apricots are labelled as not needing any soaking, but I reckon they do. Take a slice of dry or stale bread and soak it in some milk until saturated. Squeeze it out and add it to the liver and apricots and blend. Chicken liver, fried in butter as above, and blended with an equal weight of chicken breast poached in milk is another idea; use as much of the poaching liquid as you need to get to the texture you want. If you leave it thick you can spread it onto toast-and-butter fingers. When I wanted the puréed liver as a bowl-bound meal – with or without baby pasta – I sometimes stirred in some puréed carrot, too.

QUICK MEALS

What helps most is having a cache of food you can throw together easily. So you must get stocked up first. You don't need me to tell you to keep a constant supply of baked beans in the house, but I remind you simply because this is the foremost fast way to give children something sustaining to eat. I know people go on about the added salt and sugar, but I can't get worked up about it. It makes sense to watch for salt when they're tiny. I never salted any cooking water – of pasta, vegetables, anything – or added salt later, until my children were 4 years and 18 months respectively. Then I decided that, if I wanted them to eat like us, it was inconsistent to refuse to allow them to season their food like us.

BEANS AND PULSES

Just as children like baked beans, so they seem to like all pulses. Tinned chick peas, cannellini, borlotti, pinto, any bean you want, are worth keeping around for them, and if you *do* mind about salt then buy canned organic ones. Just stir some cooked chopped bacon into any of the pulses, or some prawns or fish into the cannellini. Prawns and beans happens to be an actual contemporary Italian reworking – *i ricchi e i poveri* as it's known – of the traditional *tonno e fagioli*; indeed tuna, drained, and mixed in with a can of beans, bound with a few drops of good olive oil is another meal worth bearing in mind, since canned tuna (which I detest) seems ideally suited to childish palates. Trout fillets, just poached, then roughly chopped and added to borlotti – or Pink Fish and Beans – are a particular favourite in my household, since my daughter is going through

BACON
PRAWNS
TUNA
PINK FISH AND BEANS

a deeply pink stage, which shows no signs of abating. You could use smoked fillets if you want to avoid any cooking whatsoever, or substitute smoked mackerel; this is something of a radical substitution – the taste is much stronger, the texture much oilier – but can be successful.

SMOKED MACKEREL

PASTA

Pasta is another obvious staple, as are oriental noodles. I live near a Thai shop, so buy bagfuls of fettucine-thick egg-yellow and paler thread-thin noodles (which need a minute's cooking) and fresh rice sticks, which don't need to be cooked at all – you just steep them for 5–10 minutes in boiling water. (It doesn't hurt to keep some cooked, cold-water-spritzed and drained egg noodles in a covered bowl in the fridge, either.) Any of these, with some soy sauce (as I say, I'm not salt-sensitive) lightly sprinkled over, are among the lowest-effort meals I can think of. Supermarkets sell various forms of Asian noodles now, so you don't need access to exotically stocked, stall-sized shops, shelves piled with dried shrimp and sour pastes. But going to specialist stores makes shopping so pleasurable, and it's cheaper. Sometimes I make small bowls of vaguely Japanese soup: stock, some chopped greens, manageable lengths of noodle. This, for my daughter, signals special food, partly because it's food I make for myself (see pages 425–427) and partly because it has seemed a treat ever since I took her to a Japanese restaurant and she ordered noodle soup and was given chopsticks to eat it with. She couldn't really manage them, except singly as a kind of load-bearing punt, and I ended up feeding her, ferrying food, noodle by fat noodle, from bowl to hungry open mouth like a mother bird feeding her gaping-beaked young with worms.

EGG NOODLES

VAGUELY JAPANESE SOUP

For ordinary pasta, keep bottled tomato sauce on hand and jars of pesto, both good quality. Pesto might not sound like children's food, but they like much stronger flavours than adults give them credit for. But don't buy phoney cut-price versions. How are children ever going to know how to eat well if they've been reared on inferior ingredients or ersatz foods? I don't mean – and I can't stress this enough – you must always provide them with comestibles shipped over from Peck or Fauchon, but don't pretend that an inauthentic article is the real thing. By all means cook rice and stir in peas and sweetcorn, just don't call it risotto. I speak as someone who gives her children tinned ravioli as a special weekend treat when I feel too tired even to put a pan of water on to boil, so I'm not claiming rarefied or superior status. But I don't pretend it's the real thing, or that the difference doesn't matter.

COUSCOUS

Just as children love pasta, so they seem to love couscous. This is even easier. Put some couscous in a bowl and pour over some boiling water (about 150ml water for 100g couscous). Leave, covered, for about 10 minutes. That's it. Stir in some butter and give it to them to eat.

That's the basic, baldest method. Mostly I tend to bolster couscous with vegetables and use stock rather than water: my regular standby involves chopping 1 carrot in the baby processor until it is in tiny cubes and shards, and then boiling it for 2 minutes in a pan of bubbling water to which I have added some Marigold vegetable bouillon powder. I then shake in some couscous, bring it all back to the boil, take the pan off the heat and cover, leaving it for about 10 minutes. You can fork in some olive oil or butter, as you wish, but I think you do need some fat; small children find it easier to eat when the *sémoules* are sticking together rather than fluffily, and otherwise desirably, separate. You are not making couscous a Moroccan would be proud of, I admit, but nor are you setting out to. If you want to be really brazen and British you can use frozen peas and sweetcorn in place of the carrot. Drained, canned chick peas are the easiest option. Consider cracked wheat also: my daughter loves tabbouleh (and see page 260) as well, astringent and onion-hot as I make it.

POTATO

Mashed potato is a good way to fill up a child. The easiest way to do this is the extravagant one. In other words, don't peel, cook, then mash the potatoes, but use baking potatoes instead. Bake them (½–1 per child, about 90 minutes or more in a hottish oven), eat the skin yourself (young children don't seem to cope with this) sprinkled with a good pelt of coarse salt, crunch on crunch, as you fork some butter through the fluffy-cooked flesh in a bowl for your child.

As children get older they seem to prefer the potato kept separate from other things on the plate. But up to the age of two they accept various things to make the mashed, baked potato pulp into entire, distinct meals. Add more or less milk, depending on age. Obviously, the nubblier purées are not suitable for gummy-mouthed babies. Some of the ingredients I used may sound unappealing, but they didn't appear so to my children, so may not to yours. You can add chopped ham, minced meat, strips of chicken or crunchy vegetables to the side.

WITH CHEESE

When the mashed potato is still at its hottest – don't pour in the milk to slacken it first – grate in whatever cheese you want. I started off, when they were babies, with gruyère and then went on to cheddar or parmesan or a mixture of both. They seem to like red leicester, too. Fork potato and cheese vehemently together until the fine strands of cheese start to melt. (I find a hand-held mouli cheese grater, with drum and handle, the easiest way of doing this, except, obviously, with the parmesan. But then I hate those knuckle-shaving punctured metal box graters.) Then stir in milk or milk and butter to make the mixture more liquid. If you want to boost the calorific value of this meal, add a dollop of mascarpone (or cream, of course). I sometimes beat in a raw egg yolk for this reason, too, but then I get my eggs from Martin Pitt (and see page 506) and feel confident that they are salmonella-free. I know the accepted wisdom is that the babies and small children shouldn't be given uncooked eggs to eat, but it is not a wisdom I have accepted.

WITH PESTO

From a very young age, both my children loved pesto and ate anything with it in. I add about 1 tablespoon to the flesh of each potato (½ tablespoon per child) and beat in till smoothly amalgamated. Add 1 tablespoon or so more oil. If you're being echt, which could mean being fancy, you should use Ligurian olive oil to dovetail, culinarily speaking, with the pesto. I do happen to keep this in the house (see page 506) and since it is milder than the Tuscan oil, with less of the throat-hitting pepperiness, it is probably more instantly palatable for small children anyway. Sometimes I mix in a sphere of quick-thawed and cooked finely chopped spinach, as mentioned on page 459. Go cautiously with the pesto and spinach but you can add more than the amount I've suggested if it turns out your children like this purée even stronger and greener. I'm not sure I'd try this on children before they've eaten pesto on pasta, not because I think they may not like the taste (I've not met one who doesn't) but because all children have an inbuilt caution about mixtures.

WITH EGG

If you don't like the idea of introducing raw egg (and I would recommend always using eggs that are checked for salmonella, anyway), you can just soft-boil or poach 1–2 eggs, stir in the oily yolk and then the finely chopped white. If you're worried about albumen, hard-boil the eggs and then push the dense globes of yolk through a sieve onto the potato, and think of this, archly, as mashed potato mimosa. Add milk as required and butter as desired.

WITH VEGETABLE PURÉE

A few gloopy tablespoons of puréed butternut, orange-fleshed sweet potato or carrot stirred into the potato will make a good orange bowl of mash for babies; for older children, you could grate over some red leicester and shove under a grill for a minute until scorched and almost crunchy. Substitute puréed sweetcorn, if your child doesn't mind a few rough bits, and whole sweetcorn kernels if they are beyond even gravelly purées. You could use peas (frozen peas, cooked then puréed with a knob of butter and a tablespoon of parmesan are wonderful with potatoes, whether you're a child or not), but I'd avoid other grassier green vegetables here. In all cases, consider a dollop of mascarpone for ballast and perhaps the merest, sheerest grating of fresh nutmeg.

WITH TOMATO

I don't like tomato purée: I find it invasively metallic; everything to which it's added tastes instantly, however fresh, however lovingly home-made, as if it had come out of the tinniest of tins. This, Anna del Conte tells me reprovingly, is because I don't cook the purée long enough: it needs slow, insistent simmering before that front-of-tongue dried-blood taste subsides and the flavour builds to fill the whole mouth with sweet and actual tomato-ishness. This makes sense, and I take the point and will act on it from now on, with sauces and stews, but with this kind of cooking for children, which isn't really meant to *be* cooking, I am not proposing to tend any pan for devoted hours. You have a choice: you can use tinned purée made both more gentle and more liquid by the addition of a little warm milk or a good-quality tomato sauce, strained or not as you wish. Since I aim (but don't always succeed) to keep Marks & Spencer's tomato sauce in the house, I use that. And do not hesitate – consider your constituency here – to add a good squeeze of tomato ketchup. Add grated cheese or mascarpone (or use a few tablespoons of bought, so-called fresh tomato and mascarpone sauce in the first place) if you want to provide more fuel or some protein.

WITH BAKED BEANS

This entry speaks for itself. All I'd add is that I'd use butter rather than milk to slacken the mixture.

WITH PEANUT BUTTER

Smooth, of course. Yes, I know peanut butter and potato mixed sounds disgusting and, to be frank, even I, the greediest person alive, sitting vulture-like and fork in hand, impatient to snatch the food out of my babies' mouths, manage not to pick when they're eating this. The point is that children like it (and some grown-ups do too, I've found) and it gets in extra calories and protein at the same time. I have been known – don't gag – to stir in a little coconut cream dissolved in warm milk and this went down *very* well. It's the sweetness, I suppose, and the fact that we all do seem to have an innate, inbuilt capacity to appreciate fat. Once I've gone this far, though, there's nothing to stop me throwing in a few sweetcorn kernels, too.

WITH TAHINA

As long as you don't use too much, children seem to love this pungent, soft-clay paste, diluted with a little milk or olive oil and stirred into the potato.

WITH GARLIC

Children love garlic. Bake the potato at gas mark 6/200°C (and reckon on needing 1½–2 hours depending on size: I like potatoes *really* cooked: one grain of unyielding crystalline flesh and they're ruined for me) and, ½ hour or so in, take a whole head of garlic, lop off the top so the cloves are revealed in cross-section, place on a square of foil, pour over a little oil, and wrap up the garlic so that you have a baggy but tightly crimped parcel. Cook for 50 minutes, then take out and let stand in its foil. When you mash the potato, unwrap the garlic package and squeeze in the sweet, pulpy cloves. Whip with a fork to incorporate smoothly and add butter, milk or cream to make the sort of purée you want. Heaven.

WITH FISH

Children seem to like tinned fish and you can use tuna or salmon here; with the salmon, make sure you've removed any lingering bones or slimy strips of oil-immersed skin. Add anything else you think would enhance – tomato sauce, mayonnaise, sweetcorn. And you're really halfway to fishcakes here (see below, page 491).

OTHER EASILY-THROWN-TOGETHER MEALS

If you hate the very idea of cooking, no one's stopping you from opening packets or buying ready-prepared meals. And if you're worried about salt and sugar and other additives, you'll probably be able to find more virtuous though not necessarily more palatable precooked meals at health stores. You don't want to foist your hysteria at the stove onto your offspring. Nor do you, on the other hand, want to make a cult out of cooking everything yourself, so that your children either become afraid of any alien meal or develop a terrible longing for microwaved junk food. We all know about the thrill of the illicit. Besides, it's worth keeping a stash of ready-made meals on the grounds alone that it will make your life easier. But low-level cooking needn't feel too demanding. The following suggestions occupy a culinary territory somewhere between the ideas above and the full-blown recipes below.

RICE

Rice is, in my household, just as popular as pasta and couscous. It's popular with me, too, since I've got an electric rice cooker and it is therefore one of my hands-free options. Naturally I am not presuming on your possession of such a machine, but basmati rice, cooked in a pot on the hob, is relatively low-effort. Providing you're giving the children a moderately balanced diet as it is, you don't need to add much to rice, though by all means throw in chopped meat or something that makes you feel this is more of a traditionally complete meal, if you want. I have entirely corrupted my children by letting them see how I eat my rice, which is doused in soy, so this is now how they require theirs. There's a trade-off: I happen to eat my soy-browned rice with steamed or boiled broccoli and so this is, without fuss, introduced as part of the deal.

My children enjoy rice with diced carrot, swede, peas and corn, which can be bought in bags from any supermarket, even if the mixture makes me shiver. If you want, you can make a one-egg omelette in a non-stick pan and then cut it into shreds and stir this into the rice. And while we're edging towards it, I should mention that any leftover plain cooked rice languishing in the fridge can be turned into fried rice, which always goes down well. Put some vegetable oil in a relatively deep-sided frying pan or a wok and when it's hot (with a wok you should heat the pan before pouring in the oil) stir in 2 peeled, sliced or chopped garlic cloves and 1 finely sliced spring onion if your children's digestion will

ONE-EGG OMELETTE

FRIED RICE

take them, and stir-fry for a minute or so. Add some butter to the pan. Now cook some very, very, finely chopped carrot. Then add some sliced button mushrooms and cook – pushing and prodding with your wooden spoon or spatula – for about 5 minutes. Add cold cooked rice and push around the pan for a bit longer. Cook a one-egg omelette in a non-stick pan separately, cut it into shreds and then stir it into the rice. Turn into bowls. My children like coriander, so I sometimes add that. And throwing in some cooked peeled prawns is, as far as my children are concerned, always a good move. In fact, just plain rice and prawns is a good fall-back Saturday lunch.

PRAWNS

RICE AND TOMATO SOUP

I also make an unfussy rice and tomato soup (for myself, too, sometimes, especially when I'm trying to balance out my characteristic gluttony) by diluting a good, bought tomato sauce with water, adding a handful or so of basmati rice and cooking until the rice is tender, about 8–10 minutes. With children it makes more sense to leave the soup fairly solid, but you can add water from a boiled kettle towards the end of the cooking time if you want a thinner soup rather than liquid tomato-rice stew. Grate parmesan on top and eat – with bibs.

GYPSY TOAST

This is the same thing as eggy bread or french toast. Bread, preferably stale, is soaked in egg beaten up with a bit of milk and then fried in butter. Even though I don't generally go in for making smiley faces and funny shapes out of food, as we're all supposed to do to lure a child to eat, I do cut out shapes of bread before soaking them (I normally use a star-shaped biscuit cutter for this, and I've got some otherwise unforgivably dinky aspic cutters, mini hearts, diamonds, spades and so forth, with which I stamp out shapes from bought packets of thinly sliced gruyère). The golden stars do look beautiful – until they're blooded by the required shake of tomato ketchup. My children are not particularly keen on ketchup (as I say, they're still pre-school), but here they consider it obligatory. I make gypsy toast for a late weekend breakfast or for supper, after bath and just before bedtime, to keep them sleeping longer in the morning, so that the occasional late breakfast *is* a possibility.

Mimi Sheraton, in her wonderful memoir-cum-cookbook, *From My Mother's Kitchen*, says that the best French toast is made from slightly stale challah. She's right, but away from New York you might have to substitute brioche. But whatever you have to hand is just fine. Americans tend to eat their version of egg-soaked, butter-fried bread with either maple syrup (and bacon, too, both of which I rather love) or sprinkled with sugar and cinnamon. Cinnamon toast, that's to say, ordinary toast, made with sliced white bread, and spread with a paste made by beating unsalted butter with sugar and cinnamon is tear-prickingly comforting.

POUSSIN

A poussin is about the right size for two children with leftovers or three children without, and has the advantage of not needing any effort to cook. Just smear with butter or garlic-infused-oil and sprinkle with salt or soy (or neither) before putting in a gas mark 5/190°C oven for about 45 minutes. Or throw in whole shallots and cloves of garlic, as on page 9.

LAMB CUTLETS

Chops and cutlets seem such old-fashioned food now, but they cook quickly and can be eaten in fingers. If you've got time, and aren't sure how tender the lamb is, marinate for an hour or more in the juice of 1 orange and 1 tablespoon olive oil with 1 teaspoon redcurrant jelly. Preheat the grill, line a tray with foil and cook the chops for a few minutes each side. I don't specify how many minutes because it depends how well done you want it. In my view, it's never too soon to get a child used to pink lamb and blue beef. Green beans, also eaten with fingers, are good alongside.

GARLIC MUSHROOMS

Simply cook chopped garlic in oil or butter or a mixture, and add finely sliced mushrooms. Or use a packet of ready-sliced mixed mushrooms; some are sold with a pat of herb or garlic butter already in. If I'm in a hurry or have run out of garlic, I just add some of my shop-bought, garlic-infused oil to butter and cook the sliced mushrooms in it. If I'm rich in porcini, I soak and finely chop and then bung them in, reserving the strained liquid. Even if I'm cooking for children, I like to add a slug of white wine, vermouth or sherry, too. You can stop there, so that the mushrooms have a sparse, syrupy-buttery juice clinging to them. Serve with some buttered, toasted plastic bread or buttered, toasted muffin to the side, but you could pile the mushrooms on top of either, or pour the mixture on pasta, plain rice or mashed potato. Alternatively, after adding the whoosh of alcohol, let it bubble away till the alcohol's cooked off and the liquid reduced, and then stir in a good few tablespoons of crème fraîche or double cream and let that bubble away until the mushrooms are submerged in a thick, buff-coloured creamy sauce.

QUAILS' EGGS AND NEW POTATOES

It's not surprising that children like miniature food. Quails' eggs are fiddly to peel, but my children fall upon them as if they were sweets. I buy a box of 12 for the 2 of them, but am going to have to think of increasing rations to keep up with demand. I like to balance the effects certain foods have on the digestive system, as confessed earlier, so serving boiled or steamed new potatoes (little waxy-fleshed pebbles) alongside, to form a routine culinary partnership, makes me feel better about the egg-bolting.

Put the eggs in a pan, cover with cold water, bring to the boil and cook for 4 minutes. Immerse in cold water and leave to cool for 1 minute, then peel. The eggs are slightly easier to peel if you roll them, rather heavy handedly so that the shell cracks, against the sink's draining board.

If I've got time (it does take longer than boiling) I steam the potatoes: it makes peeling them easier and, even if the skin's meant to be healthy, my children won't eat it; they either hand the unpeeled potato imperiously to me to peel for them or just spit out the offending skin. I sometimes cook some carrot batons to go with them, a few straight lines to add to the arrangement, and because I feel the presence of extra vegetables is a good thing. I have never told my children they're not supposed to like vegetables and they haven't yet worked it out for themselves, so the introduction of carrots is well received.

CORN ON THE COB

And while we're on the subject, even children who won't countenance vegetables seem to like corn on the cob. You can buy mini-sized ones (that's to say, normal ones halved) in bags, frozen, which are useful to have around. They cook from frozen.

GARLIC-FRIED POTATOES

I can see that potatoes might not constitute a meal in themselves, but the fat in which they are fried adds enough calories to overrule any hesitation on this score. Chop up garlic and give it a few minutes, stirring, in the pan before sautéeing some sliced, cooked and cooled potatoes. Try cooking them in lard or dripping; they taste wonderful and crisp up gloriously. Alternatively, leave out the garlic and just sauté the potatoes in garlic-infused oil. I have fried up bought parboiled potatoes, shaped into gobstopper-sized balls, which are found hanging limply around the prepared vegetable shelf (near salads, normally) in the supermarket. I used to give the children either egg or a slice of ham with these potatoes, but since it was the potatoes they liked, I gave up on an accompaniment, except for some crunchy green vegetables.

GARLIC ROAST POTATOES

If your children are old enough to understand about skins, and will suck the sweet roast garlic flesh from the unpeeled cloves and leave the skins on the side of the plate, I wouldn't bother to peel them. Unpeeled, the garlic steams inside its skin and grows softer and sweeter; peeled, the taste can be stronger and, if you're not careful, bitter. But just remember (if peeling) to parboil the garlic. It's not a big deal, especially since it makes the cloves easy to peel. Preheat the oven to gas mark 6/200°C. If you're using unpeeled cloves, then just scatter a few cloves (about 6 a child, but then I'm always hovering about for leftovers) in a baking tin. Chop up (don't bother to peel: when the potatoes are roasted, children don't seem to mind the skin) some new potatoes into small dice and throw into the pan, too. Pour over some olive oil and mix it all about with your hands to make sure everything's glistening and covered. Sprinkle with salt if your principles allow and roast for about 45 minutes or until cooked and golden. If you're going to peel the garlic, put the unpeeled cloves in a saucepan, cover with cold water, bring to the boil and boil for 5 minutes. Turn into a colander and run the cold tap over it, and them, and then just slip the skins off and proceed as above.

You can give your children these alone, or with roast chicken or poussin but we often eat them with a fried or poached egg and some thickly buttered white bread, with fruit after.

Perhaps here is the place to note that, as far as children are concerned, you can never have too many seedless white grapes. Fresh pear, ripe, honeyed, juicy, peeled and cut into chunks, is the everyday favourite in my household; mangoes, similarly dealt with, but with the stone to gnaw on after, is a special treat, with the status of ice-cream.

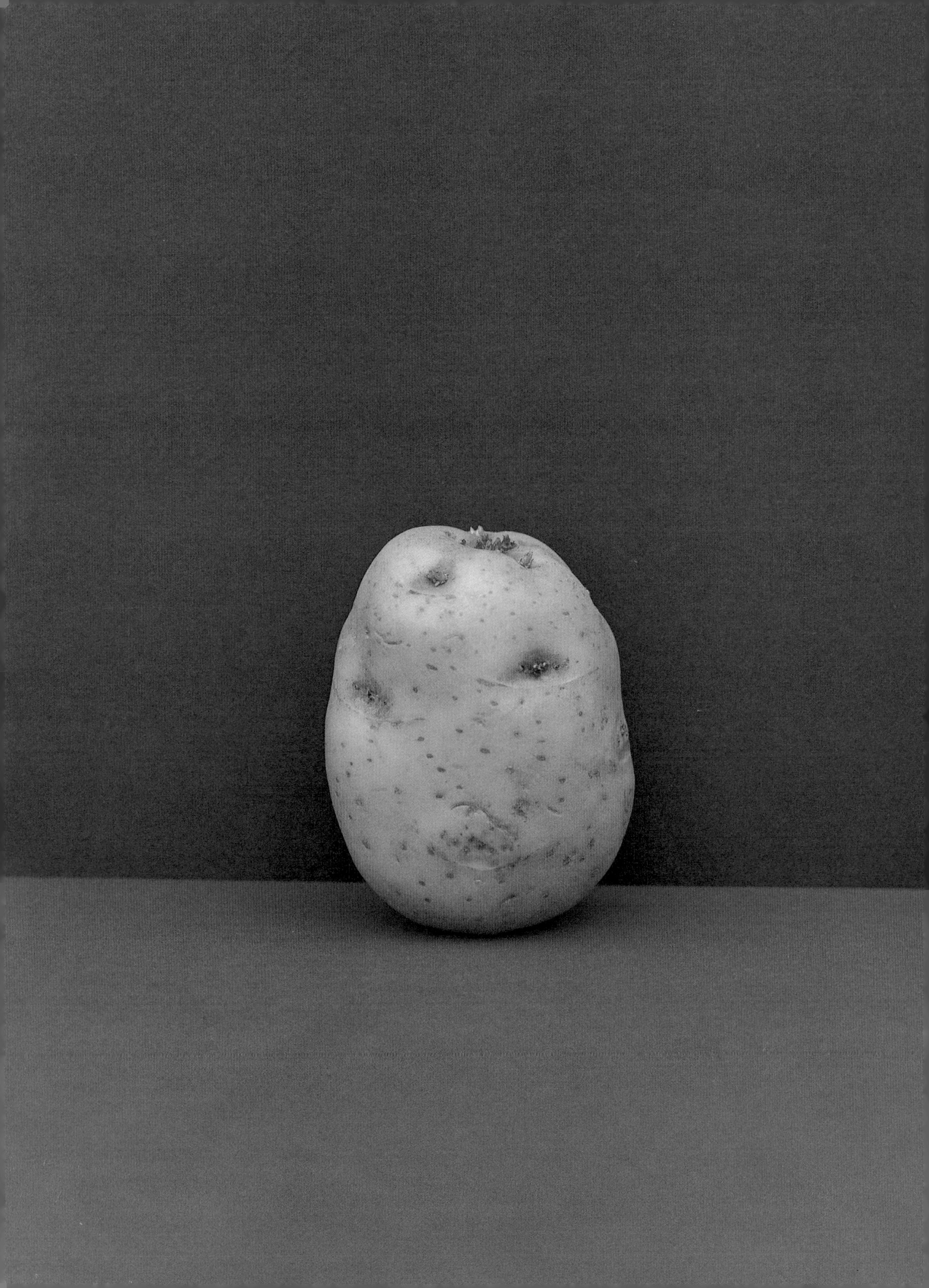

FRITTATA

A frittata is the Italian version of Spanish omelette, a fat disc of just-cooked egg, with additions, though not too many of them. I have a blini pan (see page 506) which makes a one-egg frittata that's perfect for one child (or indeed, one adult). To make a courgette frittata (it would be more linguistically felicitous to call it a zucchini frittata), heat the grill before you start. On the hob, melt a tiny knob of butter in the blini pan, sauté ½ small courgette cut into small dice for 1 minute or so, then pour in an egg beaten with 1 scant tablespoon grated parmesan and a grinding of pepper. Cook for a few minutes until bottom is set, and then place under the grill till cooked. Turn out onto a plate. Peas are also a regular filling, as are chopped, leftover, cooked potatoes. Any tiny, otherwise unusable, leftover piece of smoked salmon can be usefully dispatched here.

COD AND PEAS

You don't need, obviously, to do this as an amalgam: you can simply grill, roast or fry the cod and serve peas alongside. This recipe, though, requires nothing more complicated than standing shaking a frying pan for a few minutes. Put some butter and a drop of oil in a pan and fry in it 2 peeled cloves of garlic until they're golden brown. Then chuck them away: you want just a suggestive whiff. Then add some frozen peas, petits pois if possible, and if you've had time to thaw them earlier, so much the quicker. Turn the peas in the garlicky butter, add 1 tablespoon or so of vermouth or white wine (or water with a squeeze of lemon juice in it if you prefer; any alcohol will, however, burn off) and when they're soft, taste for seasoning, then add some cod fillet cut into bite-sized pieces. You can dredge the cod in a little seasoned cornflour first if you prefer, but just as often I leave it as it is. Turn in the pan with the peas and after 2 minutes it should be cooked through. This makes a good sauce, more of a topping really, for pasta, too. You can use trout in place of cod, wonderful and pink against the vivid Bemelmans green of the peas. This is a good way of trying out various species of fish to see how they go down. Be wary of bones. Safer to stick with fillets, and still look closely to see no bones linger.

CHICKEN STRIPS

YOGHURT AND HONEY

This is easy: get some skinned, boned chicken breast and cut into strips. Then marinate it in natural yoghurt made liquid with milk (or you could use buttermilk) and 1 tablespoon honey or soft brown sugar stirred in; 1 teaspoon soy can be added, too, if you want. 1 hour's steeping will do, but you can prepare the marinade at breakfast-time for lunch or even the night before if it helps.

Take the chicken out of the marinade and wipe dry with kitchen towel. Fry quickly in olive oil, or butter with a drop of oil, in a hot frying pan. Carrot batons, broccoli or green or runner beans – whatever you want, but it should have crunch – go well. It's worth bothering with marinade as children seem to find a lot of meat too fibrous and difficult to swallow if it hasn't been tenderised. And you can vary the marinade as you wish: adding or substituting oil, lemon juice, peanut butter, maple syrup and so on (see the drumsticks recipe on page 490, too). It's useful to keep yoghurt or buttermilk, since both make even the driest meats sweetly tender (and see page 349).

PEANUT BUTTER LEMON

RATHER MORE ORGANISED COOKING FOR YOUNG CHILDREN

If the above recipe suggestions delineate the upper limits of the amount of cooking you feel comfortable doing for your children, then stop here. Of course, I see that faffing about making pastry for children who are just as happy eating baked beans on toast might seem just one effort too far. But to that I'd say three things. First, children really do seem to like food such as pies and meatballs. Second, part of learning about food is being around its preparation, and often helping with it (and more on that later). And, third, perhaps most importantly, everything that follows is real food, the sort of food you will want to eat with your children, and to invite other adults to eat, too.

Of course, children can eat from any of the other recipes throughout the book, but these lay the foundations and delineate the best – neither fussy nor bland – sort of family food.

MACARONI CHEESE

You may wonder why I include, indeed start off with, a totally un-Italian pasta recipe, now that we are wholly won round to the authentic Mediterranean way of doing things. I suppose it is nostalgia that makes me feel the need to preserve this wholly English old-fashioned nursery staple; I worry sometimes that food like this will disappear. And it does have a certain period authenticity – if no other sort.

If you're to make it properly, observe the proprieties. Use macaroni – those little elbow shapes – rather than penne, and don't substitute any cheese for cheddar. What we are not trying to create here is some baked pasta with taleggio, however delicious it may be. A bit of grated parmesan, mixed in with the breadcrumbs to be sprinkled on top before going under the grill, could, however, be accommodated.

75g macaroni
15g butter
1 tablespoon flour, preferably Italian 00
pinch English mustard powder or cayenne pepper
200ml full-fat milk
75g cheddar, grated
1 tablespoon breadcrumbs

Since the macaroni will take about 18 minutes to cook (the quick-cook stuff is revolting), first put on a pan of water to boil. Then turn on the grill to let it get good and hot for the browning later. Butter a gratin dish or couple of little (150ml capacity) casseroles. When the water boils, salt it and throw in the macaroni.

Meanwhile, put the butter in a saucepan on medium heat and when it's melted stir in the flour and cook, stirring, for a few minutes. Italian 00 flour is good because it cooks, losing its flouriness, faster than plain flour; the French *farine fluide* is good on this score, too. (I find both at my local supermarket.) If I've only got some corner-shop-horror of fake and tasteless cheddar, I add a pinch of mustard powder or cayenne. Off the heat, pour in the milk, beating constantly. Usually, I warm the milk in the microwave in a plastic measuring jug, but you can use cold milk. Cook the sauce at the stage it is now, without cheese, for about 5 minutes, stirring all the while, then, just before the macaroni's due to come out of the boiling water, take the sauce off the heat and stir in the cheese – keeping 1 tablespoon or so back – and keep stirring. Drain the macaroni thoroughly. Add to the cheese sauce. Taste for seasoning. Pour or spoon into the dish or dishes, then sprinkle with about 1 tablespoon each breadcrumbs and grated cheese, whether it be cheddar or parmesan. Brown under the grill, but remember to let it stand and cool for a bit before giving it to the children, especially if you've made them their own little individual ones. You can fill and freeze the pots and then just sprinkle them with cheese and breadcrumbs before reheating in a moderate oven.

HAM OR FOUR CHEESE SAUCE

You can add chopped ham to this, and I often do; just as often, for a quick lunch, I cook ordinary short pasta and buy four cheese sauce (stocked in tubs in supermarket chill cabinets) to which I add some chopped ham. Chopped cooked bacon is delicious in macaroni cheese, it's just that ham is easier. But if you are frying a little bacon first, then add 1 tablespoon or so minced onion, too, and stir in both together, and be sure, as you decant, to scrape out the pan well.

MINCED ONION

Sometimes I change direction, but not shape, and leave out the cheese, but add cooked, flaked cod or other white fish instead. And I might bung in some peas, too.

PEAS

Naturally, cheese sauce can be used to cover a cooked head of small cauliflower: in other words, that other nursery classic, cauliflower cheese. I have found, though, that the only way my children will eat cauliflower is coated in egg and breadcrumbs when cooked and cooled, and fried, preferably with garlic.

CAULIFLOWER CHEESE

101 WAYS WITH MINCE

COTTAGE PIE AND SHEPHERD'S PIE

Whenever people over a certain age talk about shepherd's pie they point out reprovingly that it should be made from meat which is already cooked. And, of course, they're right. It's just that we don't go in for large roasts and hunks of meat so much any more, so we don't tend to have the leftovers to mince. But do you know what? It's better with fresh, raw, minced meat. Still, the original, leftover-meat version is useful and good enough. And wonderful, without potato topping, as a sauce.

WITH COOKED MEAT

I do sometimes mince leftover lamb or beef if the bits that linger in the fridge are too well cooked to be eaten pleasurably cold, and, as I've said, I use it often in a pasta sauce. You can cook a sauce for a long time, with quite a bit of wine, and you don't have to worry about making something semi-solid out of all those strands of dry, dry meat. Relatively small amounts of leftovers make enough for a few children.

First off, let me say none of the quantities is sensitive; use what you have. Remember to give the meat a good strong basis of flavour (with onions or shallots and garlic, plus carrot for sweetness, and herbs such as finely chopped rosemary, marjoram or thyme), and to cook it in such a way – on a low heat and with liquid – that it mellows rather than drying out even more. I throw in some semolina before adding liquid: this is to give sweetness, which children love, and texture, and to help thicken the sauce, to blend the dryish fibres of meat with the liquid it's cooking in. A bit of chopped liver would do much the same trick, as would fresh breadcrumbs.

Use whichever fat goes best with the meat: I'd use olive oil for lamb, dripping for beef, duck fat for duck (which my children particularly love, though what should this be called – pond pie?) But oil or butter, or a combination of both, is always fine. Bacon fat, if you've got it, gives real depth; or you could always just add a rasher or two of streaky bacon to the bowl of the food processor as you chop the base-line seasoning of vegetables.

I often use banana shallots in place of onions, as I like the softer flavouring of shallots, but don't necessarily want the fiddliness of peeling two or three times over. (Banana shallots are slightly bigger and longer as the name suggests.)

What follows is not so much a recipe as a suggestion, a reminder not to throw away even small amounts of meat that might be languishing, post dinner party or weekend lunch, in the back of your untended fridge.

few sprigs parsley

1 banana shallot (approx. weight 70g) or small onion

1 fat clove garlic

½ stick celery

1 small to medium carrot

1–2 tablespoons fat

100–200g leftover cooked meat (weight of edible material only, i.e. off the bone and without cartilage, gristle or superfluous fat)

1 scant tablespoon semolina

200–300g tinned chopped tomatoes in tomato purée

75ml full-fat milk

1–2 tablespoons cream (optional)

1 tablespoon butter

Finely chop the parsley, shallot, garlic, celery and carrot: I simply put them all, coarsely sliced, in the bowl of the food processor and blitz them together. Put the fat in a medium-sized, thick-bottomed frying pan and, when it's hot, add the chopped vegetables, and cook on a gentle heat for a good 10–20 minutes until soft. Remember to check especially that the carrots are cooked: since the meat is already cooked it won't need that long in the pan and you don't want the carrots to be crunchy.

When the shallot mixture is soft and unctuously cooked, but not brown, add the meat, which you have either chopped very finely by hand, put through a mincer or given a quick turn in the food processor. If the shallot mixture looks as if it needs it, add another tablespoon of whatever fat you're using before putting the meat in. Stir the meat into the sweet, taste-bolstering vegetables and sprinkle over the semolina, making sure to stir that well in, too. Add the tomatoes, just 200g at first, adding more if you think the sauce needs more liquid later. Pour in the milk, too, stirring as you do so. Cook on a low heat for about 10 more minutes, or less if all the flavours, when you taste, are coming together smoothly. If you want a creamier sauce, add 2 tablespoons of cream or more milk. When the sauce is off the heat, season to taste, and stir in 1 tablespoon butter.

If you want the children to eat this as a pie under a layer of mashed potato, obviously you don't want it too liquid: if you can be bothered, cook 2 tablespoons red lentils until dissolved into pottage and then drained, and stir into the meat to add bulk and body; baked beans (without much of their sauce) will perform the same function.

For the mashed potato topping, I work on the principle that 250g potato, weighed before cooking, mashed with a good dollop of butter, is enough to cover a small, oval pie dish, measuring 13cm at its longest point, and of about 300ml capacity. This amount of leftover-meat sauce should fill 3 such dishes, or sauce about 240g, uncooked weight, of pasta. Each dish feeds 1–2 children; work on 40g of pasta per average child portion.

WITH UNCOOKED MEAT

I tend to make cottage pie (with beef) rather more often than shepherd's pie (with lamb); but then I buy my – organic – beef from a good butcher and get it freshly minced. I wouldn't want to buy any mince, of whatever meat, that had been lying under clingfilm and the lights in a supermarket. I like to know the source of meat and I instinctively shrink from getting meat from anyone except a butcher.

The quantities as specified make enough mince to fill about 2 small oval dishes or one larger one, measuring about 25cm at its longest point. If I'm cooking a batch of mince in advance, I freeze it without the potato in bags for quick defrosting. As often as not, the children eat it then with rice rather than in a pie with potatoes; and, if you want to use it to sauce pasta, add some milk on reheating.

600g floury (that's to say, maincrop, not new) potatoes
60g butter
1 medium onion
1 medium carrot
1 clove garlic
1/2 stick celery
2 tablespoons oil
100g button mushrooms (optional)
250g beef or lamb, minced
1 tablespoon flour
50ml Marsala or apple juice
200g tinned tomatoes
1 teaspoon soy sauce or Worcestershire sauce

I start with the potatoes: peel them, cut them into chunks and put them in a pan of cold, salted water. Bring to the boil and cook till soft enough to mash easily; this could take from 25 to 45 minutes depending on the size of the chunks. Drain them and put them back in the pan over the heat for 1 minute to dry off. Then mash: the easiest way is to push them through a potato ricer and then beat in the butter; remember you want a stiff mash to top the meat, not a near-liquid purée.

Put the peeled onion, carrot and garlic clove with the celery, all cut into rough chunks, into the food processor and blitz (or chop finely by hand). Heat the oil in a medium-sized frying pan with a sturdy bottom, and preferably a lid, and stir in the chopped vegetables. Cook for a good 10 minutes until soft, then add the mushrooms, sliced thinly, if wanted. You may want to add a knob of butter at this stage, too. After 2 minutes, add the meat, pushing and breaking it up with a wooden spoon or spatula. You want it to unclump and lose its pinkness. Sprinkle over the flour and stir well, then add the Marsala or apple juice (most houses with small children seem to have apple juice in the fridge), then the tomatoes and soy or Worcestershire sauce. Stir well, cover and let simmer for 20 minutes. Uncover, prod, taste and cook for about another 10, by which time the meat should be cooked and not too liquid. You can thicken using either of the methods suggested in the recipe for already-cooked mince above, but the chances are you'll need such strategies less.

Put into the dishes and top with potato. If you want the top crispy, dot with butter and put it under a hot grill – sprinkling on grated cheese first, perhaps – for a few minutes.

VEAL, LIVER AND BACON MINCE PIE

Although this recipe includes liver, I have yet to find a child (even one who would never own up to eating liver) who didn't like it. This quantity makes enough to fill 2 little oval pie-dishes 14cm at their longest point, and 6cm deep (this is the about the right size for an older child or adult; smaller children can share one and you can freeze the other, or, if you're wise, eat it yourself). If you are opposed to veal, then this pie is a double insult since it also contains calves' liver. Not all calves, thank God, are crated: I suggest you talk to your butcher about his veal; but if you have objections, please turn over a few pages.

You could mince the meats yourself – in a food processor if you wish, since you want a gentle mush. But I buy the meat from my butcher and ask him to mince veal escalope and liver together.

I have specified whipping cream because it's what I had in the fridge (left over, as it happens, from the Marsala muscovado custard on page 367). Double cream, or indeed single, would be fine, too.

I think you do need canned, or bottled, petits pois here: that grey-green, sugary softness, just on the verge of evoking the cooking at a dusty-carpeted residential hotel, is precisely what's required. Frozen petits pois wouldn't be catastrophic, just not quite of a piece. But just use what you have to hand.

3 medium-sized maincrop potatoes (about 350–400g total weight)
1 small carrot
1 clove garlic
1/2 onion
2 rashers streaky bacon
1/2 stick celery
45g butter (about 3 tablespoons)
75g veal escalope, minced
75g calves' liver, minced and mixed with veal (see above)
1 tablespoon flour
good pinch ground cinnamon
2 bay leaves
200g tinned tomatoes
4 heaped tablespoons (drained) canned petits pois
5 tablespoons whipping cream
2 tablespoons freshly grated parmesan
nutmeg

Peel the potatoes and cut into cookable chunks. Put into a pan of cold water, bring to the boil and when boiling add salt. The potatoes will probably need around 1/2 hour, so bear that in mind as you get on with everything else.

Peel the carrot, garlic and onion, cut them into vaguely smaller pieces and put them in the bowl of the food processor. Add the bacon, derinded, and the celery, also roughly chunked. Process until you have a finely minced mess: your *batutto* or *sofritto*.

Put 1 tablespoon butter into a pan and, when it's melted, add the chopped veg and cook on a gentle but not indolent heat until more than softened; you want the vegetables cooked and mushy: 10 minutes should do it, but just keep testing. By the time they are soft enough, you will probably find they've absorbed all the fat, so put another tablespoon of butter into the pan. Add the minced veal and liver and give a good stir. Add the flour and stir in well, then add the cinnamon, bay leaves, tomatoes and peas and give another good stir. Cook over a low heat for about 5 minutes until the meats have lost their rawness, stirring and prodding with your wooden spoon every now and again. Add 3 tablespoons of cream and cook gently for another 5 minutes or so. Remove from the heat while you mash the potatoes.

Drain the potatoes when you're sure they're cooked enough. And don't be impatient: mash made with even minimally undercooked potatoes can cause instant, but justifiable, depression. Mash them (I push the potatoes through my ricer) and return to a hot, dry saucepan. Stir well, adding 1 tablespoon butter, 2 tablespoons cream and some grated parmesan. Grate over, too, some nutmeg, and taste to see if you need salt and pepper. The potato shouldn't be too slurpy.

Divide the meat mixture between bowls and cover with potato. This doesn't make a thick layer of potato for the top, but I think it's better like this. It looks mean until you start eating, and then it tastes just right.

You could dot with butter, grate over some more parmesan and blitz under a grill, although since small children don't like furiously hot food I tend not to bother. But if you're freezing one, or just keeping it in the fridge to be reheated later, you might as well sprinkle with cheese and a few shavings or gobbets of butter just before putting it into a gas mark 5/190°C oven for about 20 minutes.

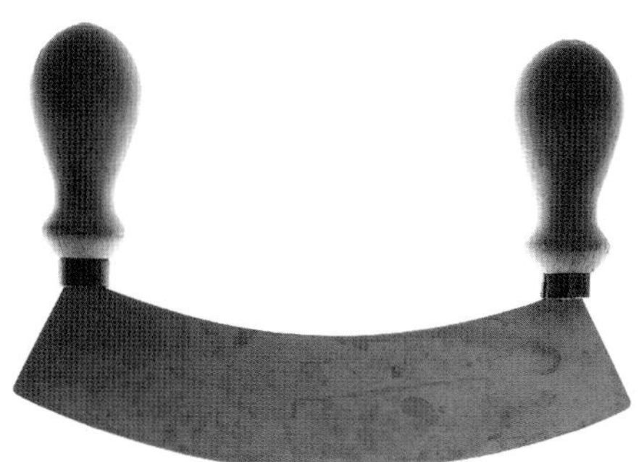

BEEF AND BEANS WITH PASTA

1 onion
1 clove garlic
1 carrot
½ stick celery
1–2 tablespoons olive oil
250g good minced beef
400g tin borlotti beans, drained
1 litre stock (see below)
1 400g tin tomatoes
2 tablespoons red wine (optional)
250g macaroni, for preference, or else gnocchetti sardi or ditalini
grated parmesan

This is all you do: put the onion, garlic, carrot and celery in the processor and turn on for a few seconds until you have a finely chopped orangey-jade mess. (If I'm chopping finely by hand I might, out of laziness or time-pressure, not bother with the carrot or celery.) Cook the vegetables in the oil in a medium-large saucepan for 5 minutes or so, until soft but not brown, and then add the beef, and turn it in the hot pan, pushing it and breaking it up with a wooden spoon, until browned. Add the drained tin, or ½ tin if you don't want too many of them, of borlotti beans. You'll need 1 litre of beef stock (stock made with a cube will do, though I keep tubs of Joubère stock in the freezer for just this sort of thing), a tin of chopped tomatoes in pulp and a slug of red wine if you've got a bottle opened somewhere. Don't put the liquid in all at once – add bit by bit, and stir. Bring to the boil, add the macaroni and cook, uncovered, for 18–20 minutes. Much of the liquid should have evaporated or been absorbed and what you'll have is a thick, busy stew of a soup. Taste for salt and pepper, grate some parmesan over, and let the eaters grate some more themselves.

If we're eating this with the children (and it comfortably makes enough bowfuls for the 4 of us) I pour over mine some fierce and glowingly orange chilli oil.

MEATBALLS IN TOMATO SAUCE

I think it's the smallness of it all, the walnut-sized balls of meat in sauce, that children like, but they also find the texture of ground meat more digestible than even the tiniest strips of unminced meat.

Since making meatballs is more fiddly than shepherd's pie (but only marginally: no potatoes to peel, remember) I tend to do a lot and then freeze them in little bags of 4 apiece. If I want to cut corners, I don't do all that chopping and gentle frying for the sauce, I just use tinned tomatoes and simmer them for a while with the chopped carrot, as below, but without the onion, and with the celery stick and garlic cloves left whole. I retrieve the bits along with the bay once the tomato and vegetables are cooked, and I give them only 10 minutes simmering before immersing the meatballs. And if you can't bear the idea of precooking the onion to go in the meatballs, just leave it out.

for the meatballs

1 onion
2 tablespoons oil
4 slices stale white bread (not plastic bread), crusts removed and broken into pieces
200ml milk
1kg minced beef
2 beaten eggs
4 tablespoons grated parmesan
1 heaped tablespoon chopped fresh parsley
flour

for the sauce

2 tablespoons olive oil
1 tablespoon butter
1 onion
2 cloves garlic
1 carrot
1 stick celery
2 tablespoons red wine or apple juice
3 400g tins best quality tomatoes or 2 700g bottles passata
3 bay leaves
200ml milk

Chop 1 onion very finely and cook it, sprinkled with salt, for about 10 minutes in 1 tablespoon of oil. When it's cooked, remove to a plate and put on one side. In the meantime, cover the stale bread with the milk in a dish and leave for about 10 minutes or until soft.

This is for the meatballs; now get on with the sauce. In a large pan or dish that will go on a hob (I use a rectangular cast-iron affair that goes across 2 hobs), put in the oil and butter with the onion, garlic, carrot and celery that you've blitzed in the processor.

Cook the onion mixture until a soft, sweet stew and then add wine or apple juice and 2½ tins of the tomatoes. Push the tomatoes around until they break up. You must use the best here, preferably those with a thick tomato sauce or juice. Then add the bay leaves. Season with salt and pepper. Cook for about 20 minutes, add the milk, then cook for a further 10 minutes, by which time everything should be thick and sweetly tomatoey.

Back to the meatballs. Put the minced beef into a large bowl. Add the bread which you have first drained of milk by squeezing in your hands. Then add the beaten eggs, the parmesan, the cooked onion, the parsley and some salt and pepper. Mix well, but gently, with your hands, or get the children to do so.

Spread a large surface with flour and have 2 large plates ready. Using your hands, form the meat mixture into small balls, about the size of a walnut. Then turn each ball in the flour and place on the plates. I make about 46 meatballs with this amount.

Heat 1 tablespoon or so oil in a non-stick frying pan (you will probably have to add more oil as you go) and brown the meatballs in it. I fit in about 11 a time and as each batch cooks put the meatballs into the pan with the sauce in. When you've done them all, throw the remaining ½ tin tomatoes into the pan in which you've been browning the meatballs and then put the contents on top of the meatballs and sauce. Cook in the sauce for about 20–30 minutes. You can test the odd one to see whether they're cooked through. Because my big, low cast-iron pot has a lid, I cook them covered. But it doesn't really matter. Remove the bay leaves if you feel like it.

We always eat these with rice.

DUCK MEATBALLS

I make meatballs out of anything, usually halving or quartering the basic recipe above. When I make duck meatballs, I use duck breasts, and just one will do. Since they're often sold in packs of two, I sometimes grill one for myself for supper and use what remains for the children. I strip the fat off and render it down to fry the onion and meatballs in. I chop the meat roughly and put it in the processor to mince, then mix it by hand with some very finely chopped orange zest, a good pinch of cinnamon, an egg and a slice of bread, as above, but soaked here in yoghurt made runny with milk (or buttermilk: either makes the fat-stripped meat more tender when it's thus ground). I often use a bottled tomato sauce mixed with some tinned tomatoes, to which I've added a good pinch of cinnamon (or I cook it with a short cinnamon stick which I remove later), another good pinch of ground ginger and, if I've got some in the larder, some gorgeous red-golden saffron.

HAM AND TURKEY

And after Christmas one year, I made some meatballs that were too moussey for adults, but which the children (and their friends) were very keen on, out of leftover ham and turkey chopped in the processor and bound with some sausage meat; that's to say, the meat taken out of some good butcher's sausages rather than that lurid pink paste you see in one vast plastic-wrapped cosh.

SPECIAL MEATBALLS

But my favourite variant is one that brings meatballs closer to Judaeo-Italianified faggots. I use 450g minced veal, 450g minced beef, 2 eggs and 1 onion as above and add some marjoram to the parsley. I use slightly less bread – 3 slices – and add 60g chicken livers, pulped in the processor. Continue as before. These are fabulous: light in texture, smokily delicate in flavour, and what I cook when I've got masses of children and their parents coming for lunch. The sauce is good if you throw in some marjoram with the onions, and use Marsala, generously, in place of wine. And sometimes I process one of the tins of tomatoes with another 60g chicken livers. In my notebook, these go by the name of Special Meatballs, and rightly so.

CLOVE-HOT CHILLI CON CARNE

In my experience, children like much stronger tastes than adults assume. When I make a chilli con carne for them – well, I'm a child of the seventies, what do you expect? – I use spices – cloves in particular – to infuse it with heat rather than chilli. I love it, too.

If you don't want to soak and cook dried beans, by all means use tinned ones and add them 15 minutes before the end. I often soak pulses at night and cook them at breakfast time, letting them cool in their cooking liquid for the rest of the morning.

And if you don't want to use porcini, use any old mushrooms or none at all. But what I *do* recommend, in that case, is that you track down some Italian-imported porcini-flavoured stock cubes.

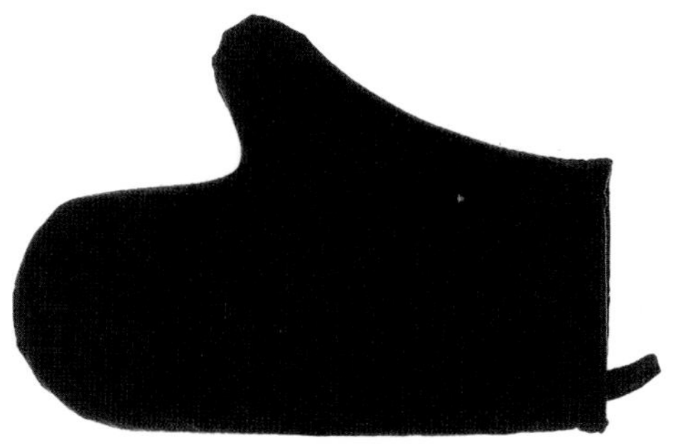

for the beans

125g borlotti beans, soaked, then next day cooked for 1 hour with:

3 cloves garlic, minced

1 stick celery

3 dried porcini

1 peeled onion, stuck with 2 cloves

1 tablespoon olive oil

for the rest

15g dried porcini

2 medium carrots

2 onions

3 cloves garlic

1 stick celery

2 tablespoons beef dripping or olive oil

1 dried peperoncino (hot, red, chilli pepper)

450g minced beef

1/2 teaspoon cinnamon

1/2 teaspoon cloves

400g tin tomatoes

2 tablespoons bottled barbecue sauce

2 tablespoons dark brown sugar

Cover the porcini with hot water. Put carrots, onions, garlic and celery in processor and chop very finely. Melt the dripping or oil in a suitable pan, cook the vegetable mixture in it, with the addition of the hot, red, dried pepper, whole, for about 10 minutes until soft. Remove the pepper: my daughter, when she was barely 3, liked it hotter by having the chilli pepper minced with the veg in the processor – but go cautiously. Add the meat and the spices and turn and push about in the pan before pouring in the tinned tomatoes and the barbecue sauce. Add the porcini. Strain and add their soaking water, pouring slowly so the gravelly, grainy bits don't gush in too. Stir in the brown sugar and the drained beans and cook for 1 hour at least.

MORE IDEAS FOR HIGH TEA

DUCK LIVER SAUCE

I suppose it's because it was dinned into me when I was a child, but I can't help thinking it incontrovertibly a Good Thing when children eat liver. Duck livers are sweeter and moussier than chicken livers, and so more child-friendly. Sometimes, when I buy a couple of ducks to roast, I use the livers either with leftover meat (in the unlikely event there is any) or some specially bought breast, diced small, to make a chunkier, meatier pasta sauce than the one that follows. For this you'd need to buy duck livers especially, I should think.

½ onion
1 medium carrot
30g lardons, pancetta or streaky bacon
2 cloves garlic
oil for frying
300g duck livers
60 ml muscat or Marsala or apple juice
1 tablespoon hoisin sauce
2 tablespoons tomato passata
½ 400g tin tomatoes

Put onion, carrot, pancetta and garlic in a processor and blitz or chop finely by hand. Heat the oil in a deep frying pan and add the chopped mix, cooking on a medium to low heat until softened, about 10 minutes or so. Add the duck livers and cook, turning often, until browned but still pink inside. Add the muscat (I had some – dark and Australian – left over in the fridge, but Marsala would do fine, and, if you don't like putting alcohol in children's food, substitute apple juice). Add the hoisin sauce, some ordinary bottled kind, and tomato passata. Cook for another minute or so and then put in a food processor and give a couple of turns, so that it is chopped, but not mushy. Put back in the pan, add the tomatoes and when warmed through taste for seasoning.

PASTA SAUCE WITH SAUSAGE

Since children seem to love sausages you should try making a pasta sauce with them (see page 482). The sausages you need for this are unbreaded Italian ones. Ask for sweet Italian sausages (to distinguish from the fiery, chilli-hot ones). I use 8 sausages in place of 450–500g minced beef, in other words substitute weight for weight. Remove the casings, and prod and push about the pan much as you do the mince, only more emphatically, to break the meat up satisfactorily. A tablespoon or so of cream or full-fat milk towards the end binds the flavours and textures of the sauce smoothly and harmoniously together.

CHICKEN PATTIES

These pale and miniature burgers take little time, require little effort and are always, at my house at least, rapturously received. To simplify matters even further, you could always substitute about 300g already-minced turkey (relatively easy to come by these days) in place of the chicken thighs; in which case use hands rather than machinery to combine everything together. If you want, you can make, cook, cool and then freeze them to be reheated quickly whenever you need a fail-safe child-friendly tea at short notice. If you're nervous about any child's reproachful sensitivity about green bits (although I've never had any complaints, even from vegetable-phobic children), then just leave out the parsley.

handful flat-leaf parsley leaves
3 tablespoons breadcrumbs
4 skinless, boned chicken thighs
2 best butcher's sausages
fresh nutmeg
oil for frying

Put the parsley into the food processor and give a good blitz. If your breadcrumbs (and see page 24 for directions as to how to make them) are on the dry side, put them in with the parsley; if they're soft, wait. Add the chicken thighs, each cut into rough chunks, and process until very finely chopped. Then squeeze the sausage meat out of their casings into the food processor, along with the breadcrumbs if not already added, and a good grating of fresh nutmeg. Process to combine and then, after dampening your hands, form into small rounds, about the size of a large walnut, and squish slightly to make small but bulging discs; you should get about 15 out of this amount.

Preheat oven to gas mark 6/200°C. Heat up some oil – a tablespoon or two – in a heavy-based frying pan. Fry the patties for a couple of minutes on either side just to brown them and then transfer them to a tin that will go in the oven. Cook for about 30 minutes.

CHICKEN PIE

When I first made this chicken pie – with some leftover meat, light and dark, from chicken roasted earlier in the week – I was going to top it with mashed potatoes, but then it occurred to me that it would be less effort and take less time just to make a little disc of pastry.

The white sauce which coats the chicken is as explained in Basics Etc. (page 21). Just a reminder: make sure the stock cube's a good one; I use Italian Knorr ones.

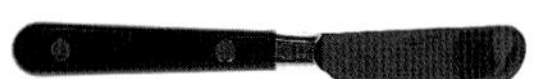

1 tablespoon butter
½ chicken stock cube
1 tablespoon flour
300ml full-fat milk
125g peas or sweetcorn or a mixture of both
200g cooked cold chicken, shredded or chunked

for the pastry
80g flour, preferably Italian 00
40g butter or butter and shortening mixed, cold and diced
1 egg yolk, beaten with a teaspoon of water and a pinch of salt

Make the pastry as directed on page 42 and put it in the fridge.

Melt the butter and ½ stock cube in a saucepan, prodding the stock cube to help it break up and dissolve. Stir in the flour and cook the manilla-coloured paste for a minute or so, stirring with your wooden spoon. Off the heat, gradually pour in the milk, stirring if not actually beating, all the while. When all is smoothly incorporated return to heat, and cook for about 10 minutes.

Meanwhile cook the peas and/or sweetcorn and when the sauce is cooked add the vegetables and the chicken, taste for seasoning – you may want a scant grating of fresh nutmeg – and then turn into a buttered dish or dishes. I make this generally in one pie, in an oval stoneware dish with an 800ml capacity.

If you're going to cook right away, just proceed, first preheating the oven to gas mark 5/190°C. But if, like me, you find it more convenient to get the pie ready in advance and warm it through when you need it, then let the filling cool before covering it with pastry. So, whenever, roll out the pastry, dampen the edges of the dish and fit on the pastry lid, cutting off excess and prinking round the edges as you like. Cut a few slashes to let steam escape. The pastry will sit somewhat on the filling. It makes the underside – but only the underside – just a big soggy. This, for me, is the best bit.

Brush with milk and cook for 25–45 minutes, depending on, among other things, whether the filling's cold or not. You can always cover loosely with a bit of foil or greaseproof after 30 minutes if the pastry looks brown enough.

A pie this size would feed 4–6 children but my children and I can polish it off in one go. Last time both of them had third helpings. I think it's the savoury saltiness of the white sauce that they especially love.

MARINATED CHICKEN DRUMSTICKS

When other children are coming for tea, I sometimes marinate chicken drumsticks. It would be foolish to be too rigid about the marinade. I might mix 1 teaspoon wholegrain mustard, 1 tablespoon honey, 2 crushed cloves of garlic and some minced onion in a glass of white wine or apple juice made slightly more acerbic with a squirt of lemon juice. You could use the marinade for the char siu (page 443 – and indeed, do the char siu itself). And I once made a marinade which, although it made me wince as I did it, consisted of creamed coconut dissolved in pineapple juice, a dollop of peanut butter, 1 teaspoon soy and some brown sugar. The children loved it. If I want to do just 4 drumsticks in a hurry, that's to say for the next day's lunch, and with stuff I've got routinely in the fridge or cupboard, the marinade is as follows: 100ml apple juice, 100ml natural yoghurt, 1 tablespoon honey, the same of soy sauce and 1 clove garlic, minced. But, normally, I tend to leave the drumsticks marinating in the fridge for some time, 24 hours say.

Arrange the drumsticks on a rack over a roasting tin and cook at gas mark 6/200°C for 35–40 minutes and then at gas mark 3/160°C for about another 20–25 minutes. Easily made, easily eaten.

You can freeze a few drumsticks at a time in their marinade (I use freezer bags rather than structured containers) and later remove them portion by portion.

MUSHROOM RISOTTO

Really, risotto does not entail terrific drudgery: I don't know why people think it does. It means you've got to stand by the stove stirring for about 20 minutes, but I find it rather calming. You can pull up a chair and get one of your children to take over. That's how they'll learn to cook; it's certainly how I did. (Remember, though, to watch them carefully, in case of accidents, but try not to nag.)

And, also, because you won't be worrying as much about how the risotto will turn out, whether it will be too claggy or too mushy or whatever, no doubt it'll be perfect.

I use dried mushrooms from the store cupboard to save shopping, but you can add, or substitute, fresh ones. As for the stock: I like to use Italian Knorr porcini-flavour stock cubes, supplemented with strained mushroom soaking water.

30g butter
1 tablespoon olive oil
1/2 onion or 1 banana shallot, chopped very finely
15g dried porcini, soaked for 20 minutes in warm-to-hot water (and/or 100g fresh mushrooms, sliced thinly)
175g arborio or other suitable Italian risotto rice
60ml white wine or vermouth or Marsala, optional
750ml hot stock, including porcini-soaking liquid
2–3 tablespoons grated parmesan
flat-leaf parsley, chopped

In a heavy-bottomed, wide saucepan put 1/2 the butter and all the oil, then cook the onion for a few minutes. Add the well-drained and chopped, soaked porcini, and stir on the heat for another minute. Stir in the rice and toss and turn well in the pan, so that every grain is covered and gleaming with the cooking fats. Throw in the alcohol if you're using it – and if you're not, this is not the place to substitute apple juice – and let it bubble away until some is evaporated, the rest absorbed.

Stir in a ladleful of hot stock (I keep it in a pan on the lowest simmer possible on a neighbouring hob) and keep stirring until the liquid's absorbed. Carry on in this vein for about 20 minutes. If I'm using fresh mushrooms, I tend to add them, sautéed with a little butter, at this stage. You may not need all the stock, you may need to add hot water at the end: bear that in mind.

When the rice is cooked, take it off the heat and beat in the remaining butter and the grated parmesan. When I make risotto for grown-ups, I sprinkle over some parsley myself, but for children I put parsley on a saucer near them on the table and let them do it. It seems to make them like it. And put more parmesan and the grater there as well.

SALMON FISHCAKES

You can make variations of this recipe, either substituting tinned tuna or crabmeat or adding peas or sweetcorn or chopped spring onion, but it stands as a useful blueprint. I find it easier to make the fishcakes in advance, store them in the freezer and then cook from frozen. Bought matzo meal is better than bought breadcrumbs.

150g drained tinned salmon
150g cold mashed potato; that's to say about 1 baking potato cooked, mashed and cooled
1 tablespoon grated parmesan
good pinch paprika
chopped zest of 1/4 lemon, optional
1 egg, beaten with 1 teaspoon milk
3 tablespoons flour
3 tablespoons dried breadcrumbs or matzo meal
oil for frying

In a bowl, mix the salmon, potato, parmesan, paprika, lemon zest if you're using, and half the beaten egg. Using your hands, form the mixture into balls, about the size of walnuts, and then flatten them slightly into fat little discs. Dredge them in flour, then dip them in the remaining egg and then in the breadcrumbs or matzo meal and let rest for 15 minutes in the fridge on a plate or tray lined with clingfilm. Heat the oil in a frying pan and fry for a minute or so each side until golden. Remove to waiting, oil-absorbent sheets of kitchen towels.

If you're making the fishcakes in advance and then freezing them, this is how you work it. Line a couple of small baking sheets with clingfilm and arrange the pre-dredged fishcakes on them. Cover with another sheet of clingfilm and put in the freezer for at least 1 hour. You want them hard. If you want to keep them in the freezer for a long time, just bag them up once they're set and completely hard.

When you want to cook them, preheat the oven to gas mark 1/2/120°C and line 2 baking trays with a double thickness of kitchen towel. Pour some vegetable oil into a frying pan and heat.

Take the fishcakes out of the freezer, release them from their plastic wrapping and dredge them first in more flour, dip them in the egg mixture and cover them in the matzo meal or breadcrumbs. Fry them for 2 minutes on each side or until golden and then put on the kitchen-towel-lined trays and into the oven. After 20–30 minutes the fishcakes will be warmed through and ready to eat, but you can leave them there for 2 hours or so without worrying.

You can fry them from frozen like this without worrying; because they're so little they'll reheat in the middle before the surfaces burn. And I sometimes dredge them in flour before freezing and fry like that, no egg, no matzo meal. The benefit of frying then oven-cooking is that you can do it in advance (which often is the only way one can cook for children).

GREENCAKES

We also make something we call greencakes, which are like fishcakes only the part of the fish is played by a variety of vegetables, chiefly broccoli and peas (though including non-green vegetables such as carrots). Cook and mash the vegetables roughly, before making them into little balls and proceeding as above.

SOUP

Children tend to like home-made soup, which has an advantage, beyond the obvious one, over canned or cartoned as it can be thicker and is therefore easier for them to spoon from bowl to mouth. When I'm feeling laid-back about mess and spillage, I make pea soup (see page 180), which can be cooked impromptu. A good bean and pasta soup has to be planned ahead, but it doesn't take great military organisation to put beans in to soak before you go to bed and to boil them for 45 minutes the next morning before you go to work.

BEAN AND PASTA SOUP

In the evening, fry up the usual onion–carrot–celery mixture, with some chopped bacon or pancetta if wished, add the drained beans, some stock, a tin of tomatoes and a potato, peeled and diced finely. Cook for about 45 minutes. Add some ditalini or other soup pasta for the last 12 minutes. Sprinkle with parmesan and eat.

Since all children seem to like both pasta and pulses, cook this when other children are coming over. You can do it all in advance bar the pasta, so it can be on the table in 20 minutes.

PUDDINGS

You may have noticed there are no recipes for puddings. It's because we don't go in for them. There's always fruit, though, and some ice-cream. And, of course, I seem to spend my life stocking up with multi-packs of fromage frais and boxes of Mini-Milks.

AN EXCEPTION: CHILDREN'S CHOCOLATE MOUSSE

I do sometimes make puddings when friends and their children come round for lunch and what I'm providing for the adults is too bitter, too rich, too alcoholic or otherwise unappealing for the children or I just want to make something that will bludgeon them sweetly into sugar-absorbed silence. And actually, I like this so much more than those dark, coffee-sharp, elegant adult versions: so, I find, does just about everyone else; you may want to make up double quantities.

100g Valhrona lacte (or other really good chocolate with 40 per cent cocoa solids)
1 ½ tablespoons water
1 tablespoon golden syrup
2 eggs, separated

In a bowl suspended over a pan of hot water on moderate heat, put the chocolate, broken into pieces, along with the water and golden syrup. When you have a smooth, melted brown puddle in the bottom of the bowl, remove from the heat. Whisk the egg whites until you have a stiff snow; it'll make it easier if you wipe round the bowl with the cut surface of a halved lemon before you start. Leave them for the moment, and beat the egg yolks, one by one, into the still warm chocolate mixture. Then take a dollop of egg whites and briskly, brutally even, stir them into the egg-yolky chocolate. This just makes it easier to fold in the remaining egg whites, which you should now do firmly but gently with a metal spoon.

Decant into a bowl and leave in the fridge for a good 6 hours before eating. I generally make this the previous day, or at least the night before. This makes enough for 4 small children, but I can't promise they won't want to eat more.

Generally, I always bear in mind Penelope Leach's advice never to use sweets as reward or solace. Chocolate is food and must be treated as such, normalised, given as part of lunch or tea. You don't want to make the main course at lunch seem like a vile duty that the child has got to wade through; nor do you want to signal that sweet food is the only comforting, treat-like food, the balm for life's ills, unless you actually want to make your child unbalanced around food later. All eating should be a natural pleasure, not just pudding-eating. Still, this is easier said than done, and my method of child-rearing often seems to be one long pattern of bribe–threat–bribe–threat.

I believe in asking children what they want to eat and in not making them sit at the table for hours, if that's what it takes, until they clear their plates. Children have likes and dislikes just as grown-ups do, and there is no reason why they shouldn't be respected. And yet, and yet. It's useful to learn to eat everything, especially when away from home; it doesn't help children to turn them into picky little brats. You've got to find a middle path. If you teach your children that if they make a fuss they will be indulged, they will just make more of a fuss more of the time. You have to put up with an amount of screaming, and to remember that if a child goes without food for one meal, even two, he or she won't starve.

So, even though you should not tell children that if they eat up those horrible vegetables they will be allowed some lovely pudding, nor should you give them any pudding if they won't eat any of their main course. (All this, of course, is so much easier said than done.) I wouldn't want to make a child clear his or her plate for the sake of it, but I'm always enchanted when it's done voluntarily. Remember that a power struggle about food is one that your child will always win; and that turning the lunch table into a battleground is asking for grief. When I was young, I was so often made, to the point of torture, to eat up every cold, congealing thing on my plate, that I now can't help but finish up everything in sight, on my plate or other people's. This might be a polite party trick, but it doesn't make for a serene life or stable weight.

COOKING WITH CHILDREN

The more that children are encouraged to help with the cooking, the less likely they are to become picky eaters. I don't say there's a magic formula to ensure they're never faddy or fussy or hampered by bizarre prejudice, but you will improve your chances of having children who enjoy food if they are part of the enjoyable process of making it. Most children like eating what they cook and are proud of doing it.

My own early memories are of wobbling on a wooden chair pushed up against the New World cooker, stirring my mother's white sauce. I often cook one-handed, with my daughter on a chair stirring or inspecting, and my still-just-baby son on my left hip, licking a wooden spoon or doing a bit of stirring with it himself. My daughter, aged three, would come into the kitchen and say, 'Lovely! Garlic!' when she smelt the cooking, or detected by the smell that a chicken had been put in the oven, or some pea-pods were being simmered into a stock on the hob. That's not genius, but a feeling for and interest in food: much more important.

Doing ordinary, everyday, real cooking with children is more to the point than making any amount of chocolate Rice Krispie cakes. If you want to cook with your children, let them help cook lunch. There's something so companionable about actually cooking with your child, rather than just letting it play with food as a toy. But of course there are times when it's nice to cook something specially, not for lunch or because you're cooking it anyway. Try to let your children do as much as possible. The results don't have to be perfect: the point of the exercise is the process.

CHEESE STARS

If you haven't got a star-cutter, do not even begin to worry. You could just as easily use a floured glass to cut out small rounds. But I find anything made out of stars beautiful, and my children do, too; I like as well the evocation of the cheese straws of my childhood, which these, in effect, are anyway.

50g self-raising flour
pinch cayenne
25g softened butter
80g finely grated red leicester
20g freshly grated parmesan, about 4 tablespoons

Preheat the oven to gas mark 6/200°C. Mix all the ingredients together in a bowl. Just using hands is most fun for children, but a food processor (let them ceremoniously press the on-button) is fine if you prefer it. You shouldn't need any liquid to bind this. When it first comes together (at least in the processor) it looks crumbly, but after a few kneads it comes together smoothly. What I tend to do is divide the finished orange-glowing dough in two, then keep one in the fridge wrapped in clingfilm, while I roll out the other. I do this partly because I've only got enough tins to bake half the dough at a time. But from the dough's point of view, it is fine without leaving it to rest in fridge. Dust a surface with flour, roll out neither very thick nor very thin – about 2½mm if you were to measure, I suspect – then put on non-stick or greased or lined trays in the preheated oven for about 10 minutes. Look after 8. The biscuits continue to crisp up while they're cooling on a rack.

If you use a 4cm star cutter and roll out to the bitter end – clumping together, reflouring, rerolling till more or less every last cheesy scrap is used up – you should get about 25 stars out of this.

DIGESTIVE BISCUITS

Since you will be required to eat whatever's cooked, you may as well try to make sure it's something you like. Although it might seem crazy to make digestive biscuits at home, I rather like them – a case of life imitating artifice. I'm not a great biscuit buyer, simply because I'm not a great biscuit eater, but when I get the urge for one of these sandy, oaty, wheaten biscuits, I brightly, in the manner of a dangly-earringed children's television presenter, suggest we make them.

Dove's Farm spelt flour is available in health stores and my local supermarket. The oatmeal, likewise, is easy to come by in health stores. Please: don't give in to the temptation to use all butter in place of the shortening and butter specified. The biscuits don't work without the shortening; they don't taste like digestives.

175g spelt flour
1 teaspoon each salt and baking powder
45g medium oatmeal
30g demerara sugar
45g shortening, lard or white vegetable fat such as Cookeen, cold and cut in approx. 1cm dice
45g unsalted butter, cold and cut in 1cm dice
milk to mix, approx. 80ml

Preheat the oven to gas mark 6/200°C.

Put the flour, salt, baking powder, oatmeal and sugar in a bowl and, using your hands, mix well. Add the diced cold vegetable shortening and rub in, using your fingertips or a convenient machine; I use a free-standing mixer here. When the shortening is about half rubbed in, add the butter. When all is rubbed in, and you have a floury, breadcrumby texture, add cold milk slowly and cautiously, by the scant tablespoon, until the mixture begins to cohere into a firm dough.

Flour a cold surface – and I use plain flour, not spelt, here – and roll the dough out, but not too thinly (about 5mm). Make the biscuits using a 6cm plain round cutter – this makes about 23 of them – and place on a non-stick baking sheet (I prick the centre, in clumsy imitation of the McVitie's original, with the tines of a fork) and cook in the oven for about 10–15 minutes. When ready, the biscuits should be golden with faintly browning edges. Watch out because they can quickly overcook, turning dusty and slightly bitter.

Transfer to a couple of wire racks, and store in an airtight tin when you're done.

FAIRY CAKES

I haven't got a heart of stone: I do realise that children sometimes like making children's food. If we're going out to tea with friends who have children the same ages as ours, we sometimes make a batch of these in the morning to take with us. They go down well with the nostalgically-minded parents; the children just pick off or lick off the icing.

I use a processor, but if you want to make the fairy cakes by hand, cream the butter and sugar, then add the beaten eggs and flour in alternate tablespoons. Use milk to bind, as usual, and you won't need the extra baking powder.

125g self-raising flour
125g unsalted butter, very, very soft but not actually melting
125g caster sugar
2 eggs
1–2 teaspoons good vanilla extract (or use vanilla sugar in place of ordinary caster, see page 82)
1 teaspoon baking powder
few tablespoons milk

for the icing
12 natural-coloured glacé cherries
approx. 200g icing sugar or instant royal icing powder
food colouring, if wanted

Preheat oven to gas mark 6/200°C.

Line a 12-bun tray with paper cases. Put all the cake ingredients except the milk in the processor, adding a pinch of salt, and blitz furiously. Then pour in 2 tablespoons milk and process again till you have a smooth, flowing cake batter. Then, using a spoon and a rubber spatula, divide it into the paper cases. Cook for 15–20 minutes and cool on a wire rack.

When properly cool, make the icing. You can use ordinary glacé icing, that's to say just icing sugar and water mixed (follow instructions on the icing sugar packet), or you can make thicker, stiffer royal icing, whipped up from a packet with a bit of water – or do the real thing and mix icing sugar with egg white. Dye as you wish: we run through the full gamut of pink ranging from ballet pink through Calpol to all-out Barbie, depending on the intensity of our mood and heavy-handedness with the bottle of colouring.

When the icing is still wet, let your child place a cherry – the natural-coloured ones gleam like poetically opaque rubies – in the centre of each. You can make double the amount of mini fairy cakes if you prefer (and then, when topping them, remember to slice each cherry in half) but make sure you've bought a mini fairy-cake tin not a mini muffin tin; you need the sloping sides for the authentic look.

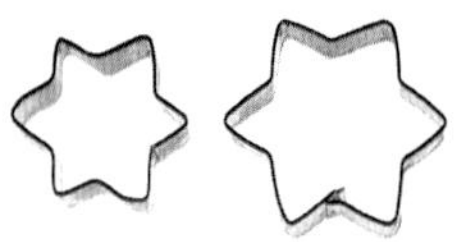

JAM TARTS

Another old-fashioned nursery delicacy, which in truth I can't remember ever having at home when I was a child, but am drawn to for the same sentimental reason my own children are: it evokes not the real but the super-real; the world of picture books and nursery rhymes. So you could say that we have a literary taste for them.

Since children like little things we make these in mini tartlet tins. (Though if you find any tiny heart-shaped tins, you will be able to create very girl-friendly pastries.) The pastry rolls out easily – the acid of the yoghurt or buttermilk makes it tenderly cohesive – so let them practise. And use cheap jam, the sort without one iota of fruit in it: it saves having to sieve it before spooning it into the pastry cases.

120g flour, preferably Italian 00
60g cold butter, cut into 1cm dice
5 tablespoons buttermilk, or 3 of yoghurt diluted with 2 of iced water
7 teaspoons strawberry jam
1 1/2 teaspoons water

Put the flour in a bowl with the butter and let stand in the deep-freeze for 10 minutes. Then, empty out bowl into processor and process until crumbly; add buttermilk or diluted yoghurt to which you've added a pinch of salt, and process again. If it's not beginning to form a dough, add some iced water teaspoon by teaspoon, with the machine running. When the dough is just beginning to come together, remove from processor, form into a fat disc and wrap in clingfilm and leave in the fridge for 20 minutes.

Preheat oven to gas mark 7/210°C.

Roll out the pastry and with a 6cm crinkly cutter stamp out 24 little circles. (Obviously, for full-sized tarts you will need a bigger cutter and will end up with fewer.) Press the pastry circles into place in the tartlet tins (if you've got only one such tin, divide the dough in two and make one batch up after another) and put back in the fridge while you heat the jam in a saucepan with the water until a syrup liquid. Put a spoonful of jam on the base of each tartlet case and bake in oven for about 15 minutes.

PERIWINKLES

This recipe, which we were shown by an American girl who stayed with us for a while and whose mom used to make these for her, is a way of using up pastry scraps.

You need cinnamon, brown sugar and honey. On each tidied-up, oblonged-off strip of pastry you – or your children – pour some honey then sprinkle over cinnamon and brown sugar and roll up, like a Swiss roll. With a sharp knife and a firm hand, cut across into slices about 5mm thick. Place them, lying down, so you can see the sweet cinnamon spirals, on a lined baking sheet and bake for about 15 minutes in a gas mark 6/200°C oven. You can cook your grown-up pie first, and then pop in the scraps when the oven's free, adjusting the heat accordingly.

PARTY FOOD

I am unhelpfully obsessive about children's parties: by that I mean I like to cook all the food myself. It gives me pleasure: it feels important. I say 'unhelpfully' because I am not as well organised as I am obsessed, so I am inevitably exhausted by the time I have to face 20 over-excited, screaming children.

I have now got wise to the general set-up, though, and there are some things you should know before you get started in this game. My comments concern themselves with small children.

1 They will be too excited to eat much. Concentrate on one or two star items – the cake, some special biscuits.

2 Your child will be more interested in the cake's icing than in the texture or taste of the sponge itself. Reserve your energies: make an all-in-one Victoria sponge, flavoured or coloured as required. And buy roll-out marzipan and roll-out icing.

3 Build a party repertoire for yourself. I now do the same biscuits party after party, but change their shape and their icing. I do the same sandwiches, provide the same sort of sausages and buy the same sort of crisps. The routine is reassuring to your children (just like the same old Christmas tree decorations coming out year after year) and helpful for you. Add to this repertoire – and see below – but keep it to provide a solid foundation.

4 Don't try to please other parents. The party is for your child.

5 Don't get agitated about the amount of sugar, food colour, salt, cream or butter. This is not the time.

Here are some ideas.

HALLOWE'EN PARTY

- Chocolate cake with green marzipan and orange icing. Put black-hatted witch on top.
- Biscuits (see page 503) shaped like pumpkins and decorated correspondingly; others to look like cobwebs.
- Jam tarts (by request: the jam to denote blood), recipe above (page 499).
- Monster's eyeballs: just use a melon-baller (for once! useful!) to scoop out a green- or yellow-fleshed melon.
- Cocktail sausages. You can't have too many. For 20 children and 12 or so adults, I make 200. You get about 65 to the kilo. Roast on trays in gas mark 4/180°C oven for 40–50 minutes.
- Sandwiches: pesto (for the green colour).
- Corn-crisps that look like bacon slices.
- Toffee apples.

A GIRL'S FOURTH BIRTHDAY PARTY

- Pink-coloured sponge cake, flavoured with strawberry flavouring, pink icing, with a Barbie sitting on the corner of the cake. (Beware: Fire Hazard.)
- Biscuits, see page 503, but stamped out with cutter in the shape of a 4, covered with bright pink glacé icing, with hundreds and thousands sprinkled over when wet.
- Hundreds of pink meringues (see Basics page 19 for recipe, adding pink food colouring in final whisk and squeezed through rosette nozzle to make flower shapes 3–4cm in diameter).
- Cocktail sausages: see above.
- Fairy cakes (see page 497).
- Marmite sandwiches (see page 505).
- Corn crisps that look like bacon slices.

A BOY'S SECOND BIRTHDAY PARTY

- Plain sponge cake, iced white, with animals clumsily made out of dyed, bought, fondant icing and marzipan, to form a circle around the edge. To tell the truth, I cannot ice, but I took the precaution of marrying someone who can.

- Biscuits, as above and recipe below, chocolate version, with grated zest of an orange added to biscuit mixture, and stamped out with cutter in shape, unsurprisingly, of figure 2. Iced yellow, made with icing sugar, orange juice and – no sleep tonight – yellow colouring, and hundreds and thousands sprinkled on top.
- Lemon tarts: following recipe for jam tarts (see above) but substituting shop-bought lemon curd in place of the jam; you need neither to heat the lemon curd nor add water to it before spooning it into the little tart cases.
- Cheese stars: following recipe above, but doubling the amounts.
- Cocktail sausages (as above).
- Several bowls of de-stalked seedless white grapes.
- Marmite sandwiches (see page 505).
- Corn crisps that look like bacon slices.

THE CAKE

In all cases use a 25cm Springform, greased and lined tin.

275g each self-raising flour, caster sugar and unsalted butter, very, very soft, but not actually melting
2 teaspoons baking powder
1 teaspoon vanilla extract
5 eggs
2 tablespoons milk

Mix everything together in the processor. With the chocolate cake I added 2 tablespoons cocoa powder mixed to a paste with 2 tablespoons boiling water. With the pink cake I added pink food colouring, and used strawberry icing. Cook in a gas mark 6/200°C oven for 20 minutes, then in a gas mark 4/180°C oven for about another 40–50 minutes. You may need to cover loosely with foil or greaseproof paper to stop it burning at the end.

Because of the sheer volume of ingredients (and lack of air in a cake when you mix it in a processor), these cakes don't rise much. You have choices: you can make the cakes in the old-fashioned way, creaming butter and sugar, adding eggs and flour and thus beating a lot of air into the batter; or you can do the cake mixture in two goes (just remember the proportions); or you can make two cakes, one after the other if you haven't got a pair of tins, and make a sandwich cake; With the pink birthday cake I made two full-size ones (so you need double the ingredients) and stuck them together with strawberry butter-cream because I felt a tall, more frou-frou-looking creation fitted the particular bill. (For the buttercream I used 350g of that compellingly vile strawberry-flavoured icing sugar you can get now and 150g butter.) But in fact the cake, though it looked wonderful, then didn't cut very well. You might decide you can live with a not-very-high cake.

On the whole that last is the wisest way of approaching it. As I said earlier, the birthday girl or boy is going to be far more interested in looking at and eating the icing. And the all-in-one processor method (see page 27, too) is easier, especially when you're up against time as you inevitably will be. Winnicott wrote about being a 'good-enough mother'; be satisfied with baking a good-enough cake.

As for the roll-out icing: for amounts needed read the packet (or ask someone in the shop) and the same goes for roll-out marzipan. For the chocolate cake, I made my own marzipan out of pistachios, but I now see that for what it was: an act of madness. Use ordinary shop-bought marzipan and dye it green; or you can buy coloured marzipan. Use the black one for cutting out a witch's hat or similarly sparky design. For the animals, let fancy, imagination or competence be your guide.

When you turn out the cake – and let it stand in the tin on a rack for 10 minutes first – just lie it domed side down so the weight of the cake flattens what will be the base and you have the nice flat bottom of the tin side to present to the world and to provide a smooth surface for the icing.

THE BISCUITS

This is the recipe I always use (it makes good Christmas tree decorations, too, if you have those special cutters and remember to make a hole at the top before baking them). It's rather like a gingerbread, only not as hot, and you can leave out the cinnamon if you like. Some fresh nutmeg grated in works well for a gentler spiciness. The dough rolls out easily. The biscuits are not frangible when cooked and take icing well. Children seem to like them, as they eat the whole biscuit rather than just licking off the icing.

If you want to make them chocolate-flavoured, use 275g flour and 25g cocoa.

300g plain flour
pinch salt
1 teaspoon baking powder
1 teaspoon cinnamon, optional (or nutmeg, see above)
100g butter, diced
100g light muscovado sugar (or ordinary soft brown sugar)
2 eggs
60g golden syrup

Sieve the flour, salt and baking powder into a bowl. Add cinnamon if using. Rub in the butter then stir in the sugar. With a fork, stir 1 egg into the golden syrup and add to the mixture, beating well. I like doing this by hand (or with a free-standing mixer) especially if I'm making it with the children, but you can just do it in the processor, mixing all but the last two ingredients and then posting those together down the chute. If needed, add the second, beaten, egg a teaspoonful at a time.

When the biscuit dough's come together, form into a couple of discs, and put one, covered in clingfilm or in a freezer bag, in the fridge while you get started on the first. Preheat the oven to gas mark 3/160°C.

Now, this dough is fairly sticky at first and there is a good reason for this: so that you can get a maximum amount of biscuits, it needs to be able to absorb quite a lot of flour without becoming too dry. Be prepared to flour the surface, the dough and the rolling pin well, and bear in mind that the dough will get smoother as you roll and re-roll. Not a shred need be wasted. Anyway, this isn't a difficult procedure, as you'll see.

Roll out to about 5mm thick and cut the biscuits out as you wish, reclumping, rerolling and recutting all leftovers till you have no dough left. You may find it easier to leave some leftovers from the first disc of dough and then add them to the leftovers from the second, in effect giving yourself three discs to roll out in total.

The biscuits take about 12–20 minutes to cook. They're golden brown anyway, so you can't tell when they're cooked exactly by colour. You don't want them to burn so keep an eye on the edges, and prod them with your fingertips occasionally: they shouldn't have any feeling of uncooked dough about them, but neither should they be rigid; they will harden as they cool. Don't get anxious about this: as long as they're not squidgy to the point of rawness they should be fine.

Let cool on a rack and, if you want, leave in an airtight tin until you want to ice them. I find this amount makes on average 60 biscuits, but naturally it depends on the shape and size of the cutters. (I don't go in for novelty-shaped or ostentatiously childish food as a rule, but I do have a huge supply of biscuit cutters in just about every form available: geometric, animals, mode of transport; all fads and fancies covered. And when I was rootling about a party shop with a specialist cake-decoration wing, I found that one of the pieces in the cutting set sold for fashioning sweet peas out of icing is the perfect shape for stamping out pumpkins.)

GLACÉ ICING

If you're making glacé icing, 300g with about 3 tablespoons boiling water (plus colouring) should do it.

Don't ask me to count the hundreds and thousands.

MARMITE SANDWICHES

You may think that giving a recipe for Marmite sandwiches shows I've lost it. I haven't: this isn't a recipe, just a helpful pointer. Unless you like spreading slice after slice of very breakable plastic white bread (and what else are you going to be using?) first with too-hard and hole-making butter and then with the filling, this is what you should do: cream the butter as if you were making a cake (use whatever machinery, elevated or basic, you prefer), then add the Marmite and beat again briefly. You will have a very soft, very spreadable brownish mass. Not beautiful, but it makes divine sandwiches. There are adults who accompany their children to parties just to get some of these special Marmite sandwiches; I know because they phone in advance to make sure they're on the menu.

I find 100g butter makes enough for a thin-sliced loaf of bread. About the Marmite I really can't be specific as it depends on whether you want a mild-tasting, buff-coloured cream or a salty-strong, sunbed-tan glaze.

If you want to make other sandwiches by this method, of course you can. Be warned, you can't offer these all-in-one Marmite sandwiches together with peanut butter sandwiches at the same party and hope to tell the difference – unless you use one loaf of brown and one of white bread.

FISH SANDWICHES

If you want to make some sort of fish sandwich, then just mix some mayonnaise, the bottled stuff, with some tinned salmon. But I have come to the conclusion that sandwiches are primarily there to placate the parents: they act as a nutritional sop, making the grown-ups feel better about all the sweet stuff that the children are really eating; it thus looks like a proper tea, not the full-on sugar orgy it is. So I wouldn't bother to do plateful upon plateful. But make sure you remove all crusts and, just this once, whatever your normal aesthetic, cut them into little triangles. Sometimes the proprieties have to be respected; a children's tea party is no place for restraint or minimalist chic.

gazetteer

It is both dangerous and helpful that most pieces of kitchen equipment you need, or indeed food you might want to eat, can now be ordered by phone. There are, I know to my cost, fewer blocks to extravagance when you're spending plastic money and not having to carry the shopping home yourself. On the other hand, it can make life easier. The list of suppliers and stockists, below, is necessarily brief; for amplification – and further information – refer to Henrietta Green's *Food Lovers' Guide to Britain* (see Bibliography).

THE HARDWARE

Buyers and Sellers

Best discount source of white goods, ovens, hobs, etc., including American fridge-freezers: 0171 229 1947

David Mellor Cook's Catalogue

Well-designed kitchenware and tableware, including mezzaluna knives and zesters: 0171 730 4259

Divertimenti

Seasonal catalogue of kitchen and tableware; also some foodstuffs, including – though not generally in its summer catalogue for some reason – Marigold Swiss vegetable bouillon powder: 0181 246 4300

Lakeland Ltd

A wide range of kitchen equipment plus a few foodstuffs, including Madagascan Bourbon vanilla extract: 01539 488 100

Leon Jaggi

Cookware and catering equipment, including traditionally shaped couscoussiers: 01233 634 635

Nisbets Chefs' Catalogue

An extensive range of kitchenware, including blini pans, mixers and heat-diffusers: 01454 855 655

Scotts of Stowe

Compelling gadgets, including Bake-o-Glide: 01451 870 087

FOR OTHER PIECES OF EQUIPMENT MENTIONED

FREESTANDING MIXER

I am in love with my KitchenAid; for stockists phone 0345 023 447

NONSTICK PANS

In Low Fat I mention the Panny and Wollpan; to find stockists for either, phone 01428 658 888.

PRESSURE COOKER

In Fast Food, I refer to the new, safe pressure cookers. There are several reliable makes. I use a Fissler and you can find out your nearest stockist by phoning 01782 565 222.

RICE COOKER

There are a wide variety on the market. I use a Zojirushi, and for stockists call 0181 998 2100.

BOOKS

Any book in print mentioned in *How to Eat*, whether published in the UK or not (and see Bibliography) may be ordered from Books for Cooks on 0171 221 1992. If you're after antiquarian or out-of-print food books, I recommend you telephone Liz Seeber on 0171 739 3031.

THE FOOD

Throughout the book, I mention certain foodstuffs which you may not be able to find easily where you live. The shops or telephone numbers for information on stockists that are listed below should be able to provide you with, or help you find, what you want. I do not include here all the shops I go to myself, simply because I have wanted to limit this list to those which will be accessible to you – in some form – no matter where you live.

MEAT

Barrow Boar

Not only boar, but a wide range of game, from peacock, emu and kangaroo to the African desert locust: 01963 440 315

Denhay Farms

Air-dried ham, bacon, Dorset Drums (cheddar): 01308 422 770

Donald Russell Direct

Excellent Scottish butcher's, which vacuum packs its truly wonderful meat so that it can be kept in the fridge for up to 3 weeks; this makes life much easier than stashing the stuff away in the deep-freeze. Also has good smoked salmon: 01467 629 666

Fletchers

Specialist venison dealers in Auchtermuchty: joints, diced meat for casseroles or stews, pâtés, burgers, mince, sausages; indeed anything made with or from venison you could imagine: 01337 828 369

Graig Farm

Welsh organic farm that will send you a variety of meats (including mutton), poultry, some cured fish and dried goods: 01597 851 655

Kelly Turkey Farms

The Kelly Bronze turkey is the best bird you can buy. Various butchers – including mine – stock it, but you can order direct on 01245 223 581.

Rannoch Smokery

All kinds of smoked meats, including wild venison and game: 01882 632 344/715

Swaddles Green Farm

Award-winning organic meat, charcuterie, pies and prepared meals. Various other items, too, including wonderful organic French cider: 01460 234 387

FISH

Cornish Fish Direct

Fresh Cornish fish sent by overnight delivery:
01736 332 112

G. B. Shellfish

Scallops, mussels, oysters, etc., from the west coast of Scotland: 01631 720 525

H. Forman and Son

Traditional London-cure smoked salmon (milder and more tender than Scottish cure), both farmed and wild, sliced or whole: 0181 985 0378

Loch Fyne Oysters

Oysters (including instructions for opening and knives), herring, kippers, salmon, scallops, langoustines, mussels and more: 01499 600 217

The Market Fish Shop

Fresh fish from Dartmouth: 01803 832 782

Quayside Fish Centre

Fresh Cornish fish and other goods sent by overnight delivery: 01326 562 008

VEGETABLES

Phone the Soil Association on 01179 290 661 for information on deliveries of organic vegetables in your area. Phone 01179 142 446 to order their full organic shopping catalogue.

CHEESE

La Fromagerie

Italian, French and British cheeses plus *pain Poilâne*, Venetian pasta, cakes and sweetmeats and more: 0171 359 7440

Neal's Yard

Cheeses from all over the British Isles:
0171 407 1800

WINE

John Armit Wines

John Armit's recommendations are to be found in the dinner chapter; you can discuss the food you're cooking and the wine you might want in greater detail as you order: 0171 727 6846

Mayor Sworder

0181 686 1155

ITALIAN FOOD

Take It From Here

Including farro and pasta di farro, cheese and chocolates: 0800 137 064

Valvona & Crolla

Huge range of Italian food, including Italian stock cubes and 00 flour; some non-Italian foods, including Marigold Swiss vegetable bouillon powder: 0131 556 6066

JAPANESE

Midori

Wide stock, including miso and instant dashi: 01273 601 460 (fax 01273 620 422)

MIDDLE-EASTERN

Green Valley

Including pomegranate molasses, powdered pistachios, sumac: 0171 402 7385

SWEDISH

Swedish Table

Various Swedish foodstuffs, plus, if you're lucky, cast-iron Plättar pans, which are frying pans with seven small indentations, excellent for blini: 0181 371 0658 or 0181 346 0996

MISCELLANEOUS

The Chocolate Society

The best: Valrhona chocolate in bars and pearls, which are good for speed of melting (and you don't have to chop them): 01423 322 230

G. Costa & Co

For leaf gelatine. I can use no other sort. Phone 01622 717 777 for local stockists.

Dove's Farm

If there's a flour you want and you can't find it in the shops, here's where you're likely to get it. Huge range, including spelt, buckwheat, organic and stone-ground flours: 01488 684 880

The Fresh Food Company

Home delivery service nationwide. Organic vegetables, meat, fish, game, dairy produce, bread: 0181 969 0351

Jekka's Herb Farm

Every herb you've ever heard of or will hear of, seed or plant, including Thai basil: 01454 418 878

Joubère

Freshly made stock – beef, lamb, chicken, vegetable, veal, game and fish – of an incredibly high standard and sold in 300ml tubs: phone 0181 992 6851 for information on stockists.

Marigold Swiss vegetable bouillon powder

Phone 0171 267 7368 for nearest stockists.

Mortimer & Bennett

Good delicatessen with a small but interesting stock, including excellent chocolate, white truffle oil, savoiardi and Italian 00 flour: 0181 995 4145

Mosimann

Mosimann's Christmas pudding is the best I've tasted yet. Phone 01628 782 254 or 0171 235 3345 for information on ordering one.

The Oil Merchant

Olive, nut and infused oils: 0181 740 1335

Martin Pitt

Excellent free-range, organic eggs: 01672 512 035

Simpole Clarke

Good deli run by professional cooks and with a stock including authentic chorizo: 01780 480646

Teesdale Trencherman

Robust list, as seems proper, including good pesto, olive paste and infused oils: 01833 638 370

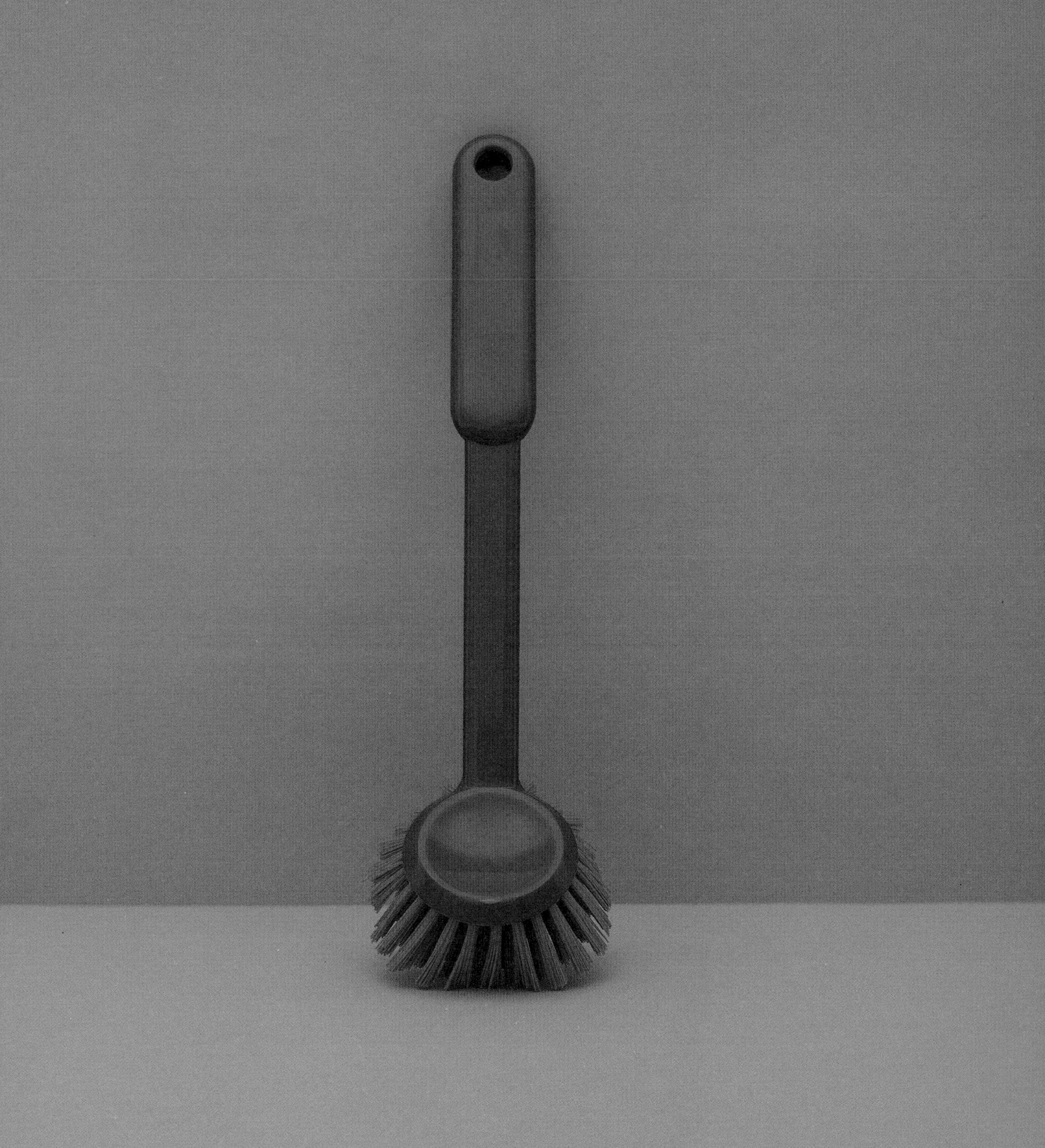

bibliography

Any book referred to in the preceeding pages should be listed below; the publishers would like to hear from authors or publishers who feel they have not been properly credited.

Allen, Darina, *Irish Traditional Cooking* (Kyle Cathie, 1995)
Alexander, Stephanie, *The Cook's Companion* (Viking Australia, 1996)

Bhumichitr, Vatcharin, *Southeast Asian Cookbook* (Kyle Cathie, 1997)
Borrel, Anne, Alain Senderens and Jean-Bernard Naudin, *Dining With Proust* (Ebury, 1992)
Boxer, Arabella, *The Hamlyn Herb Book* (Hamlyn, 1996)
Book of English Food: A Rediscovery of British Food from Before the War (Hodder & Stoughton, 1991)
Garden Cookbook (Weidenfeld & Nicolson, 1974)
Bramley, Tessa, *The Instinctive Cook* (Merehurst, 1995)

Collister, Linda and Anthony Blake, *The Baking Book* (Conran Octopus, 1996)
Coniher, Shirley O., *Cookwise* (Morrow, 1997)
Conte, Anna del, *Classic Food of Northern Italy* (Pavillion, 1995)
Entertaining All'Italiana (Bantam Press, 1991)
Costa, Margaret, *Four Seasons Cookery Book* (Grub Street, 1996)
Craddock, Fanny and Johnnie, *Coping with Christmas* (Fontana, 1968)
Crawfor Poole, Shona, *Iced Delights* (Conran Octopus, 1986)
Croft-Cooke, Rupert, *English Cooking: A New Approach* (W. H. Allen, 1960)

David, Elizabeth, *French Provincial Cooking* (Michael Joseph, 1960)

Freud, Clement, *The Gourmet's Tour of Great Britain and Ireland* (Bullfinch, 1989)

Gayler, Paul, *A Passion for Cheese* (Kyle Cathie, 1997)
Gold, Rozanne, *Recipes 1-2-3* (Grub Street, 1997)
Green, Henrietta, *Food Lovers' Guide to Great Britain* (BBC Books, 1995)
Grigson, Jane, *English Food* (Ebury, 1992)
Fruit Book (Michael Joseph, 1982)

Hazan, Marcella, *Marcella's Kitchen* (Macmillan, 1986)
Hopkinson, Simon with Lindsay Bareham, *Roast Chicken and Other Stories* (Ebury, 1994)

Kafka, Barbara, *Roasting* (Morrow, 1995)
Microwave Gourmet (Barrie & Jenkins, 1989)
King, Rani, and Chandra Khan, *Tiger Lily: Flavours of the Orient* (Piatkus, 1996)
Kreitzman, Sue, *Low-Fat Vegetarian Cookbook* (Piatkus, 1994)

Little, Alastair and Richard Whittington, *Keep it Simple* (Conran Octopus, 1993)
Lowinsky, Ruth, *More Lovely Food* (The Nonesuch Press, 1935)

MacMillan, Norma, *In a Shaker Kitchen* (Pavilion, 1995)
Morris, Nicki (ed.), *The Women Chefs of Britain* (Absolute Press, 1990)

Palmer, Leonie, *Noosa Cook Book* (The Blue Group, 1996)
Patten, Marguerite, *Classic British Dishes* (Bloomsbury, 1994)

Richfield, Patricia, *Japanese Vegetarian Cookbook* (Piatkus, 1994)
Roden, Claudia, *Book of Jewish Food* (Viking, 1997)
A New Book of Middle Eastern Food (Viking, 1985)
Ross, Rory, *Gastrodrome Cookbook* (Pavilion, 1995)
Rushdie, Sameen, *Indian Cookery* (Century, 1988)

Saleh, Nada, *Fragrance of the Earth: Lebanese Home Cooking* (Saqi Books, 1995)
Saunders, Steven, *Short Cuts* (Macmillan, 1998)
Sheraton, Mimi, *From My Mother's Kitchen* (HarperCollins US, 1991)
Slater, Nigel, *Real Cooking* (Michael Joseph, 1997)
Stuart Neil, *Pacifica Blue Plates* (Ten Speed Press, 1992)
Symonds, Nina, *Asian Noodles* (Morrow, 1997)

Taruschio, Franco and Ann, *Leaves from the Walnut Tree Inn* (Pavilion, 1993)
Thomas, Anna, *From Anna's Kitchen: Plain and Fancy Vegetarian Menus* (Penguin, 1996)

Wells, Patricia, *At Home in Provence* (Kyle Cathie, 1997)
Whittington, Richard, with Martin Webb, *Quaglino's: The Cookbook* (Conran Octopus, 1995)
Willan, Anne, *Real Food: Fifty Years of Good Eating* (Macmillan, 1988)
Wolfert, Paula, *Cooking of the Eastern Mediterranean* (HarperCollins US, 1994)

I'd like to thank all those whose recipes I've used or adapted in this book. They are mentioned by name in the text and listed in the bibliography. I'd like also to thank John Armit, Alexandra Shulman, editor of *Vogue*, where some of these recipes started off, as did my life as a cookery writer, and Rebecca Willis, my editor there.

Thanks, too, to everyone who worked on the book at Chatto & Windus, especially Penny Hoare, Caz Hildebrand and Eugenie Boyd, for whose calmness and forbearance I am particularly grateful; as I am also to Jonathan Burnham and to my agent, Ed Victor. Inés Alfillé double-checked recipes for me with serenity and efficiency, a rare combination. It's also important for me to express my appreciation of my butcher, David Lidgate; my greengrocer's Michanicou Brothers (and David) as well as Macken & Collins; and my fishmonger's, Chalmers & Gray.

Deepest thanks to Paul Golding, on whose judgement and friendship I have relied throughout; to Lucy Heller, Olivia Lichtenstein, Reggie Nadelson, Justine Picardie and Tracey Scoffield; and to Sharon Raeburn and Cheryl Robertson, without whom I could not have written this book.

To John, whose idea this book was and whose title it is, who has remained so encouraging despite being cruelly unable to eat the food. I can't say thank you enough. You know.

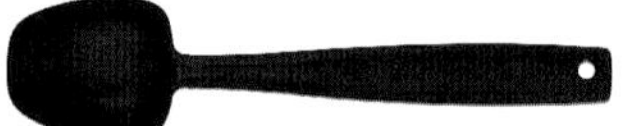

acknowledgements

index

Vegetarian recipes are marked by a green bullet point, and assume the use (which may mean substitution) of vegetable fat and stock. A pink bullet point signals those recipes which take 30 minutes or under from first move to the plate in front of you.